Key Issues in Health

Robert A. Burton, M.D. / Barry S. Ramer, M.D.
University of California School of Medicine, San Francisco

Mitchell Thomas / Scott Thurber

Key Issues in
Health

Harcourt Brace Jovanovich, Inc.
New York San Diego Chicago San Francisco Atlanta

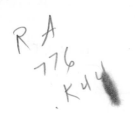

R A
776
K4

Cover photo: Heinz Kluetmeir for *Sports Illustrated,* © 1978 Time, Inc.

ISBN: 0-15-548368-4
Library of Congress Catalog Card Number: 77-94003
Printed in the United States of America

Robert A. Burton, M.D., is Assistant Clinical Professor of Neurology and Lecturer in Surgery at the University of California Medical Center, and Chief of the Division of Neurology and Director of the Neurodiagnostic Laboratory at Mt. Zion Hospital, San Francisco. He also maintains a private practice in neurology, engages in research, and has published papers in the *Journal of the American Medical Association, Archives of Neurology,* and *Annals of Surgery.*

Barry S. Ramer, M.D., is Assistant Clinical Professor of Psychiatry and of Ambulatory and Community Medicine at the University of California School of Medicine, San Francisco. He also conducts a private practice in psychiatry and is the author of numerous professional articles on emotional development, human sexuality, and drugs. Between 1969 and 1974, he directed the City of San Francisco's drug abuse treatment program.

Mitchell Thomas is a writer and journalist with a special interest in science and medicine. In 1967 he was a corecipient of first prize in the Empire State Awards for Excellence in Medical Reporting, presented by the New York State Medical Society and the New York State Department of Health. He has worked on the staffs of several newspapers, including *Newsday* and the *San Francisco Chronicle.*

Scott Thurber is a freelance writer specializing in environmental studies and other aspects of science and medicine. He has written articles on environmental affairs for the *San Francisco Chronicle* and was a feature writer for the Santa Rosa (California) *Press Democrat.* He has taught at the University of Texas, El Paso.

Preface

When we undertook the preparation of *Key Issues in Health,* we agreed on several propositions we wished the book to reflect: that it be scrupulously accurate in its presentation of scientific topics; that it be interesting to the general reader, whose background in the health sciences might be slight; and that it focus on subjects of principal interest to students in their early college years. Further, we attempted to clarify the broad term *health.*

The definition we selected is that formulated by the World Health Organization (WHO): "a state of complete physical, mental, and social well-being and not merely the absence of disease or infirmity." We also agreed on the theme of interrelatedness: mind and body; the human organism and its relationship to other people; people and their relationship to the large nonhuman environment they inhabit. Within this framework, we have attempted to address the topics that concern people of every age group and background.

Key Issues in Health consists of eight parts. Within each part, chapters encompass all aspects of health as defined by WHO and conceived by the authors: personal health; personality development and emotional problems; sexuality, marriage, and the family; drugs; sexually transmitted disease; cancer; nutrition; exercise; and health care—its practitioners and its services. We have tried to provide solid background information as well as to address the current medical and social issues involving these topics.

In addition, we have combined the standard glossary and index into one listing, in the hope of encouraging the reader to investigate a topic at length rather than stop at a brief definition.

We would like to thank the people who commented on the manuscript in its stages of development and assisted in its preparation: Gerson Jacobs, M.D.; Robert Diller, Cabrillo College; Roy E. Burkhead, City College of San Francisco; Victor Petreshene, College of Marin; Ruth Evans, Los Angeles City College.

Robert A. Burton, M.D.
Barry S. Ramer, M.D.
Mitchell Thomas
Scott Thurber

Contents

PART III   SEXUALITY

PART IV   THE MIND-ALTERING DRUGS

PART VI VITAL PARTS AND CHRONIC DISEASES

PART VII WELL-BEING

20 Food

21 Exercise

PART VIII   CARING FOR YOUR HEALTH

22 People in Health Care

23 Health Care Facilities

PART I
Wholeness

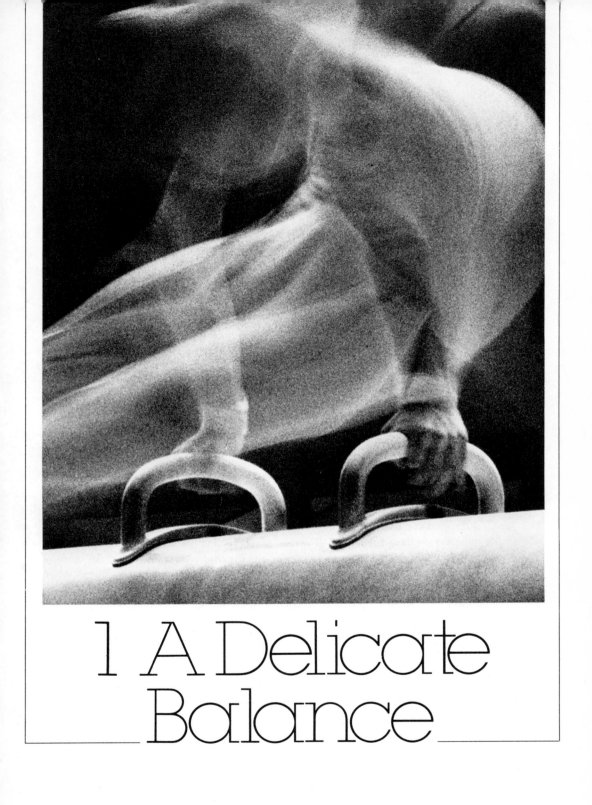

1 A Delicate Balance

Seven miles into space an airliner plies a sea of gases, hugging the curve of an orbiting planet. From earth, the jet is silent and invisible, its passing is marked only by a stream of condensed vapor, like a wake, a great white tail, a symbol chalked on blue slate.

The symbol is ambiguous. Interpreted one way, it stands for progress, the conquest of nature, the triumph of human civilization. By another interpretation, it is a reminder that progress may have its limits, that humans are bound by the laws of nature, that civilization may bear the seeds of its own destruction. From a purely scientific point of view, of course, the condensation trail has no meaning at all. It is a simple phenomenon, readily explained by any high-school physics student. Because molecules disperse when heated and draw together when cooled, hot gases tend to condense into droplets of liquid when they are introduced into cold air. Jet fuel contains water that is vaporized in the hot engines and condensed when it is expelled into the cold upper atmosphere, just as vapor from the tea kettle condenses in the cooler atmosphere of the kitchen. The condensation trail is steam, that's all.

Delving a bit deeper into physics, the phenomenon of condensation can be explained in terms of exchanges of energy between protons and electrons. Then, at a certain point, we reach the frontier of knowledge. As Sir Arthur Eddington, the British physicist, wrote some decades ago:

> We see the atoms with their girdles of circulating electrons darting hither and thither, colliding and rebounding. Free electrons torn from the girdles hurry away a hundred times faster, curving sharply round the atoms with sideslips and hairbreadth escapes. . . . The spectacle is so fascinating that we have perhaps forgotten that there was a time when we wanted to be told what an electron is. The question was never answered. . . . *Something unknown is doing we don't know what*—that is what our theory amounts to. It does not sound a particularly illuminating theory. I have read something like it elsewhere:
>
> > The slithy toves
> > Did gyre and gimble in the wabe.

Examined closely, all nature turns out to be a lot of slithy toves; but what kind of explanation is that? Lewis Carroll wrote "Jabberwocky" for our amusement, knowing that the human mind, which seeks meaning in everything, would try to make sense of his nonsense and laugh at itself for trying. But some minds fail to grasp the humor when the real world is found gyring and gimbling.

Jets crisscrossing continents and oceans, profound philosophic, economic, and political issues, science, imagination, humor, the unknown—all these, as well as food, exercise, drugs, sex, medicine, and much more are mixed up in the strangely elusive concept called health.

Health

The word *health* is derived from the Old English *hal,* which is translated into modern English as *whole.* For purposes of clarity, it could almost as usefully be translated as "wabe," that place in which Lewis Carroll's toves did gyre and gimble. Just what, in the context of healthiness, does "whole" mean?

The ancient Romans were on the right track when they defined health as *mens sana in corpore sano,* a sound mind in a sound body. At least they understood that health isn't merely a matter of physical fitness. But *sound* in this usage is just another word for *whole,* which leaves us only a little better off than we were before. We could, of course, simply agree that *whole* means unbroken, or without disease. However, modern authorities who grapple with this definition invariably conclude that health must mean more than just absence of disease. The World Health Organization, for example, defines health as "complete physical, mental, and social well-being." Unfortunately, while WHO has performed a service by expanding the concept to include our social needs, well-being is only one more way of saying health. How well is well?

The Scale of Health

Marston Bates has contributed the useful idea of health as a quantity to be measured on a scale. One can imagine a sort of thermometer on which the mercury drops from Fit-as-a-fiddle to Not bad to Rather poorly to Ghastly, then rises to Much better, thank you. At the bottom of the scale is Death. At the top is Perfect health. But while thinking of health as a relative quantity brings us closer to the mark, it doesn't solve all the problems. One problem is how to correlate physical, mental, emotional, and social health on a single scale. Another is how to define perfect health, which may be only an ideal, something that in the end would have to be described as wholeness.

It may be more helpful to think of a balance scale, suspended in space, dipping this way or that as weights are added to or removed from the bowls at either end of the crossbeam. This particular scale, however, has not just one crossbeam, but many, and the beams are intricately linked together so that all of them respond to a change of weight in any of the numerous bowls. Toss a pebble into one bowl and the entire apparatus dips and bobs in all directions. The balancing of this contraption is complicated by the fact that no standard weights are involved and no single commodity is being weighed. Into individual bowls go such disparate elements as organism and environment, individual and society, mind and body, emotions and intellect, each to be balanced individually and collectively against all the others. To get the complete picture, all of the elements, together with the machine itself, have to be imagined as a unit, a oneness. It is, perhaps, what in German is called *gestalt,* a word that has no precise equivalent in English, though *system* comes close. All of the elements are interrelated and interdependent, functioning as a dynamic whole that is characterized by a state of balance. This is the wholeness called health.

When weighing, say, gold dust on an ordinary scale, the object is to achieve perfect balance, to bring the crossbeam into absolute horizontal stability; neither buyer nor seller wants to get cheated out of a single grain. When we are dealing with health, however, the idea of absolute stability, a complete cessation of movement, brings to mind only one condition: death. What we are looking for when we seek good health, then, is relative stability, some comfortable state between absolute rest and the kind of wild gyrations that might bring our whole apparatus crashing down.

Body Rhythms

The jet cruises on. Inside its pressurized cabin, flight attendants clear away the remains of breakfast. One passenger, a rumpled man with bleary eyes, has pushed his breakfast away almost untouched. No appetite, and anyway it seems that he's been eating one breakfast after another since yesterday. Istanbul, Rome, New York, day and night turned upside down. Now, somewhere over the American Midwest, his body is telling him it's bedtime, no matter what meal is being served; but how can he sleep with all these people bustling and babbling, and with a sun that has no business being there, blazing through the window?

The man has traveled enough to recognize the symptoms of jet lag, the modern malady that plagues a long-distance traveler. His high-speed comings and goings put him out of phase with the rhythmic succession of night and day, which regulates the activities of most people. He congratulates himself on having had the foresight to schedule a day of rest in Los Angeles before his big business meeting. He isn't going to be very sharp until his biological clock, still on Istanbul time, has had at least a day or so to readjust itself.

Nature keeps its own time, measurable in the rotation of the planets, the cadence of the seasons, the ebb and flow of tides, the *circadian rhythm* of the human body. *Circadian* is from the Latin *circa,* about, and *diem,* a day. Numerous changes normally occur in the body in cycles of roughly twenty-four hours, the same amount of time it takes the earth to spin once on its axis. The changes include variations in body

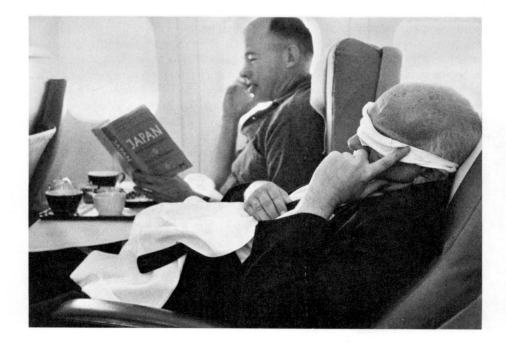

temperature and in the chemical content of the blood, as well as alternating states of consciousness. We wake, sleep, dream, and wake again. Most people can go without sleep for a night or two, but the price is discomfort and disorientation and, if sleep is postponed too long, eventual collapse. People tend to get sleepy at about the same time every day, and the body usually takes at least a few days to completely readjust to new sleeping hours. The biological clock is flexible, but somewhat stubborn.

In addition to those changes that normally take place about every twenty-four hours, certain functions follow cycles of greater or lesser duration. The heart of a person at rest beats, on the average, a little more than once every second. Every twenty-eight days, on the average, most human females within a certain age range, if not pregnant or somehow altered by chemical or other means, produce an egg that, if fertilized by a male, will become another human being.

Our biological clocks continually remind us, if we pay attention, that we belong to nature as surely as do the planets and the tides. We tend to forget this because we think of ourselves as separate from the rest, because our brains, our civilization, and our technology seem to set us apart, and because of a long tradition that pits humans *against* nature—a strange case of nature committing assault and battery on itself.

The Biosphere: A Finely Balanced System

The passengers in the cruising jet sit comfortably, enclosed in a portable environment, breathing air from an artificial atmosphere. Just outside the windows is an alien world in which the travelers cannot survive; the atmosphere at seven miles up does not contain enough oxygen to sustain human life. The biosphere, no deeper than the distance across a small city, is the only known environment in which human existence without artificial life-supporting equipment is possible. Only a handful of humans have ever been more than a few miles outside the biosphere. The airline travelers are merely skirting its outer limits.

The biosphere is a finely balanced system energized by radiation from the sun. Plants, in the process of photosynthesis, capture solar energy. Humans and other animals get their energy by eating plants or by eating other animals that have eaten plants. The energy, locked in the bonds of molecules, is released in the cells of animals through chemical reactions that require a steady supply of oxygen. Waste material from the conversion process is exhaled by animals as carbon dioxide. Plants absorb this carbon dioxide and break it down, using the carbon to make new cells. They release oxygen, which replenishes the atmosphere, thus making animal life possible. The decayed remains of dead plants and animals provide nourishment for the growth of new plants, which nourish animals, which, in turn, provide nourishment for plants.

Organisms

It is thought that all life on earth evolved from simple one-celled organisms formed billions of years ago as a result of chemical reactions in a warm sea. The word *organism* is derived from *ergon,* which is Greek for work. An organism is a physical structure in which the parts work together as a special kind of system. This system is capable of exchanging matter and energy with its environment without losing its physical identity. It is also capable of reproducing itself and manufacturing additional structures with the basic qualities of the original. An organism is composed of molecules that, like everything else, are made up of atoms, which are made up of protons, neutrons, and electrons. The protons, neutrons, and electrons in all of the atoms in the universe appear to be interchangeable. Basically, stars and clouds and rocks and flowers and people are all made of the same stuff, the differences among them being a matter of structure.

Cells

The human body is made up of some sixty trillion individual cells, each one a complex structure. Each cell takes in food and oxygen, expels wastes, manufactures various products, and, in most cases, reproduces by splitting into twin cells. Within the human body the cells exist in a watery environment much like the sea from which our distant ancestors are supposed to have come. The individual human cell, as scientist Walter B. Cannon pointed out, lives under much the same conditions as any one-celled organism attached to a rock in the bed of a stream. Those relatively simple organisms depend on the flowing water to bring them food and oxygen and to carry away their wastes; if the stream dries up, they die. The cells of our bodies depend on the flowing streams called blood vessels and lymph channels.

The fact that we are not fastened to rocks or rooted to the ground, that we carry our own life-supporting streams around inside us, frees us to hunt, to flee, to board a jet, and to fly around the planet. It also helps to create the illusion that humans are somehow separate from the rest of nature. Our internal streams, however, must be replenished continually from the larger environment. Cut off from oxygen, we die within minutes; without water, we may last a few days, no more. Deprived of food the human body begins to consume itself and usually expires in a matter of weeks. We are as dependent on our environment, and as much a part of it, as those one-celled organisms in the stream beds. The shallow biosphere we inhabit is our sea, our stream.

Adaptation Within the Biosphere

The fuel that drives the transcontinental jet might once have been lunch for one of the dinosaurs that abounded on the earth long before humans evolved. Jet fuel, like the fuel that powers cars, most factories, and electricity-generating plants, is produced from the fossilized remains of long-dead animals and plants that have been converted over millions of years by physical and chemical processes into oil, gas, and coal.

Dinosaurs appeared on our planet about 230 million years ago and existed for perhaps 150 million years. Although they were the dominant beings on the planet, they eventually died out because they were unable to adapt to the changing environment.

Humans have existed for only a few million years, and many authorities doubt seriously that our species will last nearly as long as the dinosaurs. By evolutionary standards, after all, it would not be surprising if we went the way of *Tyrannosaurus Rex,* since extinction is the rule rather than the exception. Two-thirds of all species have become extinct, because of an inability to adapt to changing environmental conditions. If we do disappear, leaving the planet to the durable sharks, ants, viruses, and crab grass, it will probably be because we failed to adapt to changes of our own making. Paradoxically enough, what finally causes our destruction may be our remarkable success in improving what we usually think of as health—physical, if not mental and emotional.

During the last few centuries, advances in science and technology, including farm machines, fertilizers, and pesticides, have enormously increased the world's capacity to produce food, dramatically reducing the number of deaths from starvation and from the diseases that accompany unrelieved hunger. At the same time, advances in medicine, improved sanitation, and better control of disease carriers, such as mosquitoes, have made it possible to prevent, cure, or virtually eliminate diseases that used to be major killers. In many parts of the world, the average life span has doubled or trebled and the death rate, particularly for children, has fallen dramatically.

Consequences of Adaptation

As a result, we now have a population explosion. In 1900 there were about 1.6 billion humans on the planet. By 1940 the world population was estimated at 2.25 billion. The figure passed the four billion mark in the mid-1970s, and, by then, was doubling at a rate of about once every thirty years.

It is obvious that if the population keeps growing, it must eventually reach a point at which a small planet with limited resources can no longer support all of its people. Already, the strain is showing.

More people need more factories, cars, planes, and houses, which cause more wastes and more pollution of air and water. Pollution of one kind or another has killed great numbers of plants and animals, consequently threatening some human food sources. It has also caused sickness and death in people, although the numbers are sketchy and the overall effects have still to be calculated.

In Africa in the 1970s, humans starved by the tens of thousands as the Sahara Desert crept southward, claiming what had once been grasslands that supported large animal populations. The grasslands were destroyed when the expanding human population brought in herds of cattle and allowed them to graze unchecked until there was no vegetation left. The cattle died, the people died, and so did many of the wild animals that formerly occupied the region.

In other parts of the world, once-rich agricultural lands dried up after forests on nearby mountain ranges were cut down. The leaves and needles of trees collect large amounts of water from passing clouds, even when no rain is falling. The water drips off the trees, collects in streams, and runs down the mountains to water the valleys. When the trees are cut down the water supply fails.

Dwindling deposits of fossil fuels, which created the well-known energy crisis, also created a shortage of fertilizers made from natural gas, thereby reducing crop yields in some parts of the world and adding to the problem of trying to feed the increasing population.

Overpopulation: The Most Serious Problem

The problems resulting from the population explosion are so numerous, and so immense, that they go far beyond the scope of this book. What is important in the present context is the way in which everything is interrelated, a gain in one area being offset by some unexpected setback in another.

Many of the problems could be solved, of course, if only the population growth could be halted, but intensive efforts in that direction have had little worldwide effect. A majority of the world's people are illiterate and superstitious, all but unreachable by programs intended to teach them simple birth-control methods. Furthermore, throughout history, people have been indoctrinated into believing that they should have large families; in earlier times, many people were needed for work forces and armies and to consume the flood of goods turned out by increasingly efficient production methods. It is hard to convince people that what they have always been taught is right has suddenly become injurious to world survival.

In major industrial nations, where people are relatively well educated and materially well off, population growth has slowed in recent years. However, in poor countries, which have the worst problems, populations are growing faster than ever. For traditional, religious, and economic reasons, children are regarded in those countries as wealth; they are extra hands in the fields, and they also assure a comfortable old age for their parents.

TABLE 1-1 Estimated World Population: A.D. 1000–A.D. 2000

Continent	Population at Given Times (In Millions)						
	1000	1600	1800	1900	1960	1977 (midyear est.)	2000 (est.)
Asia and Oceania	165	279	599	921	1,700	2,347	3,639
Europe, including Russia	47	102	192	423	641	737	853
Africa	50	90	90	120	244	423	811
Americas	13	15	25	144	407	576	902
Total	275	486	906	1,608	2,992	4,083	6,182

Source: Statistical Abstract of the United States, 97th ed., 1976; Population Reference Bureau, 1977 World Population Data Sheet.

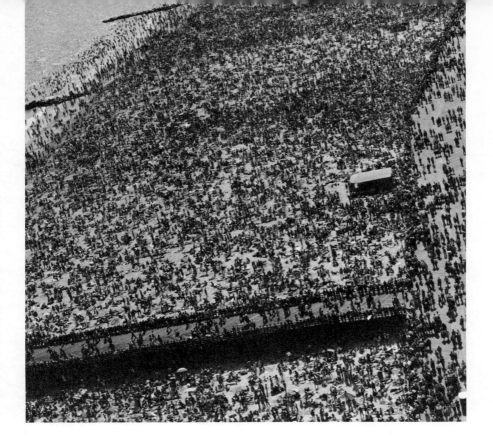

Why don't the wealthy nations simply look after their own interests and leave the rest to starve? Aside from questions of humanity, there are global politics and economics to be considered. Some poor countries control the natural resources needed for the industries of the rich countries. Despite their poverty, the poor nations also provide markets for many of the goods manufactured by the industrial countries, which produce more than even their own affluent populations can consume. Then, too, the industrial nations are bitterly divided among themselves, politically and ideologically, and they compete not only for resources and markets, but for military and diplomatic alliances with poor countries that might otherwise ally with the other side. Finally, the populations of the rich nations are outnumbered by those of the poor; with nuclear weapons falling into more and more hands, the poor nations may soon be in a position to enforce their demands for a larger share of the world's wealth.

It may be difficult to grasp the fact that all of this is related to the personal health of individual humans, but, then, the individual dinosaur probably didn't see the approaching glacier as any great threat, either. The human species appears to be facing a problem of adaptation in which the outcome is not foreseeable. What it amounts to is a health problem on a global scale, and it involves not only physical resources but politics, economics, ideology, religion, morality, ethics, education—a whole made up of many disparate elements, all interrelated, all in need of balancing.

A Sense of Security

Tom Wolfe, the journalist, wrote about a conference at a midwestern university at which one expert after another presented a gloomy view of America and the world and forecast an increasingly dismal future. Finally, after an ecologist had declared that environmental conditions in the United States might become so bad that life wouldn't be worth living by the year 2000, a student raised his hand. "I'm a senior," he said, "and for four years we've been told by people like yourself and the other gentlemen that everything's in terrible shape, and it's all going to hell, and I'm willing to take your word for it, because you're all experts in your fields. But around here, at this school, for the past four years, the biggest problem, as far as I can see, has been finding a parking place near the campus. . . . What I want to know is—how old are you, usually, when it all hits you?"

> And suddenly the situation became clear. The kid was no wiseacre! He was genuinely perplexed! . . . For four years he had been squinting at the horizon . . . looking for the grim horrors which he knew—on faith—to be all around him . . . and had been utterly unable to find them . . . and now he was afraid they might descend on him all at once when he least expected it. He might be walking down the street in Omaha one day, minding his own business, when—whop! whop! whop! whop!—War! Fascism! Repression! Corruption!—they'd squash him like bowling balls rolling off a roof!

In his own hyperbolic fashion, Tom Wolfe put his finger on a problem that, to one degree or another, affects everyone's personal health. The name of the problem is anxiety.

Anxiety

Strictly speaking, anxiety is usually regarded as an emotion distinct from fear, the latter being defined as a response to some immediate and identifiable threat, something concrete, such as a charging rhinoceros or a thug with a knife. Anxiety is a response to something abstract, intangible, uncertain, often experienced as a vague foreboding of impending disaster, sometimes as intense uneasiness (dis-ease). Anxiety is associated with specific but unrealized threats ranging from global war to personal misfortune, such as failure in an important examination. It is also associated with the nonspecific, abstract potential for pain, failure, and disappointment in everyday life and with the basic insecurity of human existence and the certainty of death. Semantic considerations aside, anxiety *is* fear—fear of the unknown, of potentially painful futures, probable and improbable.

Anxiety seems to be that which has been described as a disease of adaptation. As a species, humans are faced with the problem of controlling our population and protecting our environment, both of which are endangered as a result of our own ingenuity—the problem of adapting to changes arising out of the evolution of the human mind. As individuals, we are faced with the problem of adapting to the workings of our own minds.

A large part of this problem lies in the fact that the human organism has not completely learned how to differentiate between the concrete and the abstract, between the flesh-and-blood hoodlum with a knife and the imaginary mugger who might or might not be waiting in the next alley. The human organism long ago evolved a marvelous mechanism for dealing with real, immediate threats. The first sign of danger sets off a burst of reactions among nerves, hormones, and muscles, preparing the body to fight or run. It is this physical response that produces, initially, the feelings associated with fear. The sudden surge of fear serves as an alarm, putting the mind on guard, which is why the word *alarm* is often used as a synonym for fear.

Instinctual Response

Unfortunately, the body responds in precisely the same way to an imagined threat or to a real but distant threat that poses no immediate danger. A piece of disturbing news sets off the interplay of nerves, hormones, and muscles, that, as a popular writer put it, "is the caveman's response when the shadow of a pterodactyl falls over him. Adrenal secretions increase and muscles tense and the coagulation chemistry gets ready to resist wounds. Fight or flight. But what pterodactyl is this? They tell you: the market is down twenty points, or, the vice-president wants to see you, or, this whole operation is going to be shut down and moved to Chicago. Blam, pterodactyl time." The alarm goes off. The guard goes up. But the pterodactyl doesn't attack because there's no pterodactyl there, only a shadow that keeps circling ominously. The alarm keeps jangling away, and, though it may fade into the background, it keeps nagging at the mind, the emotions, the body. Too much of this can result in excessive stress (see Chapter 19), which can lead in time to serious physical as well as mental illness.

Boredom

The stress associated directly with anxiety is only one manifestation of the problem. Anxiety brings uneasiness, unhappiness, depression. People try to escape with alcohol and other drugs, or to find comfort in overeating—escape routes that lead only to worse problems. Since thinking and feeling are bodily functions, abuse of the body brings further deterioration of the mental and emotional life, which may lead to further body-abusing escape attempts—a vicious circle. Many people try to escape in other ways, by repressing anxiety, pushing it into their unconscious minds and refusing to think about anything that might threaten their imagined security. Then they find that the world, stripped of adventure, has become bland, arid, sterile—in a word, boring. Boredom is often the reverse side of anxiety, and, like anxiety, it often drives people into unhealthy attempts to escape.

The Way to Health

Anxiety and boredom, the twin roots of so many of our health problems, make many people's lives so joyless that they wonder whether anything is worthwhile. Life looks so drab, the future so uncertain, that they can't find within themselves the motivation necessary to change unhealthy habits, to seek the kind of life-style that offers the best chance for a long and relatively happy life. Others can't see any reason to make changes because, whatever the future might bring, they're having such a good time—frequently a temporary state achieved through one or another unhealthy escape route—that nothing else seems to matter. Of course, what everyone really wants is happiness, but the healthily happy want to enjoy their happiness for as long as possible. A test of one's personal state of health is the desire to live as long as possible and the will to take the reasonable steps that appear most likely to lead to longevity.

Many of us find even the most elementary steps—those aimed at keeping the basic equipment, the body, in good working order—extremely difficult to follow. Eating properly, exercising adequately, getting enough rest, avoiding smoking and excessive use of alcohol and other drugs—these are the fundamentals of any personal health program, and yet many of us know from frustrating experience that they are not easily achieved. What is needed is motivation and purpose, and that means finding enough satisfaction elsewhere in our lives to repay us for our efforts.

Personal Goals

People seek satisfaction in work, in love, friendship, and family life, in games and in the arts, in learning and exploring, in social and civic activities. Within these areas, life is given purpose and direction by the establishment of personal goals. In establishing these goals we create our own purposes. But what of The Purpose, the great question that everyone ponders at least once in a while: What's it all about? What is the meaning of life? Somehow, everyone must come to terms with the unknown, with the fundamental mystery of the gyring, gimbling universe, in order to lay some kind of foundation for a healthy, whole existence. Many find their meaning in religion, others in one philosophical system or another. Some make the search for meaning a goal in itself, delighting in the search and taking much satisfaction from their sense of wonder at the mystery of it all, their repeated confirmation of the proposition that "knowledge itself can be defined as detailed awareness of unsolved problems."

Take a moment to look around you. You can, if you try, see yourself and your surroundings as a whole, a single pattern of shapes, colors, and textures. You are in the middle, a part of the pattern, a sensing, feeling, experiencing concentration of molecules, atoms, and electrons. And here you are, at this moment, spinning and spiraling through space and time on a small planet near the edge of a minor galaxy that is among billions of galaxies making up a universe wherein space curves and wherein, eventually, everything may collapse into a black hole—but probably not in the near future.

It is a special kind of enlightenment, a modern philosopher wrote, to have this feeling that the usual, the way things normally are, is odd—uncanny and highly improbable.

"I don't like to think about it," a young woman told one of the authors. "I get weirded out."

Reality made her feel insecure and anxious, so she refused to think about it. But, while she could repress her anxiety, it didn't go away. It was still there in her unconscious mind, nagging, making itself felt in one way or another, building up stress. This particular young woman had, since childhood, sought refuge from anxiety in food—which was her greatest comfort. She overate and became fat, which not only exposed her to the numerous physical ailments associated with obesity, but damaged her self-image and her social life, making her feel even more insecure and anxious.

The refusal to face disturbing realities is a denial of important parts of life. It leaves one unwhole. But, while looking squarely at reality may make one uncomfortably aware that absolute security is an illusion and that one can be only relatively secure at best, a clear-eyed appraisal of immediate reality can also bring surprising relief from anxiety. Recall, for example, the student who investigated his immediate environment for signs of approaching calamity and could detect no problem more serious than finding a place to park. For most of us, most of the time, that's pretty much the way life is. The immediate reality turns out to be not very threatening after all. The threat is in some potential future, uncertain and unreal.

Potential dangers, of course, are not to be ignored. Initially, anxiety serves as an alarm. Once alerted, what can we—as insignificant individuals—do about the growing threat of an overcrowded and dangerously polluted planet? We can arrange our personal lives so as not to add to the problem. And we can, if so moved, vote, circulate petitions, join organizations, run for office, perhaps find a career in a field in which important personal contributions are possible. We can do, in other words, as much as we can do, and that's all. Once we've become aware of a problem and decided to act or not to act, anxiety serves no further purpose. We have responded to the alarm. Now it needs turning off. One way to turn it off, or at least to make it quieter, is to focus on the present, where we are most likely to find relative security. We can't, obviously, live entirely in the present and still make the plans and pursue the personal goals that give us direction. We need to learn to see life as a whole in which present and future are among the many elements that require balancing. Seeing life as a whole, we may then have a clearer idea how to go about balancing the rest of the elements of health.

The Individual's Pattern of Health

The jet begins its descent, approaching its destination; the passengers collect their belongings and their thoughts. Here and there someone removes the plastic earphones through which the sound system has been piped over various channels, rock, jazz, country-and-western, classical, and mood music—different rhythms for ears attuned to different drummers.

They are a diverse lot, these people who have spent a few hours crossing a continent together. They are male and female, young, old, and in-between—a colorful mixture of styles and expressions, complexions and accents, mannerisms and demeanor. They are returning to their homes or visiting friends and relatives; they are going to see sights, to look for jobs, to honeymoon, to study, to make speeches, to close deals, to escape from something. No two think the same thoughts or feel quite the same emotions in exactly the same way. There are, among these people, some who feel healthy and happy only amid the clamor and hustle of the city, others who thrive best in the quiet countryside. Some live contentedly on wholesome diets, while others seesaw continually between overrich, overabundant foods and the misery of self-denial. Even their circadian rhythms are different; there are ''day people'' and ''night people,'' some who feel terrible if they don't get at least nine hours of sleep, others who get along fine on six.

No one can lay down a simple formula that will meet all of the health needs of all of the people. The needs vary too much. A book like this can offer some understanding of the workings and interrelationships of body, mind, and emotions; it can offer some general guidelines, a very few specific rules, and perhaps here and there a helpful bit of insight. We can define health, pointing out that it is much more than a matter of food and exercise and medicine, that it is also a matter of perspective, of ways of thinking, of styles of life.

In the end, however, personal health is a matter of personal responsibility. One must find one's own formula, one's own special balance.

Summary

Perfect health might be defined as a wholeness. It might best be measured on an intricate scale that weighs and balances, individually and collectively, such disparate but interdependent elements as organism and environment, individual and society, mind and body, emotions and intellect. Man's biological clock and other regular cycles in his life show he is a part of nature. He is dependent on his environment for survival, and must adapt to its changes.

World population continues to grow: More people are being born, and people are living longer. The end result could be a planet so overcrowded it can no longer sustain us. So we face a global health problem, too, that involves more than personal health and a healthy environment; it also involves politics and morality and ideology, among other things—and these, too, must be balanced on an intricate scale. They can cause anxiety by threatening our sense of security. On an individual basis, one must overcome anxieties, face realities, and try to view life as a whole. We must remember that good health isn't just physical well-being—it is also a way of thinking and of living.

References

p. 4   Arthur Eddington, *The Nature of the Physical World* (London, 1935), pp. 180–81.

p. 4   Benjamin A. Kogan, *Health: Man in a Changing Environment,* 2nd ed. (New York, 1974), p. 3, quoting the World Health Organization.

p. 5   Marston Bates, "The Ecology of Health," in *Medicine and Anthropology,* Iago Galdston, ed. (New York, 1959), p. 59.

p. 8   Walter B. Cannon, *The Wisdom of the Body* (New York, 1932), pp. 27–28.

p. 12   Tom Wolfe, "The Intelligent Co-ed's Guide to America," *Harper's* (June 1976), pp. 27–29.

p. 13   Adam Smith, *Powers of Mind* (New York, 1975), p. 5.

p. 14   Attributed to "an English Absurdist writer" in a review by John Weightman, *New York Times Book Review* (May 23, 1976), p. 31.

p. 15   Alan Watts, *The Book: On the Taboo Against Knowing Who You Are* (New York, 1966), p. 6.

PART II
The Person

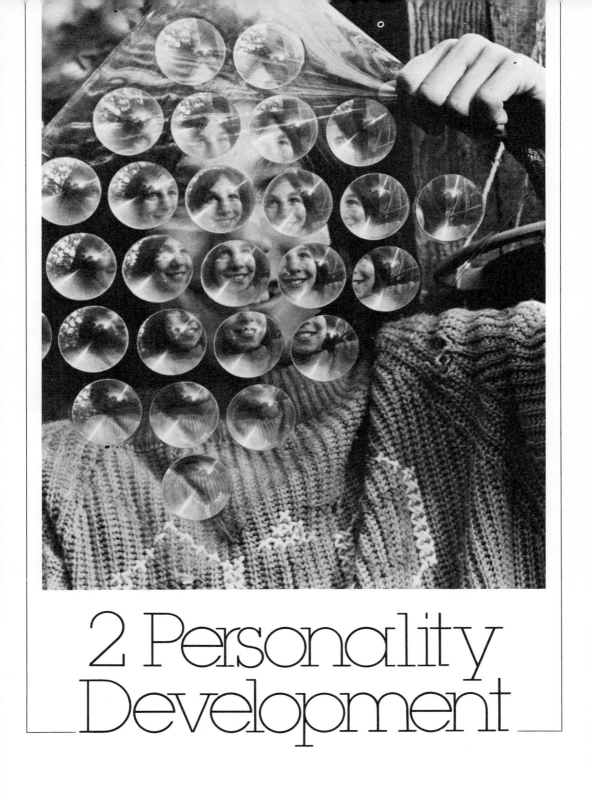

2 Personality Development

Larry is four and spends a lot of his time imitating his father. He lugs around a battered old cardboard file-folder which he calls "my briefcase." From time to time he puts the folder on the coffee table, extracts a sheaf of grubby papers, and examines them with a frown. Sometimes, with a grunt and a nod, he scrawls something illegible on the papers. Then he stuffs them back into the folder and lugs it away. The boy also hugs his mother frequently (Daddy likes to hug Mommy). And just the other day he caused a mild flap by picking some choice flowers from a neighbor's garden so he could bring her a bouquet. (Daddy often brings flowers and gifts to Mommy.)

Larry wants to be like Daddy—who is a busy and important man and a nice man who thinks of others. To use an overworked household term, the boy is "going through a phase." The phase he's in now has a lot to do with how Larry fits into the small but expanding world around him—with his own perhaps unconscious responses to the way this small world has treated him during his short life. His behavior reflects the way in which his needs for warmth and affection and sustenance have been met by the important people who occupy his world: his parents, his brother and sister, even the family dog. More important, four-year-old Larry's feelings during this particular phase— his sense of love or rejection, for instance—are going to be reflected in things this same Larry says and does perhaps fifteen or twenty years later: in the rituals of dating and courtship, for example.

Theories of Freud and Erikson

Each of us goes through a set of developmental stages. Sigmund Freud (1856–1939) discerned five distinct stages of development from birth to maturity. Later, the Vienna-trained psychologist Erik H. Erikson (1902–   ) expanded that list to eight—including three stages in adulthood.

Freud's phases were said to be *psychosexual*—that is, they focused on sexuality. Erikson took a broader, *psychosocial* approach, emphasizing the social rather than the biological problems of development. In broad terms, his earlier stages roughly correspond to Freud's.

Viewed from either perspective, young Larry's development obviously has passed beyond what Freud calls the *oral* and *anal* periods and has entered the *phallic* or *Oedipal* phase. In the oral stage, the infant's world focuses on oral gratification, nominally in the period of breast or bottle feeding. Anal gratification is usually associated with the rituals of toilet training.

In the phallic or Oedipal phase, the main area of erotic focus has become the penis in the boy, the clitoris in the girl. A child in this phase customarily experiences strong sexual attraction toward the parent of the opposite sex. In the Freudian view this is coupled, at least at first, with a desire to be rid of the other parent of the same sex—who has become a rival. Sometimes it's complicated by the fear that the rejected parent might somehow retaliate—a fear which can make the child repress his sexual and possessive feelings toward the preferred parent. Generally, however, the child takes a more realistic course: he decides to please Mommy by being more like Daddy; to win a woman like her by becoming a man like him.

The phase which Freud called the phallic or Oedipal period is regarded as critically important in personality development. The growing child's experiences in this period, and his ability (or inability) to cope with them, set the pattern for dealing with other persons in adulthood. Little Larry obviously has made this adjustment well, and his success in coping with the demands of this and other phases of childhood development are going to be reflected in his attitudes and conduct as an adult.

The same conclusions apply, in a negative sense, to little Charley, who is Larry's age and lives just down the block. There are big differences at Charley's house, though—and their impact may be every bit as lasting. Charley lives with his older sister and younger brother in a fatherless home: his mother was widowed shortly after his brother's birth. He has never had the fatherly attentions, or examples, that Larry has. He is uncertain of his role as a male, and when he reaches the ages of dating and courtship his underlying insecurity may be of crucial—perhaps painful—significance.

Stages of Development

Freud's stages deal with the growing child's mostly erotic repsonses to the stresses of childhood. In any of the five stages, he reasoned, the child could react adversely to stress and develop subconscious emotional problems that might not emerge until adulthood. Freud was dealing with the *libido,* a broad concept of sexual drive and desire, which he considered a major motivating force in all human behavior. He theorized that the libido was focused in different parts of the body during the progressive stages of personality development. Proper development of the personality, he contended, required that the critical tasks peculiar to each stage be met and resolved at the right time and in the right order.

Erikson, building on and expanding Freud's theories, refined and defined the concept that each step was a "task" that the child must master before moving successfully to the next step. The name of each of his phases is based on what results if the task is successfully resolved—and what results if it isn't.

Basic Trust Versus Basic Mistrust   Corresponding with Freud's *oral* stage, Erikson's first phase is called *basic trust versus basic mistrust.* This first phase involves an infant who is totally self-centered—the center of the universe—yet at the same time totally dependent. The infant's basic needs (nursing is uppermost) are almost entirely satisfied (or frustrated) by the mother. As the infant grows, and becomes more aware of the world around him, the quality of his relationship with his mother plays a major role in helping him decide how much, or how little, he's going to trust that world and feel safe in it.

Significant emotional problems in later life are often traced by psychologists to "fixations" dating back to the earlier phases. Freud regarded fixation as a state of arrested development in which the libido got "stuck" in one developmental area.

Erikson maintains that there's no abrupt dividing line between one phase and the next. The child who has entered one of the later stages may well continue to resolve (or fail to resolve) the problems of earlier stages.

Autonomy Versus Shame and Doubt   About the time he begins to walk, the infant toddles into the second stage of development. Freud called it the *anal* period. The child usually is subjected to toilet training during this period, which Erikson calls *autonomy versus shame and doubt*. The now ambulatory infant has achieved greater control over most of his muscles. He learns that he can consciously control his bowels and bladder—sometimes stubbornly withholding when it serves his attention-getting purposes. The anal area has, in this phase, become a major source of erotic gratification. If the parents are patient, tolerant, and understanding during this phase, the child achieves a lasting sense of *autonomy* (control of self) and pride. Parents who are rigid and overdemanding, or who tend to ridicule, may produce enduring feelings of shame and self-doubt in the growing child.

Initiative Versus Guilt   This stage of development is the one Freud called the *phallic* or *Oedipal*—the one in which we encountered young Larry and his neighbor, Charley. Erikson calls this preschool phase *initiative versus guilt*. The youngster who has coped successfully with the tasks of the earlier stages should enter this one with a strong sense of security (from the first stage) and of self (from the second stage). He is aware now that he is a person, and he wants to know more about himself and the *kind* of person he will become. In this phase, the parents—consciously or not—assume critical roles as models, because the child now tends to imitate them: little Larry wants to be like Daddy; his sister Susie wants to be like Mommy. Poor little Charley down the street is confused.

The child in the third phase is both aware of and curious about sex: Larry knows he's a boy, Susie knows she's a girl. But they want to know more—and are likely to spend some time examining themselves and others. Stern parental disapproval of this can make a child feel that his genitalia are something dirty, thus he must be dirty too. This can produce the kind of lasting guilt feelings that may lead to the psychiatrist's couch in later years.

Complicating the problems of the child in this phase are the strong attractions toward the parent of the opposite sex, coupled with rejection, for a time, of the same-sex parent. The attraction, discussed earlier, is an expression of the *Oedipus complex* (named for a tragic king in Greek mythology who unknowingly murdered his father and married his mother; when he discovered what he had done, he blinded himself). Guiding a child through this period of ambivalence can provide a severe test of the parents' sympathy and understanding. But if these feelings aren't handled with skill and compassion, the child may develop emotional problems based on guilt, which may provoke serious inhibitions in later life.

Industry Versus Inferiority   After the Oedipal conflicts are resolved, the child goes into the fourth stage—called the *latency* period by Freud because it usually coincides with

TABLE 2-1 Erikson's Chart of Developmental Phases

	Infancy	Early Childhood	Play Age	School Age	Adolescence	Young Adult	Adulthood	Mature Age
I. Infancy	Trust vs. Mistrust				Unipolarity vs. Premature Self-Differentiation			
II. Early Childhood		Autonomy vs. Shame, Doubt			Bipolarity vs. Autism			
III. Play Age			Initiative vs. Guilt		Play Identification vs. (oedipal) Fantasy Identities			
IV. School Age				Industry vs. Inferiority	Work Identification vs. Identity Foreclosure			
V. Adolescence	Time Perspective vs. Time Diffusion	Self-Certainty vs. Identity Consciousness	Role Experimentation vs. Negative Identity	Anticipation of Achievement vs. Work Paralysis	**Identity vs. Identity Diffusion**	Sexual Identity vs. Bisexual Diffusion	Leadership Polarization vs. Authority Diffusion	Ideological Polarization vs. Diffusion of Ideals
VI. Young Adult					Solidarity vs. Social Isolation	Intimacy vs. Isolation		
VII. Adulthood							Generativity vs. Self-Absorption	
VIII. Mature Age								**Integrity vs. Disgust, Despair**

Eight crucial stages in psychosocial growth and development, each consisting of unique themes and conflicts that the individual must deal with throughout life. *Source:* E. H. Erikson, "Identity and the Life Cycle: Selected Papers," *Psychological Issues* (International Universities Press, 1959), I:1. Reprinted by permission of W. W. Norton & Co., Inc.

sharply reduced sexual interest. (There's some question as to why this happens. It could be a biological dropoff of the libido, or perhaps a subconscious repression of sexual impulses that the child feels somehow endanger him.)

Industry versus inferiority is Erikson's name for this new stage, which generally begins about the time the child first enters school. What he learns in the classroom (and on the playground) will teach him more about who he is and who he will become. Achievement is of considerable importance here—and the child gains satisfaction from knowing that he's accomplishing something. Parents, again, should attempt to handle these new developments with intelligence and understanding. They should give warm praise *when and if* it is due—but they shouldn't praise something they know is unworthy. On the other hand, unwarranted criticism from the parents—or a lack of interest on their part—may well engender a strong sense of inferiority in the child and make him feel inept, inadequate.

Identity Versus Self-Diffusion Puberty, the fifth phase of personality development, is one of complex emotional problems. Freud called this the *genital* phase. In this period the libido asserts itself again more strongly than ever. (Freud said the focal point is again

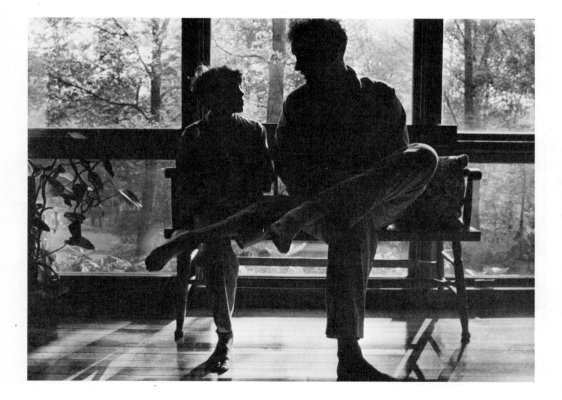

the penis for the male, but that it becomes the vagina rather than the clitoris in the female.) A person who has successfully resolved the challenges of the earlier stages should be able to achieve mature sexuality in this one, the Freudian theory contends. But more than sexuality is involved in this developmental phase; the young teenager is neither child nor adult, and he sometimes feels as though he's the object of a struggle between two worlds, two identities.

He has come to terms with his childhood. He is safe there. But now—in the perplexing turmoil of adolescence—he must push away from this haven of the known. He must, ready or not, enter a dangerous world he knows only from imperfect observation: adulthood. The teenager's conflicts during this trying period are many. He experiences pressures from the world at large, or so it seems to him; he is frequently in conflict with his parents, with society at large—and with himself. In all too many cases, the teenager finds that his parents are applying a double standard of behavior and performance: he finds he is expected to perform like an adult in some areas (responsibility, work habits, mature judgment, for example) and as a child in others (obedience, curfews, school attendance, household chores).

This parental ambivalence is one of many things that can bewilder the youngster entering this phase, which Erikson calls *identity versus self-diffusion*. The physical changes that occur with the onset of puberty sometimes cause emotional upsets. Intellectually, the teenager begins to question some of the standards—political, moral, social, religious—that society and his parents represent, and which he has previously taken for granted. He is searching for answers just as surely as he is seeking his own identity. His journey into adulthood is a difficult one, and he requires sympathetic understanding from the adult world.

Erikson's Adult Phases

Freud's list of development stages ends with the transition from adolescence to adulthood, but Erikson has gone beyond that point to three adult phases.

Intimacy Versus Self-Absorption   At this stage, adolescence is over, the search for self-identity largely resolved. It's now possible for the young adult to seek and form mutual relationships with others—to fuse his identity with theirs in partnerships, close friendships, sexual unions, love. He has not only the ability to commit himself to these relationships, but the ethical strength to abide by them.

Generativity Versus Stagnation   In this second phase of postadolescent personality development, the mature adult is ready for the kind of rewarding give-and-take called creative sharing. It can involve the sharing of ideas as well as material things. Generativity, as the word itself suggests, also involves a desire to share the experience of parenthood—to bring a new generation into being. A person who emerges from the first adult stage with strong feelings of isolation or self-absorption will find such creative growth difficult; his personality growth may stagnate.

Ego Integrity Versus Despair   Erikson says that in this final phase the adult personality, ideally, is like a fruit that has gradually ripened through time and experience. This ideal state comes to someone, he says, who has made the adjustments of the earlier stages; to a person who has learned to live with triumph and defeat, who has learned to love and be loved, to give and to receive, to lead and to follow.

Death holds no particular terror, Erikson says, for a person who has achieved this accrued integrity of the ego; but the lack or loss of ego integrity is signified by fear of death. The person who has achieved this quality accepts that he has but one life-cycle, that it is the ultimate in life. His life holds neither disgust nor despair. Indeed, Erikson suggests that if adults have the ego integrity not to fear death, their children will have the trust not to fear life.

Piaget: Intellectual Development

Related to the personality development stages of Freud and Erikson are the intellectual development stages of the noted Swiss psychologist Jean Piaget (1896–   ). His revolutionary concepts of the *cognitive* (knowledge acquisition) development periods in children are the product of studies begun more than half a century ago. Piaget's theories were highly controversial and drew sharp attacks from other psychologists with more traditional ideas. However, his concepts are now widely accepted.

Piaget outlined four stages of intellectual development. Each has been described in exhaustive detail by the scientist, who subdivided each stage into its own internal phases of progressive development. The four major stages are presented here in simplified form. All age brackets are approximate.

The Sensory-Motor Stage   This covers the period from birth to age two. Throughout the stage, the infant remains *egocentric* (totally self-centered), but he gradually becomes aware that he and the entire world are not one and the same. He begins to distinguish between himself and objects (he knows his foot is part of him and the crib-railing he kicks is not). He masters *object permanence*—he knows that something hidden from him or in another room continues to exist out of his sight.

The Preoperational Stage   This covers the years from two to seven. The child is still egocentric, thinks solely in terms of his own viewpoint. His linguistic skills develop and expand along with his ability to use symbols and images to represent objects or events. He hasn't yet mastered the concept Piaget calls *conservation*—that given quantities of a mass remain the same even though their shape is changed. For example: If two identical glasses of water are placed before a child in this stage, he acknowledges that they are "the same." If the water from one glass is emptied into a taller but narrower glass he will say it has "more water." He is unaware that if the water from the tall glass is returned to its first container, it will resume its original height.

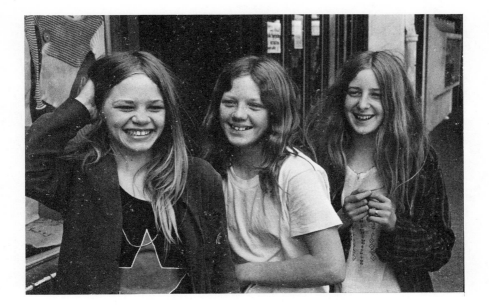

The Concrete Operational Stage In the early part of this stage (ages 7–11) the child usually masters the conservation concepts outlined above. The perceptions of the preceding stage have progressed into intellectual operations—logical thought processes begin to emerge. The child is no longer egocentric—he can take the viewpoint of another. He has acquired what Piaget calls *seriation,* the conceptual ability to arrange things by some dimension such as size, weight, or shape. This is necessary for the development of early mathematical thinking.

The Formal Operational Stage This stage (ages 11–15) is marked by the adolescent's ability to think, to reason, in purely abstract terms. He is capable of the kind of reasoning that Piaget calls *hypothetico-deductive*—he can consider a specific problem in terms of a number of possible but unproved solutions (hypotheses) and, by trial and rejection, proceed to a logical and provable answer. It is only in this stage that he achieves the ability to think, and to worry, perhaps, about possible future events in distant places; to hypothesize their resolution.

Summary

Sigmund Freud traced five successive stages of personality development, from birth through adolescence. Later, Erik Erikson built on and expanded Freud's theories, and extended them to include another three development stages in adulthood. Erikson conceived (and named) each stage as a task completed, or failed. For instance his first phase (Freud's "oral" stage) is "basic trust versus basic mistrust" and his final phase is "ego integrity versus despair."

The Swiss psychologist Jean Piaget has spent his adult life studying intellectual development, the growth of the ability to acquire knowledge, in children. He has evolved four stages, birth to about age fifteen. His ideas, once highly controversial, are now widely accepted.

References

p. 22   Theodeore Lidz, *The Person* (New York, 1969), pp. 76–80.

p. 23   Erik H. Erikson, *Childhood and Society,* 2nd ed. (New York, 1963), pp. 247–69; *Identity, Youth and Crisis* (New York, 1968).

p. 28   Richard Isadore Evans, *Jean Piaget, The Man and His Ideas,* trans. Eleanor Duckworth (New York, 1973).

p. 30   Lawrence C. Kolb, *Modern Clinical Psychiatry* (Philadelphia, 1972), Chap. 4.

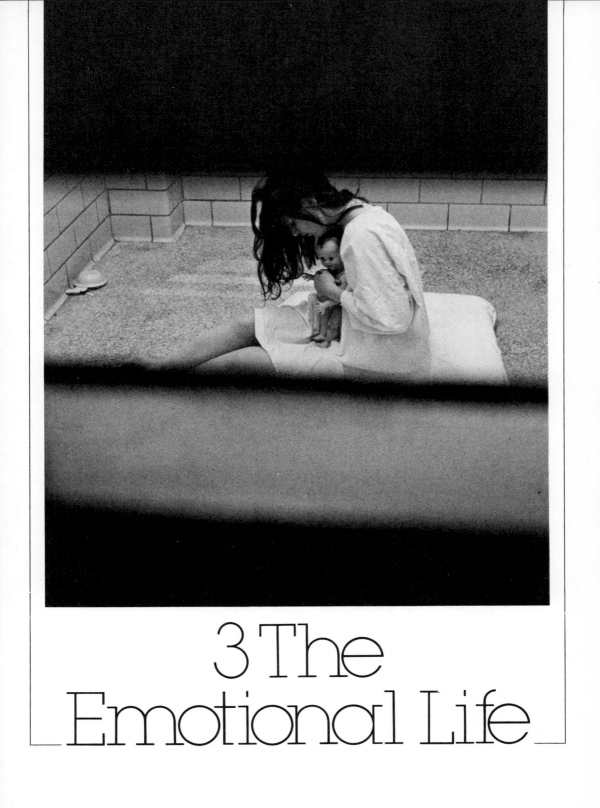

3 The Emotional Life

After the first call George slammed the phone down and said he was "just mad as hell!" After the second, a few minutes later, he hung up gently, almost reverently. He was smiling broadly, and said he was "delighted—just on top of the world!"

Same person, same telephone, same day—but different messages. The first call was bad news—about a business deal that went awry, or a horse that came in last, or an expensive breakdown of his car. The second was good news: the deal went through, the horse came in, the breakdown was covered by the warranty.

George was reacting just as we all do. Most of us don't travel that far, that quickly, but when we do, it's entirely normal. Feelings like anger, fear, disappointment, happiness, pride are with us all the time. These are the ordinary emotional reactions we have to outside stimuli. They are not the artificial kind of high you get from something you swallow or smoke, or the low from a pill called a "downer." They are not the extreme kind of feelings and reactions that stem from illnesses called *psychoses* or *neuroses*. These natural highs and lows are caused within us—when we react to things around us: to people, to events, to things we experience, see, hear, or hear *about*.

Everyone becomes angry once in a while—sometimes even to the point of rage. Once in a while someone is "overjoyed." But mostly our ups and downs are milder. They are routine: being "glad" at someone's good news; having to say you're sorry about a minor misfortune; getting irritated when the pencil point breaks at the wrong time, amused at a mildly funny story. Or perhaps just feeling good.

"Feeling" is an unscientific word used to describe some of our daily emotional gear changes. Whatever you call them, these changes are happening, these feelings occurring, all the time.

The Positive Side

Exhilaration is a word that bounds immediately to mind as a kind of emotional high. But *contentment* is also a high. Between them are a variety of moods and feelings, shaded a bit differently here and there, which we try to convey with words.

Both contentment and exhilaration are variations—in shading and extreme—of a number of emotions we tend to classify under the general heading of *happiness*. You might tell everyone you're "happy" about your new job assignment but "extremely happy" about your vacation plans. Words such as *joyful* and *delighted* and *overjoyed* convey upward-ranging intensities of the same emotion. They are emotions experienced by people who have something to be *pleased* about.

Love, as a word, is used casually by many people these days. Love, as an emotion, is one of the most powerful feelings known to mankind. Its intensities range from the quietest kind of tenderness to the strongest of passions. Other emotions which express degrees of love include, on a downward scale, *affection, fondness, liking. Hope* and *pride* are two other emotional highs which rate with love at or near the top of the scale.

A moderate "high" reaction involving something funny is called *amusement,* and if whatever amuses is especially funny, the reaction might be an exhilaration-scale high: *hilarity.* Both extremes connote *enjoyment,* but the stimulus doesn't have to be funny to be enjoyed. It might also be a tragic drama, a good meal, or a walk down a country lane.

The Negative Side

Rage is perhaps the strongest version of the general emotion we call *anger.* It takes a strong provocation to enrage a person, and somebody who "flies into a rage" often, and with little or no seeming reason, isn't experiencing normal emotional reactions. There may be a neurotic or psychotic cause.

Our language seems to have more words for negative emotions than for positive emotions. Many of them are kinds or degrees of anger. *Displeasure* is a down-the-scale reaction in this sense. Frustration can be another, although frustration doesn't necessarily involve anger. *Irritation* is considerably stronger. Even angrier is *annoyance. Impatience* is another decidedly negative reaction that often teams with frustration. If persons

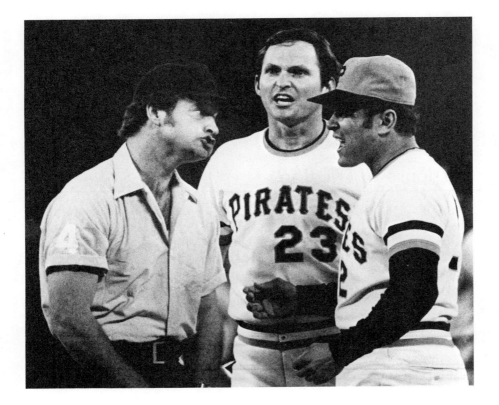

or events somehow damage your ego, your pride, you may just suffer a mild reaction we call *hurt feelings.* Or the emotion you feel may be *embarrassment, shame,* or at the extreme end of the scale *humiliation.*

We have many emotions reflecting different kinds of *sorrow.* If a close friend suffers a death in the family, your reaction might be *regret* if the deceased is a distant relative, but *grief* for someone very close, someone you know. A feeling of sorrow somehow coupled with a feeling of guilt would be *remorse.* An extreme kind of grief, near the breaking point, would be *anguish.* If something goes wrong at school or office the unhappiness you feel may be *disappointment, distress,* or *dismay,* but rarely *despair.* Despair is a sense of futility. It is often associated with *loneliness,* with feelings of *isolation,* sometimes of *melancholy, gloom,* and *depression.*

Depression in its severe states is a serious ailment. So is *anxiety.* Everyone suffers now and then from the milder forms of anxiety—a vague, disquieting sense of *unease, apprehension,* and *uncertainty.* Anxiety isn't the same thing as *worry,* which surely is one of the most common emotional reactions humans experience. Worry is a troubled *concern* about something or somebody: about a relative out driving on a stormy night, about tomorrow's tasks, about bills.

Two other emotional reactions can be particularly strong—those involved with *hate* and those involved with *fear.* A simple *dislike* or *distaste* for a person or a thing is common enough. *Disdain* is a somewhat stronger reaction that tries to turn the offending stimuli aside. *Disgust* is considerably more serious and involves not only a strong dislike but something that offends the sensibilities. An even stronger reaction in this direction is *repulsion.* An intense, active dislike that ranks with *hatred* is *loathing.*

When you enter a darkened room and have a vague feeling that something's wrong, it's probably just *unease,* or some other minor gradation of anxiety. But a series of unexplained noises can lead to emotional reactions such as *trepidation* or *foreboding,* which in turn can be propelled to *fear* or even *terror* or *panic.*

Bodily Response to Emotion

Everyone has this experience: At times of strong emotional stress—particularly an extreme such as anger or fear—the body's various mechanisms take measures to cope. Heartbeat and breathing quicken sharply, blood pressure rises, blood sugar increases. Blood from other portions of the body (the intestinal tract, for instance) is diverted to the brain and muscle tissue. These activities, coupled with a sharpening of the senses and the pumping of *adrenalin* into the bloodstream, mean the body is arming itself for physical exertion in its own defense.

Defense Mechanisms

Our built-in defense mechanisms involve more than just the preparation for combat or flight. There are also built-in weapons designed to protect us from environmentally induced stresses such as anxiety, and some of the other strong emotional reactions discussed earlier in this chapter.

All known forms of animal life have developed some kind of *adaptive* processes for protection from environmental threats. Lower species try to camouflage their bodies in order to hide from predators. In the same sense, man often masks or suppresses his true feelings to hide from anxiety or to reduce internal conflicts. These unconscious defenses are at work within all of us, and psychologists say when used in moderation they are essential to the evolution of a healthy personality. If they are relied upon to excess, the result may be the abnormal personality or personality disorders.

Most of the time we resort to these unconscious defense systems to reduce or eliminate anxiety and other uncomfortable emotions such as guilt, hostility, aggression, resentment, or frustration. Conflict between our basic drives and what we consciously know is right produces anxiety that must be controlled if we are to remain emotionally healthy.

Repression   We use this defense to force disturbing ideas or memories out of our conscious thoughts—pushing them temporarily into our subconscious. As adults we tend to forget the terrible embarrassment we felt as a child when we were caught stealing a candy bar from the corner grocery. The memory is still buried there; even today, if it bobs to the surface, it disturbs us. But our facility for repression keeps it pretty well hidden most of the time.

Rationalization   This has nothing to do with rational thought. It involves, rather, an attempt to make our irrational thinking or behavior *seem* rational. In a sense, it's our way of defending our largely indefensible thoughts and actions; it's self-serving self-justification. We rationalize our failures: an employee who is passed over for promotion convinces himself that he didn't want the new job in the first place.

Reaction Formation   We defend ourselves against guilt-provoking impulses by leaning strongly and publicly in the other direction. It's sometimes called "overreacting." Someone uncomfortably titillated by sexually explicit pictures and books, and torn by his own internal sexual conflicts, might react by donning a prudish manner and by publicly denouncing all kinds of pornography and nonconformist sex. Or a man beseiged by strong feelings of hostility and aggression might become a public leader in campaigns to wipe out antisocial behavior through aggressive "law and order" stances.

Emotional Extremes

It was on the morning of August 22 that Rita, a thirty-two-year-old housewife and mother of four, dropped a prize china platter onto the kitchen floor, where it shattered. A minor event, in itself, but in Rita it triggered a kind of bomb. Methodically, tearfully, she took all the other dishes out of the sink and smashed them, one by one, into small pieces. Then she fled to the bedroom, slammed the door and locked it. She was still there when her husband got home from work.

Rita had reached a breaking point—pushed there by a morning in which everything had gone wrong, following a series of bad mornings and a chain of bad weeks. Rita was no longer able to cope.

This is hardly an unusual case. Most of us are able to manage most of our emotional stresses most of the time, but we all feel a little overwhelmed once in a while. In Rita's case the emotional pressures—she felt she was trapped, inadequate; resented her husband's freedom; felt he and the children "used" her—became more than she could handle. Her battered defense mechanisms finally collapsed. She exploded—and then withdrew into a sullen, inconsolable state. It took several months of therapy, and some long and sympathetic talks with her husband, to coax her back out of her self-imposed shell. Rita's problems, the real and the imagined, had combined to force her to an emotional "low" well below the norm. She was emotionally ill.

Emotional illness is the term widely used to describe emotional states that exceed in intensity and duration the normal balance of emotions. They are afflictions that make it difficult, if not impossible, for the individual to function as a normal and healthy adult. The milder disorders are called *neuroses,* the more severe ones, *psychoses.* A number of different disorders are grouped under each of those headings. Many psychiatrists and psychologists object to these categories as overly rigid—but because they are still widely used we will include them here.

Neuroses

A *neurosis* or *neurotic disorder* is a relatively benign personality disturbance, often with its roots in childhood experiences. A person becomes neurotic because of an inability to cope with anxiety.

Anxiety Neurosis   This is a much stronger, harder-to-shake variety of normal anxiety. A person suffering from anxiety neurosis experiences strong feelings of restlessness, agitation, and fear. He has a profound but unexplained sense of impending doom. Physically, the neurosis may show itself in heart palpitations, rapid pulse, lightheadedness, dizziness, nausea, or tingling sensations over the body. Many people try to cope with anxiety neurosis by numbing its symptoms with alcohol or drugs.

Phobias   These are fears that are factually irrational but, to the sufferer, terribly real. Some of the more common phobias include *claustrophobia* (fear of confined spaces), *acrophobia* (fear of heights), *agoraphobia* (open spaces), *hydrophobia* (water), *nyctophobia* (darkness), *xenophobia* (strangers), and *ailurophobia* (cats). Some of these phobias—notably those involving enclosed spaces or extreme heights—obviously limit the circumstances under which a person can work.

Hysteria   The explosive outbursts of rage or weeping that most of us associate with the word hysteria have nothing to do with hysteria as medical science defines it. Hysteria, sometimes called *conversion hysteria,* amounts to neurotic imitation of physical disease: the hysterical person might develop a paralyzed arm, partial blindness or deafness, or some other physical symptom for which physicians can find no organic cause. The problem is all in the patient's mind rather than due to physical disability.

Obsession/Compulsion The compulsive neurotic tends to be fastidious, meticulous, rigid, and formal to the point of ritualism. A hardworking person with a compulsive personality often becomes so preoccupied with the mechanical rituals of his job that he loses sight of its purpose. *Obsessive* thoughts are unwelcome thoughts, or memories, which intrude on the individual to his discomfort and affect his behavior. For instance, a person with *obsessive* (and negative) thoughts about clutter and disorganization may so *compulsively* overorganize his work that his efficiency is impaired.

Depressive Neurosis This is the most common of all neuroses and is characterized by feelings of helplessness, hopelessness, and despair. Sufferers lose weight, are unable to sleep, complain of inertia and blue moods. The illness is often caused by a major loss, such as a loss of friends, job, or possessions. Mourning a deceased loved one is, however, a common form of normal depression.

Psychoses

There are two kinds of *psychotic disorders—organic* and *functional.* An organic psychotic disorder is one that has some physical cause—as distinct from emotional. Injury, disease, malnutrition, and hereditary factors are often involved. *Senility* or *senile dementia* is perhaps the most commonplace of the organic psychoses. It is caused by the deterioration of aging brain cells in the elderly, and usually shows itself in a dimming of the memory and a general slowing of thought-processes.

The psychotic disorders classified as functional are those that stem from no discernible physical cause. They are characterized by an inability to see life in realistic terms and, usually, by a stubborn insistence that there is absolutely nothing wrong. Normal functions—job performance, family and other interpersonal relationships—are severely impaired.

The most common of the psychoses include schizophrenia, manic-depressive psychosis, and paranoia.

Schizophrenia Commonly known as the "split personality" syndrome, schizophrenia is the most prevalent of the psychotic disorders. The chief characteristic of the disease is the sufferer's mental withdrawal into his own private fantasy world. Delusions and hallucinations are commonplace. Outwardly, the schizophrenic appears lethargic and dull, disoriented. Sometimes his behavior is inexplicable, probably because he is so involved in his own private world.

For many years, schizophrenia was considered incurable, and its victims were institutionalized. In recent years, new drugs have been developed to cope with the illness, and the general prognosis for its victims is greatly improved.

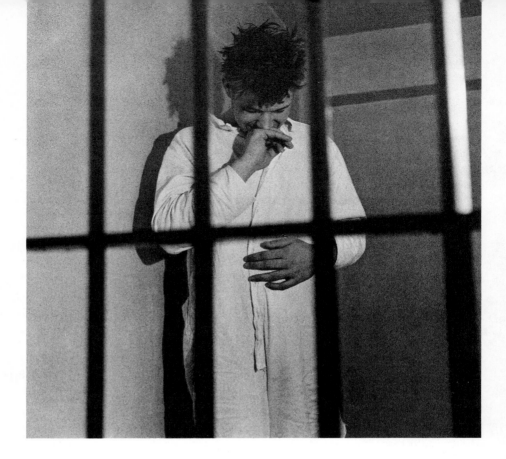

Manic-Depressive Psychosis This is an extreme exaggeration of the normal emotional highs and lows. The manic-depressive may swing wildly from extreme elation on the one hand to profound depression on the other. Sometimes an attack will involve one extreme, but not the other.

Paranoia Often considered a kind of schizophrenia, paranoia is associated, in the public view, with feelings of persecution: the victim feels that someone is out to get him. It may also involve delusions of grandeur.

Other Disorders

Psychosomatic illnesses often involve stress and anxiety manifesting themselves in the form of physical ailments. The most widely known form is *hypochondria*. A person with high anxiety levels often develops various kinds of symptoms of physical disease that send him in frantic pursuit of doctors and medicines to effect a cure. Other psychosomatically induced illnesses may include ulcers, migraine headaches, asthma, and some forms of hypertension.

The psychopathic personality is ascribed to some people who, because of strong emotional dysfunctions, are unable to get along with others. Extreme selfishness is one characteristic of the psychopath; total irresponsibility is another. Many hardened criminals have been diagnosed as psychopaths.

Character disorders is a catchall term used to describe persons who show a number of nonconformist, sometimes antisocial, traits. The alcoholic and the drug addict are sometimes included in this group. Some psychologists believe that homosexuality is also a character disorder.

Treatment

Neurotic and psychotic disorders are illnesses and are treated as such. In general, diagnosis and treatment are made by a *psychiatrist,* a medical doctor trained in the techniques of *psychotherapy* and *psychoanalysis.* A thorough physical examination precedes any treatment. The therapist—who may also be a *psychologist*—often confines himself to a listening role, and lets the patient talk his problems out.

Treatment—depending on the diagnosed problem—may range from prolonged talk sessions to various kinds of drug therapy. Often, psychotherapy is practiced in groups. The trend today is toward treatment closer to home, and many states have closed their large mental hospitals.

Summary

Every day, each of us experiences a variety of emotional responses—varied in kind, shading, and intensity. These are the ordinary feelings, ups and downs, with which we react to events, to people, to things we see or hear or even eat. Negative responses might range from irritation to rage, or from disappointment to grief. On the positive side, the range might be from contentment to delight, from amusement to hilarity.

Our bodies respond automatically, subconsciously, to extreme emotional stimuli such as terror or rage. We have built-in defense mechanisms, such as repression and rationalization, to protect us from heavy stress, from emotional extremes.

Most of the more severe emotional reactions—mental responses which exceed the "ordinary" in intensity and duration—are called either neuroses or psychoses. Neuroses are relatively benign. They include extreme anxiety, phobias, and obsession/compulsions and depression.

Psychoses, the more serious disorders, include schizophrenia (the so-called split personality disorder), the manic-depressive psychosis of extreme highs and extreme lows, and paranoia. These and most other psychoses are functional—they have no discernable physical cause. Other psychoses are called organic because they are caused by physical injury or other disorder. Senility, caused by brain cell deterioration in old age, is an example. Psychoses and neuroses should be treated professionally by psychiatrists or psychologists.

References

p. 33   Anna Freud, *The Ego and the Mechanism of Defense,* rev. ed. (New York, 1966).

p. 35   Lawrence C. Kolb, *Modern Clinical Psychiatry* (Philadelphia, 1972), Chaps. 5, 6.

p. 37   Karl Menninger et al., *The Vital Balance* (New York, 1963).

p. 39   Alfred Freedman and Harold Kaplan, *Comprehensive Textbook of Psychiatry* (Baltimore, 1967).

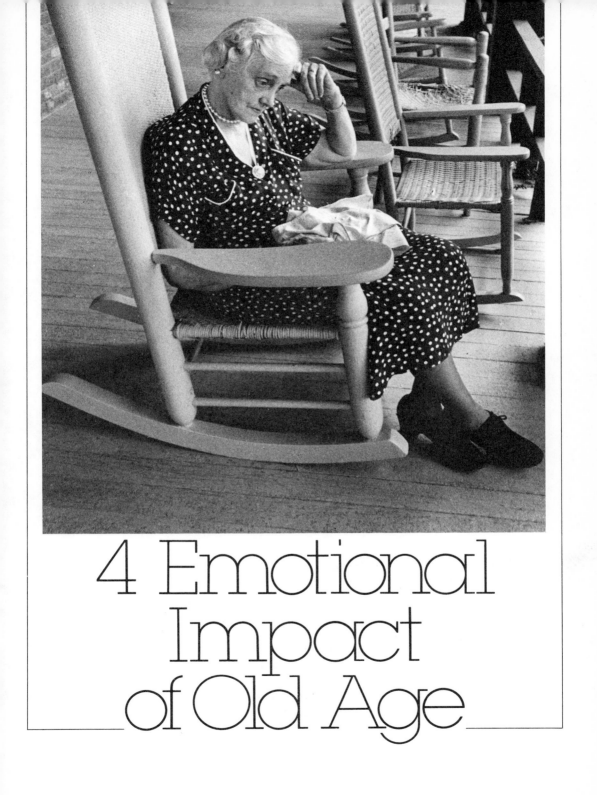

4 Emotional Impact of Old Age

I am twenty-nine years old, and I know that this is the end of a part of my life, the end of youth. . . . But it is also the beginning of a new phase of life, and the world we live in is so full of swift change and color and meaning that I can hardly keep from imagining the splendid and terrible possibilities of the time to come. . . . My future life will not be what it has been. And so I want to stop a minute, and look back, and get my bearings.

John Reed's thirtieth birthday had a significance to him far beyond mere numbers. It was the end of youth. Most of us seem to assign a terrible importance, a milestone status, to certain steps in the aging process. When we're very young, we contemplate these approaching milestones with eagerness, anticipation, even impatience. At six, we'll be able to start school. At twelve, we can join the Boy (or Girl) Scouts. At eighteen (in many states) we can cast our first votes. At twenty-one, we become full-fledged adults and can, among other things, walk into a bar and order our first legal drink.

After twenty-one, we begin to regard these approaching milestones with more than a little reluctance, some uneasiness, and, in some cases, even a bit of trepidation. After thirty, we aren't pursuing the milestones with such eagerness any more. Indeed, they seem to be pursuing *us,* relentlessly and all too swiftly. To deal successfully with the later milestones—forty, fifty, sixty, seventy—the individual must be comfortably at home within himself and with society. He must be aware of inevitable changes, and must be willing and able to cope.

Middle Age: A Transition

There are no scientific boundaries to what we call middle age. To an eighteen-year-old, middle age is thirty. To somebody in his or her mid-forties, middle age is something ten years or more in the future. The "youth cult" aspect of our contemporary culture makes it difficult for many of us to accept the simple fact that we're getting older. Middle age is that vaguely defined period between the time you stop being a "young adult" and the time you become a senior citizen. In middle age, you're probably too old to take up tennis but you think jogging or bike-riding might be a good idea. You're concerned with various aspects of your health and general condition.

In middle age you may get a bit thicker around the middle, despite regular exercise.

Your doctor tells you to stop eating fats and start watching your weight. In middle age your hair turns gray or your hairline recedes.

From the positive point of view, middle age can be the prime of your life. Most people in their forties and fifties—and well into their sixties—are usually at their career peaks. Their earning power is at its all-time high. People at middle age are a power group—and know it. They run many things including small businesses, labor unions, big businesses, and governments. Socially, too, this is usually the prime of life: friendships—from casual acquaintances to intimate friends—are well established. Social and recreational habits—clubs and the pubs, the weekly bridge game or poker session or round of golf—have caused you to settle into a familiar and comfortable pattern.

Of course, middle age isn't without its turmoil. By the time parents have passed the age fifty milestone, their children usually are grown—and have left the nest for school or jobs. They may have married and begun families of their own. To the woman who has devoted some twenty-five years to the role of housewife and mother, the departure of the children can pose some bedevilling questions about what to do with all that vacant time. Many women busy themselves with clubs and civic activities. Many approach their new freedom with relish, and resume their educations or begin new careers.

Physically, both men and women must recognize that their body—marvelous machine that it is—is showing signs of wear and must be given the kind of care it deserves. Women must cope with menopause and the realization that it means an end to the role of childbearer. Men—sometimes uncomfortably aware of emerging competition at work from the eager and ambitious younger generation—are often even more uncomfortable about their diminished sexuality. They have to accept the fact that arousal takes a little longer, that sex just isn't going to happen as often. Most probably come to terms with this. But some middle-age men really can't accept it, and try to "prove" themselves in liaisons with other, usually younger, women. As a result, the divorce rate often peaks in this period, and suddenly old friends are dying off—from heart attacks, cancer, strokes. The names in the obituary columns are suddenly familiar, not strange. Coping realistically with these situations is an important challenge in middle age—and old age.

Old Age

We hear and read a lot about old age in terms of contented senior citizens strolling hand-in-hand toward the sunset of their golden years. Beautiful, but terribly euphemistic. Old age exists; it won't go away. But, at its best, it *can* be a time of contentment, of satisfied contemplation of the past, of restful and even zestful enjoyment of the present, and calm acceptance of the future. At its worst, old age can be a time of illness, loneliness, financial problems, anxiety, even despair. However, the elderly—those who are sixty-five or over—are becoming an increasingly potent political force in the United States. And well they might: people are living longer today, and people over sixty-five now comprise more than 10 percent of our population. Of twenty million Americans over sixty-five, more than half are over seventy-three. And with improved health care, diet, and general understanding, the life-expectancy rate continues to rise. Many people in this elderly group are vital, active, and aggressive. Small wonder, then, that they have tended more and more to organize into lobbying groups in order to seek the things they believe society should help them with. They have campaigned actively for improvements in the Social Security System and Medicare. Their lobbying efforts also have been directed at changing the laws allowing corporations (and government agencies) to impose a mandatory retirement age. The elderly contend these laws make it possible to put useful, vigorous people "on the shelf" for no real reason except that they have attained a certain chronological age.

Problems of Old Age

There are other problems that must be faced by the elderly, and these can be confusing, distressing—and sometimes seemingly impossible to cope with.

Futility The older person often has a sense of uselessness, of disengagement from society. Mandatory retirement at an age like sixty-five cuts many people off in what they regard as midstride. Still in their prime, they feel, they are suddenly forced to give up the career they've pursued for all those years. Many find the readjustment hard to take. But

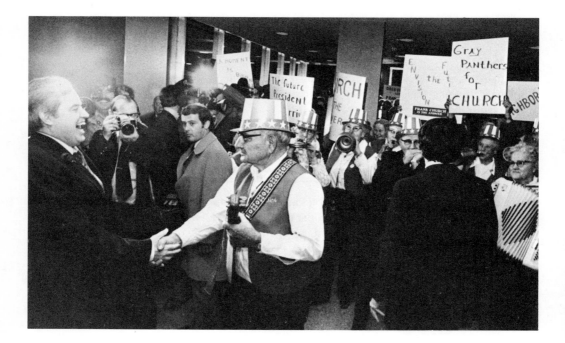

the person who has, during his active working life, developed outside interests may find the resources he needs to keep himself physically and mentally active.

Loneliness   The sometimes agonizing loneliness facing the elderly and retired transcends simply missing all the activity at the office. Without fail, there's going to be the genuine deprivation caused by the death of friends and—inevitably in a marriage—the loss of a mate.

Many lonely elderly people spin out their last years sitting in bleak little hotel lobbies, or in institutionalized "rest homes." Many governmental and private agencies try to ease the problems of loneliness by activity programs—ranging from circulating libraries to arts and crafts instructions, from dancing classes and chess tournaments to group tours of the neighboring countryside.

Money, Housing, Medical Care   It's difficult to separate these three subjects because decent housing and medical care cost money and, for all too many of the elderly, there simply isn't enough money to go around. Pensions—Social Security and private plans— generally have fallen far behind the cost of living. Indeed, the Social Security system has been beset by financial problems of its own. Government-backed health care programs, such as Medicare, consistently fail to cover all the necessary medical costs of those in an age bracket which faces increasingly frequent and severe health problems. Spokespeople for the elderly have noted the irony of the situation: While working, and in normally good health, the employee often is covered by the employer for almost all medical needs—including surgery and prolonged hospitalization. But this coverage disappears on retirement, when health problems are beginning to get more frequent and more serious.

There's a particular irony in the housing situation. Countless elderly citizens have, by the time of retirement, paid off the mortgages on the homes they've lived in for many years. Yet, because of steadily increasing taxes—fueled by real estate speculation that forces values and assessments upwards—many elderly people can no longer afford to live in their own homes. On their limited incomes, they can't even afford to pay the taxes. So they must sell.

The alternatives can be grim: a small apartment with none of the amenities of the old home; a tiny room, for some. Living with their children and grandchildren is not uncommon, but to a large degree it's considered less than ideal by all concerned. Most "rest homes" are impersonal, some say "dehumanizing." There are "retirement communities" with many amenities, group activities, and the like, but most of them are quite expensive.

Loss of Loved Ones   Typically, the loneliest among the elderly is the aged widow. Women commonly outlive their husbands, and today there are four times as many widows as widowers. After dealing with the emotional trauma of her husband's death and funeral, the widow sometimes must face the prospect of living out her days alone. She might have to exist at the poverty level since quite often her husband's pension and Social Security ceases at his death.

"These things shouldn't happen," said one spokesperson for the elderly. "It's a shame the way we callously put our senior citizens out to pasture—in pastures without grass."

Death

Each of us will die someday, and each of us knows it. But accepting that fact is one of the most difficult mental and psychological adjustments any of us will ever make.

Erik Erikson contends that to accept death on its inevitable terms, one must first have managed to cope, on a comfortable and realistic basis, with life. He calls this "ego integrity." In youth, in the exuberance of well-being, one sometimes feels immortal—capable of living forever. Later in life the aches and pains of even a moderately serious illness can create a terrible feeling of vulnerability, of mortality. Still, inside each of us there is an urgent, recurring whisper that says, "Surely this can't happen to *me*." But it can, of course, and it will.

Our strongest realizations of death normally involve a loved one—a parent, brother or sister, son or daughter, intimate friend. Even when death follows a lingering illness there is shock and grief although we accept the loss, and, eventually, we get back to the business of living.

Suicide

The inability to cope with life often culminates in death by self-destruction, or *suicide,* an act that so fascinates psychologists that more than 7,000 books and articles about it have been published. Suicide is believed to result from profound depression, although the actual act sometimes occurs almost on impulse. Many unsuccessful suicides are regarded as attention-getting gestures, cries for help from troubled minds.

Studies show the suicidal person is somehow alienated from society, self-derogating, with strong feelings of hopelessness, helplessness, rejection—and often loneliness. Suicide (more than 20,000 are recorded each year) is, after accidental death, the number two cause of death among students in the twelve to twenty-five age group. The rate is also quite high among college students. Many colleges and cities have established "suicide prevention clinics" with widely publicized telephone numbers. Persons who are contemplating suicide are encouraged to call and talk things out before taking that final and irrevocable step.

Responses to Death

Although suicides, as well as accidents and homicides, account for many deaths, most of us expect a natural death, whether from a totally unexpected heart attack or from the erosions and attritions of old age. And, admit it or not, everyone nurtures a fear of death. Taming that fear, reshaping it from an irrational terror into a calm and rational acceptance, is the goal of many groups in a growing movement which involves counseling the dying. The movement's concepts are beginning to spread into the community at large—the idea being that *everybody,* not just the terminally ill, should learn to accept the fact of death in its proper perspective.

In her book, *On Death and Dying,* Dr. Elisabeth Kübler-Ross reports on her work at a Chicago hospital with terminally ill patients and their families. She says there is much the dying can teach the living about impending death. In her Preface she states that her book is neither "a textbook on how to manage dying patients" nor "a complete study of the psychology of the dying."

"It is simply an account of a new and challenging opportunity to refocus on the patient as a human being, to include him in dialogues, to learn from him the strengths and weaknesses of our hospital management of the patient. We have asked him to be our teacher so that we may learn more about the final stages of life with all its anxieties, fears and hopes . . ."

Chapter by chapter, the book traces the stages of a patient's awareness of a terminal illness:

Denial and Isolation   The patient refuses to believe the diagnosis and then, particularly in a hospital, develops a strong sense of loneliness and isolation.

Anger   After "it *can't* be me" the patient's emotions focus on "*why* me?"

Bargaining   An almost childlike promise is made, sometimes to God, to behave nicely in exchange for a little more time, a little less pain.

Depression   The terminally ill patient can no longer deny his illness, nor laugh it off. More surgery is needed, or extended hospitalization, or the physical ravages of the disease become more pronounced. Resentment and rage are replaced by a deep feeling of loss.

Acceptance   If the patient has been helped through the earlier stages and has expressed his anger at his fate and his envy of those who don't share it, he may reach a stage where he is neither depressed nor angry. He may "contemplate his coming end with a certain degree of quiet expectation."

Threading its way through all these stages, Dr. Kübler-Ross writes, is a single emotion: hope. " . . . even the most accepting, the most realistic patients left the possibility open for some cure . . . it is this glimpse of hope which maintains them through days, weeks, or months of suffering . . ."

Summary

Significant chronological ages are treated as milestones by many people: school age is one, voting age another. After the twenty-first birthday we are more wary, less eager:

thirty, forty, fifty, sixty, and beyond mean moving from youth and young adulthood into middle and old age.

In middle age, most of us are at our peaks of career attainments and earning power. We are part of the age group that runs things. We are settled into comfortable habits and routines and circles of friends. If we have children they are usually grown and away at jobs or school. We're reminded of middle age by weight problems, graying hair, less frequent sex, and the annoying presence of ambitious younger people who'd like to succeed to our jobs.

Old age, ideally, can be a time of contentment and happiness. But it also can be—and often is—a time of despair. The loss of a loved marriage partner, loneliness, and illness often are combined with a serious lack of money for food and housing. Social Security and other pension services lag far behind the rising cost of living. Programs such as Medicare and Medicaid fail to pay major parts of our medical expenses.

Each of us will die someday and each of us refuses to accept it and fears it. Dispensing irrational fears and learning to cope with the fact of death on a calm, rational level can be a major achievement of adult personality development.

References

p. 42   John Reed, a legendary intellectual-activist-writer, covered Pancho Villa's Mexican Revolution in 1913 and in 1917 went to Russia as a supporter of the Soviet Revolution. His book, "Ten Days That Shook the World," is considered a classic. Reed died in Russia in 1920. He was almost 33. "Almost Thirty" appeared in the *New Republic* posthumously in 1936.

p. 44   Silvano Ariete, *The American Handbook of Psychiatry,* 2nd ed. (New York, 1974).

p. 45   Ariete, "The Problems of Aging," in *American Handbook of Psychiatry,* Chap. 43.

p. 45   Alexander Leaf, "Getting Old," *Scientific American* (September 1973), p. 44.

p. 46   Alfred Freedman and Harold Kaplan, *Comprehensive Textbook of Psychiatry* (Baltimore, 1967), Chap. 33.

p. 47   Elisabeth Kübler-Ross, *Questions and Answers On Death and Dying* (New York, 1974).

p. 47   Robert S. Morison, "Dying," *Scientific American* (September 1973), p. 54.

PART III
Sexuality

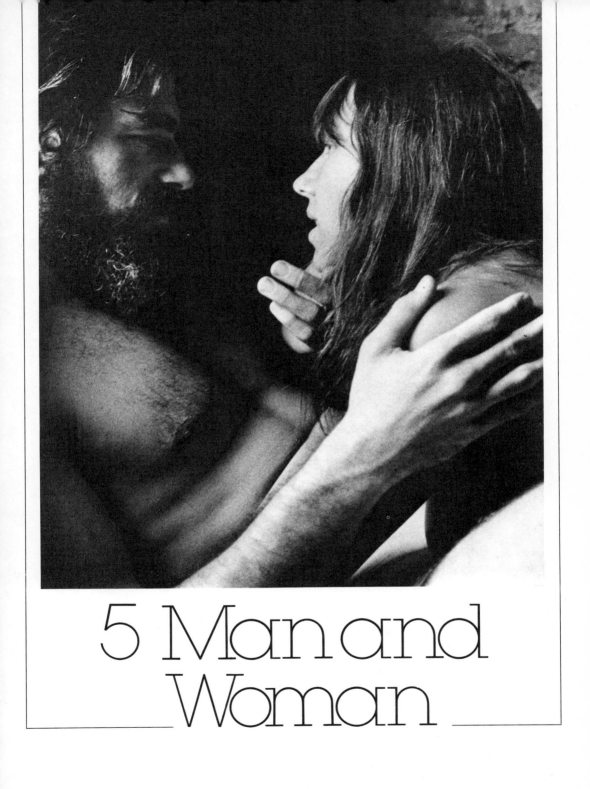

5 Man and Woman

Saturday morning; Henry exulted in the quiet luxury of awakening at his own pace. He could feel the warmth of the sun on his head and shoulders. He stretched, yawned, and looked at Jennifer. She's pretty, he thought—not for the first time. He reached toward her, stroked her cheek, then tousled her hair.

Jennifer opened her eyes, turned toward him, and smiled. His hand was still on her head and she cupped it in hers. "Good morning," she said. He drew her toward him and kissed her—gently at first, then with decided fervor. His hand began to massage her shoulder, then her back. Her hand encircled his waist, then moved down and began to stroke his leg.

"Why don't we make love?"

"I'd love to."

A handsome dude, Sally told herself as she changed clothes. She'd told him she'd "slip into something comfortable." He was waiting in the living room with the drink she'd made him. She daubed some perfume behind her ears and debated—briefly— what to wear. She picked the sheer, filmy robe.

Mike. That was his name. Seemed intelligent—he was an account executive for an ad agency she'd never heard of. They'd met about an hour ago in that quiet little bar near her office—a place she dropped into sometimes after work. She'd come in with friends, and so had he, and they'd sort of gravitated to each other. A casual conversation became increasingly intimate. The second drink led to a third, and then to dinner, and then to the overwhelming question: "Your place, or mine?" It turned out to be hers, which was closer and had no roommate complications.

Sally checked herself in the mirror, not without satisfaction, and walked into the living room.

Diane smiled and squeezed his hand. "It's been a *wonderful* evening Keith," she said. "Everything. The dinner, the movie . . ."

"I'm glad," he said in a half-whisper. He put a hand on each shoulder and drew her closer. God what a lovely creature, he thought, subconsciously aping a line from the movie they'd seen. He kissed her. He was sure she liked it. He kissed her again. She snuggled closer and his arm encircled her waist. Another kiss.

"Diane, I love you," he said. She smiled: "I think I love you too, Keith." Her voice was a bit breathy, he thought. Gently he put his left hand on her shoulder, then slowly let it slide down until it touched, then cupped, her right breast. She frowned slightly and moved his hand away with her own. "Don't."

He did it again and this time she let it linger. Emboldened, he moved the hand slowly down to her waist. She stiffened. "Don't," she commanded. "Please don't."

"But Diane . . ."

"No, Keith. Maybe sometime. Not now. I'm not ready. I guess I want it but I'm not ready. Please. Now I've got to go in. Walk me to the door."

Sexual Desire

These three scenes have one thing in common: sexual desire—fulfilled or frustrated. Two of them share something else: love. Each scene depicts a common human experience: sex with love, sex without love, love without sex. Each involves powerful emotional and instinctual urges. The scenarios might well have ended differently: Jennifer might have told Henry to forget it, she wasn't in the mood and, besides, she wanted another hour's sleep. Mike—for physical causes keyed to an excess of liquor— could have suffered temporary impotence: the incredibly embarrassing inability to maintain an erection.

And these same scenarios, involving the same drives and emotions, could well have involved homosexuals of either sex.

However these scenes ended, they all involved urges and emotions that, while not unique to humans, show themselves most dramatically in human actions and interactions. Affection and, indeed, lifetime mating are not unknown among many species, particularly the higher primates. But with most creatures, sex is entirely for reproduction. The when and how of its occurrence are dictated by powerful, deep-seated hereditary instincts. Mankind has these instinctual drives, but nature has added another factor: It has made sex an exciting, titillating, enjoyable experience that transcends the simple procreative urge.

Human sexuality is a highly complex thing. To understand it, one must explore all its aspects. And there is no better way to begin than with a discussion of the physical mechanisms that make it work.

The Human Reproductive System

Basically, the elements of human reproduction are simple: The female carries an egg that is fertilized by the male sperm or seed. The resulting embryo is nourished and sustained within the mother's uterus until it has reached "full term." The mother then begins "labor," and the baby is born.

In practice it is much more complex than that. So let us consider the physical systems which make reproduction possible.

Male Reproductive System

The male reproductive system is mostly external. Its visible parts are the *testicles* or *testes* and the *penis*. The testicles are a pair of walnut-shaped organs contained in a protective sac called the *scrotum,* which hangs between the upper thighs at the base of the penis. They produce the male seed, or *sperm*. The sac containing them is located outside the body in order to keep them at the proper temperature for sperm production (lower than the body temperature itself). The scrotum moves up closer to the body when

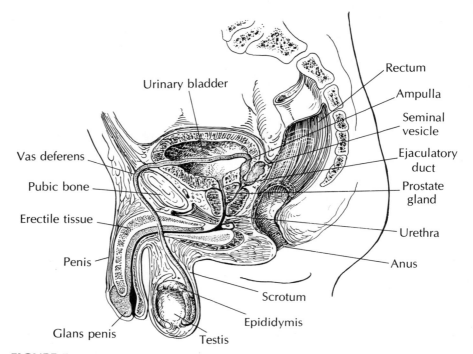

Urinary bladder

Vas deferens

Pubic bone

Erectile tissue

Penis

Glans penis

Testis

Epididymis

Scrotum

Rectum

Ampulla

Seminal vesicle

Ejaculatory duct

Prostate gland

Urethra

Anus

FIGURE 5-a *The male reproductive system: cross-section.*

the man is cold, and drops down when he is warm. Both the scrotum and the testicles are highly sensitive and rough handling can be extremely painful.

The testicles also produce the hormone *testosterone,* which is responsible for the development of male characteristics—including genital growth, body size, and beard growth. The tiny coiled tubes *(seminiferous tubules)* of the testes convey the mature *spermatozoa* (sperm) into a larger tube, at the back of each testicle, called the *epididymis.* Most sperm are stored there and in the spermatic cord *(vas deferens),* which leads to abdominal sacs or glands called the *seminal vesicles.* During sexual excitation, and before ejaculation, the sperm are augmented by secretions from the vesicles and the *prostate gland* to form a fluid called *semen* that is expelled from the *penis* during intercourse.

The *penis* is the principal male copulatory organ. It is a fleshy cylinder consisting of *erectile tissue* and the *urethra,* a canal that leads from the prostate and ejaculatory ducts to the tip of the penis. (This canal also serves to discharge urine from the bladder.) When the male is sexually stimulated, the vascular spaces in the erectile tissue fill with blood—pumped in faster than the veins can pump it out—with the result that the tissue distends. The ejaculatory ducts at the base of the organ contract and propel the semen into, through, and out of the penis by way of the urethra.

The female reproductive system is considerably more complex than the male. The external genitalia of the woman are located anatomically about where the base of the penis is in the man. The pubic bones are covered by a soft layer of fat called the *mons pubis*. This area, covered with hair, is above the *labia majora,* two rounded, hair-covered folds of flesh that form the external boundaries of a vertical opening known as the *vulva*. Within this cleft are two narrow lips (the *labia minora*), which have at their apex the *clitoris*—a tiny protuberance similar to the penis in structure and sensitivity. The area between the labia minora and below the clitoris is the *vestibule*. In its upper portion is the exterior opening of the urethra, leading to the bladder. Below that is the opening of the *vagina,* the principal female copulatory organ.

The vagina is a muscular tube extending inward about three and one-half inches. Its inner walls are highly elastic: it can accommodate a penis of almost any size, and it stretches tremendously in childbirth when it functions as the birth canal. The lower part of the vaginal opening is covered by a protective membrane, the *hymen,* which usually is ruptured or stretched during first intercourse. The area between the vulva and the *anus* is called the *perineum*.

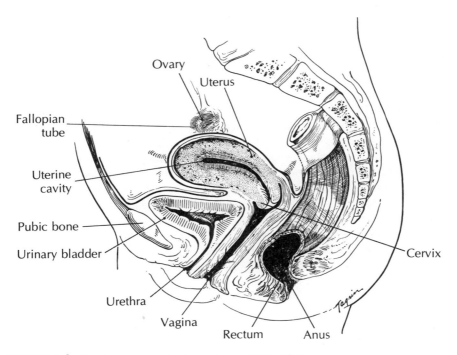

FIGURE 5-b *The female reproductive system: cross-section.*

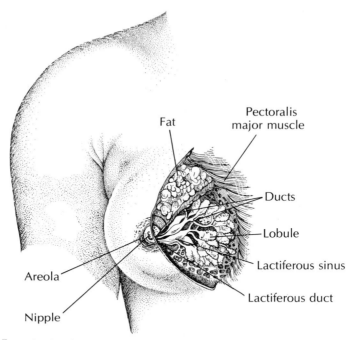

Fat

Pectoralis
major muscle

Ducts

Lobule

Lactiferous sinus

Areola

Lactiferous duct

Nipple

FIGURE 5-c *The female breast, showing the duct system.*

The *breasts,* or *mammary glands,* are also part of the external reproductive system. They are located in the pectoral area of the chest, one to a side, between the second and sixth ribs. Males have breasts, too, and they are not discernably different until puberty, when the female breasts start to develop. Although her breasts are an important source of erotic arousal, their main function comes after childbirth when they produce milk. At the apex of each breast is the *nipple,* surrounded by a circular pigmented area called the *areola.* The interior of each breast consists of the glands and lobes (the *mammary gland lobules, lactiferous sinus* and *lactiferous duct*) which are the *lactation* (milk-producing) system. In pregnancy, the breasts secrete a thin yellowish substance called *colostrum.* This nourishes the new infant for several days until milk production begins, stimulated by an onrush of hormones that had been feeding the placenta. The milk-producing capacity ceases in several weeks if the infant is not breast-fed.

Internal Genitalia The largest of the internal female reproduction organs is the *uterus* or *womb,* a pear-shaped organ which acts as a "nest" for the embryo after conception, and which must expand greatly during pregnancy to accommodate the growing *fetus.* The uterine walls contract to expel the infant when the time for birth arrives. On either side of the uterus are the *ovaries*—almond-shaped glands about one and one-half inches in length and one-half to three-quarters inch from front to back. They are *gonads,* as are the testicles, and their function is basically parallel: as the testicles produce *sperm* or seed, the ovaries produce *ova* or eggs. With periodic regularity (about every twenty-eight days) one of the ovaries produces a mature egg and expels it into one of the *Fallopian tubes,* from where it descends to the uterus. This process is called *ovulation.* If conception occurs, the egg usually is fertilized at the top of the tube. These slender tubes, about three to five inches in length, open into the uterus at their lower ends. The upper ends, lying close to the ovaries, have fringed, finger-like openings called *fimbria.* These grasp the ovum and guide it into the tube, where tiny hairlike cells push it toward the uterus. If the ovum isn't fertilized within about two days, it disintegrates within the uterus and is discharged through the vagina and *menstruation* begins.

Menstruation   The onset of the menstrual period is "day 1" in a woman's recurring cycle of interrelated menstrual and ovulation periods. The start of menstruation is taken to mean conception has not occurred.

Menstruation begins with the onset of puberty, usually about age twelve. It continues with cyclic regularity until about age fifty. The unfertilized egg expires in the Fallopian tube and the uterine lining—which had been ready to nurture the egg if

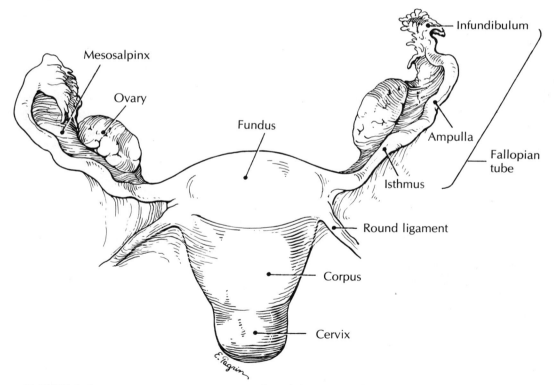

FIGURE 5-d *The female reproductive system: frontal view.*

fertilized—begins to break down and slough off. The result is a vaginal discharge, marked mostly by blood, which continues for four or five days. Some women experience abdominal cramping, especially during the early days.

Vaginal deodorants and *douches* are not necessary and could be harmful: the vaginal orifice is self-cleansing, and the deodorants may cause tissue irritations.

Menopause Menstruation continues from puberty until *menopause,* which usually occurs after a woman reaches forty. It signals the end of ovulation, the end of fertility but *not* the end of sexual interest, activity, and enjoyment. Many women experience distressing physical symptoms during menopause, and many suffer periodic depression, sometimes sufficiently serious to warrant psychiatric care. The most common physical symptoms of menopause are the so-called "hot flashes"—often uncomfortable flushes and feelings of unusual warmth.

The Erogenous Zones

Sexual intercourse doesn't—or at least shouldn't—just happen. Ideally, it should occur only when partners are ready for it, physically and psychologically. Or, to put it another way, sexually aroused.

Arousal is a natural response to sexual stimuli and usually occurs during a period of preliminary lovemaking—ideally a mutually enjoyable period of intimacy which should heighten mutual enjoyment of intercourse when it occurs. This period of arousal is called foreplay, and its essential ingredient is touch—the tactile stimulation of the most sexually sensitive areas of the body: the *erogenous zones.* Different people respond to different stimuli, of course, and certainly not all of them are physical. The sexual response of many persons is enhanced by stimulation of the other senses—by music, for instance, by a heady perfume, by the immediate environment (the comfortable room with subdued lighting, the summit of a hill bathed by moonlight).

Also, different people "turn on" to different degrees, and the buildup of sexual desire takes longer in some than it does in others. As a general rule, the male will be aroused more quickly than the female: the man's response curve is comparatively sharp and precipitous—his passions are aroused quickly and subside quickly. The woman generally builds more gradually to her responsive peak, and her erotic feelings subside more gradually after sexual fulfillment (or the lack of it).

Male Erogenous Zones

The penis, particularly the rim and underside of the *glans* or head, and the underside of the shaft, are most susceptible to erotic stimulation. Erection, the obvious sign of male arousal, usually follows light but persuasive stroking of the penis. Erection occurs when heightened excitement pumps more and more blood into the shafts of spongy erectile tissue, which run through the penis to its head. Blood flows into this tissue faster than the veins can carry it out, and the organ enlarges and stiffens.

Many men are unduly concerned with the size of their penis. The experts say its size has nothing to do with sexual performance, or masculinity, or the ability to satisfy a sexual partner.

Female Erogenous Zones

The clitoris is considered the most erotically sensitive single part of the female body. Most of the time only the tip of the organ is visible, but during sexual arousal the clitoris enlarges in a manner similar to a male erection. Unlike the penis, the clitoris has just one function: sexual stimulation. It has no role in procreation except as a tool in the sexual process that can lead to conception. Some women, however, react to clitoral stimulation only after their overall arousal has begun. And, according to some studies, many women have complained about lovers who concentrate on clitoral stimulation to the exclusion of other and perhaps more subtle means.

The inner lips of the vulva (the labia minora) are quite sensitive to stimulation, as are the vaginal entrance or cuff, the *mons veneris,* the perineum, and the anal area. The breasts, particularly the nipples and the surrounding area (the *areola*), are a major source of arousal in the woman and, to a lesser degree, in the man.

Sexual Arousal

In both sexes, sexual arousal may be accomplished through stimulation of such areas as the ears (the lobes and the rest of the external structure) and the nape of the neck. Of particular erotic significance are the lips, the tongue, and the interior of the mouth. In kissing, these sensitive regions provide strong sexual arousal.

Men and women both are responsive to external stimuli such as erotic books or movies.

There are many outward signs of sexual arousal. Some (notably the man's erection) are more obvious than others. Both the man and the woman experience faster pulse rates and quicker breathing as arousal proceeds to and through intercourse. And their skin often acquires a deep flush as arousal continues.

Oral and Anal Sex

Oral and anal sex, particularly the former, are widely practiced by heterosexual couples—although both practices have been historically associated, in the minds of many, with homosexuality.

Many people say oral-genital stimulation (*cunnilingus* and *fellatio*) are a regular, essential—and highly enjoyable—part of their erotic foreplay leading to "conventional" intercourse. Many continue it to orgasm. Others practice oral stimulation on occasion—to add some exciting variety to their lovemaking. Some people avoid the practices because they regard them, variously, as unnatural, immoral, unhealthy, or illegal. (They *are* illegal in some states, although many states have adopted, or are considering adopting, laws that legalize oral and anal sex practiced in private by consenting adults—homosexual or heterosexual.)

Cunnilingus is the oral stimulation of the vulva. The kissing and licking usually is concentrated on and around the clitoris and the vaginal opening. *Fellatio* is the oral stimulation of the penis. Sometimes the glans and shaft are taken deep into the mouth, and sometimes the lips and tongue concentrate on the highly sensitive rim and lower tip of the glans.

Anal sex—the substitution of the anus for the vagina in sexual intercourse—has historically been denounced by society. But the act *(pederasty)* is widely practiced by homosexual, and to a lesser extent by heterosexual, couples. Some heterosexuals practice it occasionally for the sake of variety, others use it as they would oral sex—as an erotic prelude to vaginal intercourse. Doctors warn that the penis must be lubricated before insertion, to prevent injury to delicate anal tissue. If vaginal intercourse is to follow anal intercourse, the penis should first be washed thoroughly.

Criminal statutes against anal intercourse customarily call it *sodomy*. Any form of the practice, even in private by consenting adults, is illegal in many states. It is universally illegal in cases involving force or minors.

Masturbation

Masturbation is the manual manipulation of the sex organs, usually to the point of orgasm. Although the term is customarily associated with self-manipulation of the penis or the vulval area, it isn't uncommon for two people to manipulate each other's sex organs in this manner (mutual masturbation).

Although masturbation is commonly associated with teen-age boys, the practice has its rudimentary beginnings in infancy, is commonly performed by females, and is hardly unknown to married couples. Sometimes a husband or wife will masturbate to orgasm when alone; mutual masturbation as a prelude to intercourse is a normal component of erotic foreplay.

In generations past, disapproving parents used any manner of scare tactics to dissuade their children from masturbating. The act was incorrectly described as the cause of such assorted maladies as pimples, falling hair, insanity, and eventual impotence. Today's parents seem more inclined to accept masturbation as a natural state of affairs—and well they should, since repeated surveys indicate most of them have practiced it at one time or another.

Some people are able to achieve a quicker and more intense orgasm by masturbating than they can when their partner stimulates them. This seems particularly true of women. The logic, of course, is that the woman can feel what the manipulation is doing to her, and can adjust her "target" to heighten her response. She can only *tell* her partner that such-and-such a pinpoint area excites her the most.

The Sex Act

The basic mechanics of sexual intercourse consist of insertion of the penis into the vagina, and a mutual pelvic thrusting that continues until the partners achieve orgasm.

Intercourse

In terms of postural positions, however, intercourse (or *coitus*) is a theme with many variations. Most of the people, most of the time (if the various sex surveys are to be believed) have their sex lying down, in bed, with the man on top of the woman. But there is a wide variety of other positions—not only reclining but sitting and even standing—and the general rule seems to be that there isn't any "wrong" position, or even any universally accepted "right" position. The correct one is the one that's right for you and your partner.

The basic man-atop-woman posture is called "the missionary position," a term apparently applied by derisive Polynesian natives to the sexual habits of the missionaries who came to their islands. (The islanders apparently employed a sort of sitting position for their sex.) Other commonly used positions are woman on top, side-by-side, and rear-entry (with the penis inserted into the vagina from the rear, usually with the woman on all fours). Mutual satisfaction is the aim of the sexual partners when they opt for any of the many possible coital positions.

Orgasm

The sensual climax of the sex act, the moving culmination to all that has preceded it is the orgasm. It has been described as emotional and physical fulfillment, and it has also been called release.

Orgasm in the male is relatively simple. The production of sperm, and its combination with other fluids to form semen, has already been described. As intercourse proceeds, the already erect penis becomes *tumescent* (swollen, full) in preparation for ejaculation. The orgasm begins as the sensations of approaching ejaculation are felt. It reaches its peak with ejaculation itself, then subsides, and the penis begins to relax back into its limp, unexcited state.

In the female, there's some dispute about just what happens—and precisely where—during orgasm. Surveys have shown for years that women were harder to arouse, and less likely to achieve orgasm, than men—but more recent studies have shown a change. Today's woman is likely to respond more quickly and fully to erotic foreplay, and is more likely to achieve orgasm. This change is attributed to two things: the growing personal, social, professional, and economic emancipation of women—as advocated by members and supporters of the feminist movement—and the sexual emancipation brought about by the development of more sophisticated and foolproof methods of birth control, principally "the Pill."

There is another school of thought that contends a woman can experience two different kinds of orgasm—the clitoral and the vaginal. There are those who say the former is more intense, and there are those who say the opposite. In addition, there are those who say the two are actually one and the same. The orgasm consists of muscular contractions in a regular rhythm (said to be at the same pace as the male's ejaculation— the spasms 0.8 seconds apart) in the vaginal and clitoral areas and the uterus. Unlike the man, the woman does not ejaculate, although vaginal secretions increase as the intensity of response heightens.

Despite all that is written about simultaneous orgasm, many studies indicate that this kind of fortuitous timing is the exception rather than the rule, and that it isn't necessary for complete mutual fulfillment.

Multiple orgasm is another subject about which much has been written. Many women seem to experience repeated orgasm during a single act of intercourse—but it often depends on the man's ability to prolong the erection by delaying his own orgasm and the resulting return to flaccidity.

Younger males are indeed capable of having a number or orgasms in a brief period—although having several during just one act of intercourse would seem unusual. The male's recuperative and restorative powers diminish as he gets older. He has to wait for a longer time after intercourse before he is capable of repeating the act. This period may vary considerably in an individual because of changing external forces that might heighten or lessen his sexual response.

The final phase of intercourse has been called "afterglow." It is a period of warmth, tenderness, lassitude—a time when many couples simply like to cling to each other.

Frequency of Intercourse   This can be a source of difficulty when the sexual appetites of the partners are markedly different. There probably is no "normal" frequency in any relationship. Our contemporary mythology would have it that young couples spend most of their time making love, and older couples virtually none at all. Both positions are, no doubt, exaggerated. It is likely that most couples have sex more often when they are younger and less frequently in later life, but surveys have shown that many couples are still enjoying regular sex (perhaps once or twice a week) when they are in their seventies.

Conception

Nature's desire to perpetuate the various species seems to approach the point of excess in some instances. And people—whose methods of fertilization are hardly as haphazard as fish—are no exception.

The typical male ejaculation, which might fill a large teaspoon, contains perhaps 500 million spermatazoa. Each of these microscopic organisms, with bulbous head and wriggling tail, is *motile* (capable of self-locomotion) and propels itself unswervingly toward its target, the female egg, though only one sperm will fertilize the egg.

The human female is born with the nucleus, of about 400,000 to 500,000 eggs, half in each ovary. Of these potential eggs—the woman's lifetime supply—only about 400 will leave the ovaries as mature ova during a full and productive life.

Conception is to a large degree a matter of timing. The passage of the spermatozoa from penis to cervix is usually a matter of seconds. But it may take hours for the steadily diminishing army of sperm to invade the uterus and (in even smaller numbers) the Fallopian tubes. Estimates vary, but apparently the number of spermatozoa that survive the acidic secretions of the vaginal canal and reach the uterus are numbered in the tens to hundreds of thousands, and the survivors that actually enter the tubes range from a few hundred to a few thousand. For conception to take place, a mature and viable sperm must unite with a mature and viable ovum. The spermatozoa survive for perhaps three days, at the most, after being deposited in the vagina. An ovum probably survives for two days after it leaves the ovary. But since the ovulation (and menstrual) cycles of different women may vary considerably, deciding when a particular woman will ovulate is largely guesswork.

Ovulation and Menstruation

Ovulation and menstruation are different occurrences, but they are interrelated and interdependent, and must be considered together. Ovulation has the dual functions of producing a mature ovum to be fertilized, and of preparing the uterus to receive and nurture it. Menstruation disposes of the egg—and the preparatory material—if fertilization doesn't take place.

The ovarian and menstrual cycles are generally said to occur during a 28-day period. That is average, although for many women the overall period is longer, or shorter. The first day of menstruation is generally regarded as the first day of this overall cycle, or "day 1." Menstruation normally lasts four or five days. Ovulation, which is quite difficult to detect because of the dearth of outward physical signs, is believed to

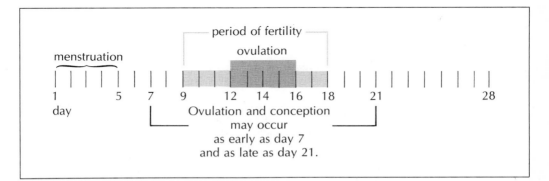

FIGURE 5-e *The menstrual cycle.*

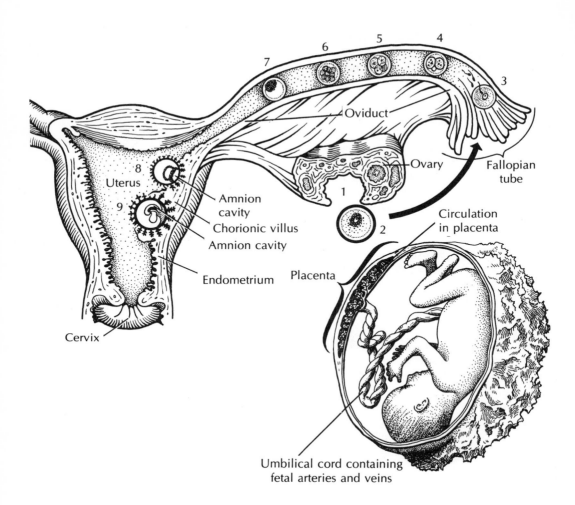

FIGURE 5-f *Human reproduction: fertilization, implantation, and the placenta (schematic). Upper drawing: 1, 2. Liberation of an egg from a follicle in the ovary, which shows corpora lutea. 3. Fertilization of the egg in the oviduct shortly after it has entered (during ovulation the ovary is pressed closely to the mouth of the oviduct). 4–7. Cleavage stages. 8, 9. Embryo, with its amnion cavity already clear, implanting on the endometrium of the uterine wall. The chorion of the embryo has developed fingerlike villi that burrow deep into the endometrium and serve as the embryo's agents of exchange of nutrients and wastes with the maternal tissues of the placenta. Lower drawing: An advanced fetus in the uterus, with the umbilical cord leading to and from the placenta and carrying the fetal circulation.*

start midway in the cycle, or about day 14, although it may begin as early as day 7 and as late as day 21. Considering the presumed life-span of the spermatazoa and that of the ovum, then, conception might result from intercourse as early as day 4, or as late as day 22 or 23.

Fertilization

When fertilization occurs, it is because just one sperm enters the egg, as previously noted. But getting that one sperm inside is something of a team effort. The mature ovum is surrounded by a thin inner membrane, which in turn is covered by a tough transparent layer or belt called the *zona pellucida*. This in turn is covered by a cellular layer called the *corona radiata,* which is held together by a kind of acid. The assault wave of sperm detach this corona, allowing other sperm to attack the zona pellucida. One manages to penetrate, the zona is closed, the membrane thickens, and all other sperm are excluded.

The male pronucleus in the head of the sperm that gained entry then fuses with the female pronucleus in the egg and fertilization takes place. The combined cell is called a *zygote.* It takes two to four days for the zygote to travel down the Fallopian tube into the uterus, and it does not implant itself in the *endometrium* (the mucous membrane lining the uterus) for several days. But, from the time of fertilization, the zygote has been dividing: one cell into two, two into four, four into eight, and so on. By the time the zygote reaches the uterus, it is a many-celled structure surrounding a fluid-filled cavity. The whole mass, called a *blastocyst,* implants itself in the uterine wall. The sex of the embryo was determined at the moment of fertilization; the irregular spacing of the multiplying cells presages the development of all the various components of a human being.

Genetics

The interactions of the sperm and the egg at the moment of fertilization do much more than determine the sex of the embryo and start its growth. They also decide many things about its physical characteristics, such as body size and bone structure, color of hair and eyes, thickness of lips, size and shape of nose. They determine whether the child will or won't be color blind, and whether, in later life, he or she will be afflicted by such inherited afflictions as diabetes, heart disease, or (especially in the male) early baldness. And the elements that combine at conception have a lot to say about a person's intelligence, creativity, personality (extroverted or introverted), conduct (aggressive or nonaggressive) and disposition (mostly sunny or mostly sullen). But traits of personality, intelligence, creativity, and behavior are also influenced and perhaps modified by interaction with the environment, with parental attitudes, diet, and education.

The components of the sperm and the egg that produce these physical characteristics and behavioral traits—which literally pass them along from one generation to the next—are the work of microscopically tiny organisms called chromosomes, and of infinitesimal components of the chromosomes called *genes.*

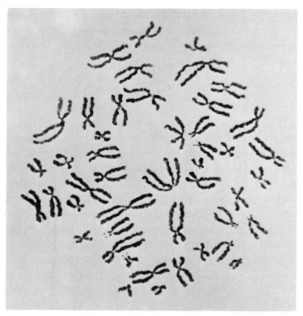

Chromosomes of a normal human male.

Except where rare abnormalities exist, the ovum contains 23 chromosomes, the sperm 23, so that the beginning zygote has 46 chromosomes of 23 pairs. Within each of the threadlike chromosomes are many (perhaps a thousand or so) of the genes that carry the imprint of the hereditary influences. The genes also occur in pairs—one from the father and one from the mother.

Mitosis

Growth of the zygote, the embryo, the fetus, and, ultimately, of the living human is through a process of cell division called *mitosis*. In the earliest stages of division (one into two, two into four, and so on), mitosis produces new cells identical to the original. But they soon begin to differentiate according to the tasks they will perform: the creation of muscular tissue, for instance, or bone structure, or the nervous system. Yet one thing remains constant: The chromosomes within each new cell, and the genes within each chromosome, are precisely the same, and the hereditary messages are the same.

Meiosis

There is one exception to the rule that cell division always produces new cells with 46 chromosomes (23 pairs). This is the cellular division occurring only in the testicles and ovaries. The dividing process in these areas is called *meiosis*. The cells it produces have only 23 chromosomes each, and are capable of surviving only for a short period if they aren't united (sperm and egg) by fertilization to produce a cell (the zygote), which survives and reproduces.

Cell Structure

Despite differentiation and specialization, most cells are basically similar in structure. Each consists of a living substance called *protoplasm,* encased in a membrane. This chemical substance consists of carbohydrates, proteins, fats, inorganic salts, and vitamins, and enzymes necessary to sustain the life of the cell. The protoplasm of the cell contains many *organelles* (a specialized part of a cell that resembles and functions as an organ). The principal organelle is the spherical *nucleus,* which is responsible for the reproduction of the cell, among other things. The nucleus contains protoplasm, the chromosomes and genes, and a smaller spherical organelle called the *nucleolus* or "little nucleus." Sometimes several *nucleoli* are present in the nucleus. The precise functions of these small nuclei have not been determined, but they may have an important role in the production of the key component of the genes called DNA.

The protoplasm existing outside the nucleus is called *cytoplasm.* This living fluid contains a number of tiny organelles, and is responsible for such functions as digestion, respiration, secretion, and excretion of the cell.

Sex Determination   The 23rd pair of chromosomes in the zygote determines the sex of the embryonic infant. Whether it is male or female depends on the father—or, rather, on which of his sperm penetrates and fertilizes the ovum. The sex chromosome within the egg is always what is called an X chromosome. The sperm, however, will contain either an X or a Y chromosome. If the fertilizing sperm has an X chromosome, the combination (XX) means the child will be female. If fertilization is done by a sperm with the Y chromosome, the combination (XY) will produce a male child.

Abnormalities   Sometimes, abnormal conditions produce mutations of the basic XX and XY combinations. Rarely, some malfunction in cell division can produce a female child with just one X sex chromosome (such children generally are physically but not mentally deformed). On occasion an XXY combination of sex chromosomes will result (the child usually develops with physical signs of both sexes—small breasts, small penis, and small, unproductive testes).

More frequently, abnormal conditions produce a male with an XYY combination. The XYY male is said to be larger in physical size and to possess a stronger-than-normal sex drive. Earlier studies, now largely refuted, held that the XYY male was also unusually aggressive, with a propensity for violence. The general thinking now is that if the XYY male is abnormally aggressive, the trait probably stems from environmental conditions associated with large physical size.

Mutations or abnormalities in the 22 nonsexual chromosomes (usually called *autosomes*) may cause various mental and physical deformities. For instance, the mental condition called Mongolism or Down's Syndrome can result from the production of an extra autosome on Pair 21. (In most cases where the fertilized egg receives more or fewer than the normal 46 chromosomes, it will develop abnormally and die early.) Maternal illnesses, such as German measles, also can cause genetic mutations.

The Genetic Code and DNA   Genes are made of *deoxyribonucleic acid* (abbreviated to DNA). This substance contains all the genetic information that will imprint various hereditary traits on all the developing cells within the embryonic being. Each infinitesimal DNA molecule consists of a chain of nitrogen bases in varying combinations which encode the necessary information for various hereditary traits.

The DNA molecules are capable of duplicating themselves with each cell division, but they can't get out of the nucleus of the chromosome. And to dictate the formation of the kinds of proteins necessary for the creation of cells of various functions, the DNA's stored information must be imparted to amino acids in the cytoplasm outside the nucleus. This is done through the creation of molecules of *ribonucleic acid* (RNA), which are able to get out of the nucleus in the proper form, and impart the genetic knowledge from the DNA molecules. In all, a highly complicated process, performed by elements so tiny as to defy imagination. Consider: A normal male ejaculation produces perhaps a teaspoonful of semen which contains roughly 500 million sperm. Each sperm contains 23 chromosomes, and each chromosome carries a chain of perhaps 1,000 genes.

"Recombinant" DNA   A scientific controversy has sprung up around the subject of so-called recombinant DNA. In 1972, molecular biologists discovered a special class of enzymes that could cut portions of the double-stranded DNA molecules in such a manner that they could be joined with strips of DNA from a different organism. The resultant, restructured DNA molecules can then reproduce.

Science, it is agreed, can learn much about the genetic code from these man-synthesized organisms, but many scientists (and even government officials) believe this kind of research could be hazardous to man if not rigorously controlled. Most of the experiments have involved DNA from a strain of bacteria commonly found in the intestines of human beings, and some scientists fear the research might lead, inadvertantly, to the creation of new human infections for which there are no known cures.

In 1974, a group of eleven prominent molecular biologists proposed a temporary ban on this kind of research, and a year later, one hundred forty molecular biologists from sixteen countries proposed strict guidelines for the research. Their stated goal was to allow beneficial experiments to continue, under restrictions that would prevent medical risks to man. Since then, the legislative bodies of some states and cities have debated, and in some cases passed, new laws restricting the kind of genetic research that can be conducted, and limiting the places it can be done.

Dominant and Recessive Genes   For each trait embedded in the chromosonal pattern, there are two genes, paired. Sometimes they express the same trait in the same way. Genes of this sort are called *homozygous,* and they may be *dominant* or *recessive.* If they are dominant, the trait they dictate will be manifested in the person. If they are both recessive, their form of the trait will also be expressed. Often, two genes relating to a certain characteristic will express it differently (technically they are *heterozygous*). In such pairings, one gene will be dominant and its version of the trait will be shown by the person. But the recessive trait will be carried, and will show itself in some way in the next generation. Red hair, blue eyes, thin lips, diabetes, hemophilia, and colorblindness are examples of recessive traits.

Colorblindness is one of a number of inherited traits said to be "sex-linked." The most common variety of this affliction—the inability to distinguish between red and green—is common in men but unusual in women, yet the trait is the product of a recessive X gene. Thus a colorblind father and a woman with normal color perception would produce sons (XY) with normal vision. Their daughters (XX) would carry the trait as a recessive, and might produce colorblind sons (but not daughters) if the sons receive their mothers' recessive rather than dominant X genes.

Some human traits, including intelligence, are the product of a number of sets of genes, rather than just one. They are described as *polygenic*.

Pregnancy

When the fertilized egg (zygote) starts its journey down the Fallopian tubes toward the uterus, it begins the cell-division process (mitosis), which will result about nine months later in the birth of a child. During this cycle the single cell that began it all will divide and redivide, differentiate and specialize, in a remarkably precise manner.

By the time the tiny mass of multiplying cells (the blastocyst) is ready to plant itself in the prepared uterine wall (endometrium), the action of hormones has converted the endometrial cells into nutrient-enriched cells called *decidua*. These surround the growing organism (called an embryo after the first week) and nourish it until that function is taken over by a specialized organ called the *placenta*. This organ forms in the decidua between the embryo and the uterine wall. It consists of a complicated network of blood vessels. It is an exchange area of sorts through which the mother supplies food and oxygen to the embryo, and the embryo discharges wastes that ultimately are released through the mother's own excretory system.

The embryo is attached to the placenta by the *umbilical cord*, which acts as a conduit for incoming nutrients and outgoing waste. The embryo has by now become encased in a double-membrane sac filled with amniotic fluid. It will remain in the sac, floating in and bathed by the fluid, until birth.

Within three to four weeks after fertilization, the heart has formed and has begun to beat, pumping blood through a rudimentary but still-evolving vascular network. By the end of eight weeks the tiny embryo is recognizable as a human form. It is only about an inch long, but its evolving eyes, ears, and nose are visible, as are its arms and legs. Its hands and feet and external genitalia are beginning to form. From this point (the beginning of the third month) until birth, the developing child is called a *fetus*.

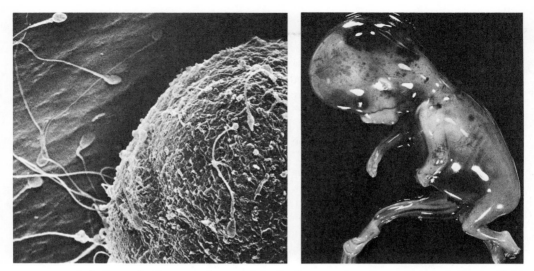

Left: Sperm floating around ovum. Actually, the ovum is as tiny as the head of a pin. Right: Human fetus at approximately 12–16 weeks.

By the end of the twelfth week (after the third 28-day lunar month or first trimester of pregnancy) the fetus weighs about an ounce, is three inches long, and has tiny, soft nails on its newly formed fingers and toes; its eyes (under closed lids) and its ears are clearly recognizable; its kidneys are working; it moves, but isn't yet felt by the mother although a physician can feel the uterus protruding above the pelvis into the abdominal cavity.

After 16 weeks, the fetus weighs four ounces, is more than six inches long, and is starting to grow a small bit of rudimentary hair on the scalp. At 20 weeks the eight-ounce, 10-inch-long fetus has a heartbeat that can be detected by a stethoscope. The fetus has become increasingly active, and its movements are emphatically (although not painfully) felt by the mother.

By the 28-week mark (the end of the seventh lunar month) the fetus is about 15 inches long, weighs about 2½ pounds, can open its eyes and distinguish light from dark. More important, if born at this premature stage, the infant has a fair chance to survive because of the development of its lungs and intestinal system. A month later, development has reached the point where the chances for survival in premature birth are considered good.

The fetus reaches "full term" and usually is ready for birth after the ninth lunar month—usually about midway into the 10th lunar month (roughly 265 days from conception and, on the average, 280 days from the end of the last menstrual period preceding conception). The newborn infant may be about 20 inches long and weigh about 7.5 pounds—but these figures are rough averages.

Detecting Pregnancy

The complex but orderly sequence of events that begins with fertilization may have been taking place for some time before the woman knows that she's pregnant. The missed menstrual period is, of course, the most common indicator. Others include nausea ("morning sickness") and tenderness in the breasts along with enlargement of the nipples. But any of these signs may have causes other than pregnancy.

Laboratory tests directed by a physician will detect pregnancy in its early stages. Customarily they involve injection of the woman's urine into immature laboratory animals, especially rabbits, mice, and frogs. If the woman is pregnant, her urine will contain a special hormone which appears after the ovum is implanted. This hormone causes ovarian changes in female mice or rabbits. It causes spermatogenesis—the creation of sperm—in the male frog.

These are the most common tests, and they are considered mostly but not wholly accurate. Detection of pregnancy as it progresses is easier, as the growing fetus makes its presence known.

The Expectant Mother

From the time pregnancy is detected until the time the child is born, the mother-to-be must take certain steps to insure her own good health and that of the fetus she's carrying. She should visit her doctor at regular intervals for a physical examination and a variety of laboratory tests. She should adjust her diet: pregnant women need more calories, protein, carbohydrate, and fat, as well as vitamins and minerals. Deficiencies in prenatal diet—inadequate supplies of protein, calcium, calories, and certain vitamins can cause a number of medical problems—including diminished physical and neurological development, and lower resistance to disease—in the child. The expectant mother may expect to gain something close to 20 or 25 pounds during the course of normal pregnancy.

She must also avoid exposure to some diseases—particularly Rubella (German measles), which may lead to fetal deformity if the mother gets it during the first three months of pregnancy. A number of effective vaccines against German measles are now available. Infant blindness is the major Rubella-linked deformity.

Other serious fetal afflictions may result from syphilis or other venereal diseases. Overexposure to X-ray radiation can kill or deform a fetus. Chemical food additives can reach the fetus by way of the placenta. Many physicians counsel against the use of alcohol or tobacco, at least in large quantities, during pregnancy. Use of any drugs is strictly controlled by the physician.

Sexual intercourse during pregnancy, particularly in its later stages, used to be considered dangerous. Today, many physicians allow their patients to have sex during the entire term of pregnancy. But physical conditions that would make sex either permissible or unwise will vary from patient to patient, and decisions about sex during pregnancy should be made individually, upon the advice of the responsible physician.

Childbirth

The physical process that culminates in the birth of the baby is called *labor*. When it begins, the cervix starts to open and dilate, and rhythmic contractions commence in the upper portion of the uterus. As labor progresses, and birth (or delivery) gets closer, the contractions occur at a faster pace, are of longer duration, and are felt by the mother with greater and greater intensity.

The pressure of the contractions usually ruptures the amniotic sac at the onset of the delivery phase of labor. If the fetus is in proper position for a normal delivery, it will leave the uterus head first. The intensifying uterine contractions force it out through the cervix and through the vaginal canal. Often the delivery process is aided by the mother's own body pressures.

When the baby is entirely out of the mother's body, the attending physician gets it to breathe on its own, and the newborn infant customarily utters its first cry. The umbilical cord is severed and tied off close to the body. The placenta (commonly called "afterbirth") is expelled from the uterus by renewed contractions that begin a few minutes after childbirth. The distended uterus begins to contract to its normal size.

Breech Birth   This is the term used for a delivery in which the baby emerges buttocks first. It can involve serious complications, and the physician who determines that the fetus is facing the wrong way often attempts to reposition it by manipulation before the mother is ready to start labor.

Forceps Delivery   A delivery in which the physician uses a mechanical device to grasp the head of the fetus and pull it gently through the vaginal canal. This method is used when complications slow the normal delivery, or when medical reasons dicate that delivery should be speeded.

Caesarean Section   This is a surgical procedure by which the infant is removed through an incision in the abdomen and uterus. Caesareans are employed for a number of reasons when the labor is not proceeding normally. The most common cause is that the infant is too large to be delivered through the uterine canal. This kind of surgery may be used to terminate a prolonged labor that threatens the life of the mother, or child, or both.

Natural Childbirth

Is childbirth an intensely painful experience that should be eased with drugs? The answer you get to that question depends on who you ask. In recent years there has been increasingly widespread acceptance of the theories of "natural" childbirth. Advocates of the method believe labor may be accomplished with relatively little pain, and without drugs or with a minimal dosage. In many cases they go beyond that, and urge programs of education that also involve exercises in breathing, in muscular control, in relaxation. Natural childbirth programs also sometimes involve the husband who will in many cases be at his wife's side during labor and delivery.

There are, of course, many safe medicines to reduce whatever pains may occur in labor, and the ultimate decision as to whether they will be used must be made by the mother-to-be and her physician.

The Post-Natal Period

The new mother's principal concerns naturally center on the newborn baby and its needs. The infant's very presence—whether it is the first child or the third—means many changes in the day-to-day household routine for all family members, but particularly for the mother. And the woman must also cope with certain post-natal changes in her own body.

Many of these changes involve the process of a return to normal in the woman: the uterus and vagina begin to contract immediately after delivery, and within six weeks they are almost back to normal. There is weight loss, of course, as part of the delivery and post-delivery processes. The mother should be back to her prepregnancy weight in about a month and a half. When her menstrual periods resume they may occur with some irregularity and at first they may involve a copious flow.

Lactation

One significant change in the mother is the beginning of milk production in her breasts *(mammary glands.)* Physical changes during pregnancy prepare the breasts for *lactation,* and by the time of delivery, the mother is physically equipped to nurse the infant.

Nursing is believed to heighten the close physical and emotional rapport of mother and child, and to pass on the mother's immunities. But some mothers prefer, for various reasons of their own, to bottle-feed their babies instead. And in some cases there are medical reasons which cause a physician to recommend against nursing.

Birth Control

Al and Lucille Miller want a family but they don't want to start it yet. They've been married just a year, and are just barely getting by financially. She works as a librarian and he's in law school. He has two years to go, and they don't want children until he starts earning a salary too.

Peggy and Gary Nelson have five children now and would love an even bigger family, but feel they've reached the limit: even one more, and they'd outgrow not only their present house but their combined income from Gary's job as a department store clerk and the work Peggy does at home typing manuscripts.

Judson and Edna Marston can afford nearly anything they want, but one thing they don't want is children. They simply don't like them.

Emily and Norman Rutledge have a small boy who's their constant delight. They'd like to give him a brother or sister, but they've decided they won't, if they can avoid it. As concerned as they are by their personal problems, they are even more concerned about the world at large—about the problems of overpopulation. They feel strongly that people everywhere must limit the sizes of their families if civilization is to survive on an increasingly overcrowded, resource-depleted planet.

The concerns of these people, ranging from highly personal to global in scope, reflect at least some of the reasons that people in all walks of life, in all economic strata, take steps of some kind to limit the size of their families. What they are doing is variously called "family planning" (actually a broader term which also includes counseling for couples having trouble conceiving), or birth control, or contraception. Contraception is perhaps most germane to this discussion, because what we're discussing is the prevention of conception by whatever means: abstaining entirely or at timed periodic intervals; taking pills; using various devices and/or chemicals; or, with more finality, through surgery.

During the past decade there has been a dramatic increase in public awareness, through most of the world, of the dangers inherent in this combination of factors:

1. The birthrate has continued to grow in most parts of the world, and people are living longer.

2. Overconsumption has continued the alarming depletion of many nonrenewable natural resources, including the fossil fuels.

3. The amount of land suitable for food production—at best no more than 25 percent of the earth's land surface—has been inexorably reduced by such factors as erosion, overplanting, and the conversion of farmland to other uses, including industrial and residential developments.

4. Many living species, including some important links in the natural food chain, have become extinct, or nearly extinct, for reasons that include the destruction of their natural habitats and the poisoning of their food supplies by pollution.

5. In many parts of the world, pollution has made the water unfit to drink, the air unfit to breathe.

Surely, it is argued, on a planet of finite size, with finite and diminishing resources, the long-range-survival odds are pretty grim for seemingly infinite future populations. Not just logic but the survival instinct itself, it is argued, dictate that the world must reverse its upward population spiral or, at the very least, cut its rate of growth to zero. But however frightening the overpopulation arguments may be, they are no more serious, to individual families, than such strong personal concerns as those noted above.

Today there are many approaches to birth control. Some involve high risks, some are hit-and-miss, and still others are relatively safe and effective. But some of the more effective methods carry the risks of potentially serious illness, or even death. And most of the widely used methods are opposed by large segments of the world population on religious grounds. Couples who are seriously concerned about effective birth control are advised to consult a physician or a local family-planning clinic.

TABLE 5-1 Birth Control Methods

Contraceptive Methods Requiring Consultation with Physician		
Method	**What It Is, How It Works**	**Effectiveness and Acceptability**
Oral Contraceptives (The Pill)	It is generally accepted that the synthetic hormones contained in oral contraceptives (estrogen and progestogen) inhibit ovulation. There are two oral contraceptive pill methods. The most commonly used method is often referred to as the "combination" or "balanced progestogen-estrogen" method. This method is by far the one most commonly prescribed (more than 90 percent). Each pill contains a combination of both synthetic estrogen and progestogen to assure inhibition of ovulation. When no egg is released from an ovary a woman cannot become pregnant. In the other one, called the "sequential" method, two different pills are used each month. When this method is used, a pill containing synthetic estrogen is taken daily for the first 14, 15 or 16 days of the cycle. This pill inhibits ovulation. The second pill, containing a mixture of synthetic estrogen and progestogen, is then taken for 4, 5 or 6 days to assure orderly bleeding within 3 to 5 days after the last pill is taken in each cycle. The pills are now usually taken for 21 or 28 consecutive days in each cycle. Original schedules were for 20 days.	Except for total abstinence, or surgical sterilization, the combination pill is the most effective contraceptive known today. Failures, even when occasional pills are omitted, are extremely rare, numbering less than one per 100 women per year. The sequential pill method, when used correctly, is only slightly less effective, with failures of about 1.4 per 100 women per year. No woman should take the pill until she has had a physical examination by a physician who knows her medical history and has approved use. Reexaminations are usually performed at six- to twelve-month intervals. Initial and refill prescriptions must be authorized to obtain the pills from a pharmacy or clinic. There are definite warnings and precautions to both the user and the prescriber, as well as a number of side reactions reported to be associated with the use of the pill. Some of these are not dangerous, including tenderness of the breasts, nausea, weight changes, spotty darkening of the skin, especially of the face, and unexpected vaginal bleeding or changes in the menstrual period. Other reactions, not proved to be caused by the pill, may be dizziness, changes in appetite, loss of scalp hair, and changes in sex drive. After discontinuing use of the pill, there may be a delay before the woman can become pregnant. Resuming use of the pill too soon after childbirth could affect the nursing mother's milk supply. The most dangerous side effect is abnormal blood clotting. It has been estimated that about one woman in 2,000 on the pill each year suffers a severe blood-clotting disorder. Blood clots are about three

TABLE 5-1 Birth Control Methods continued

Contraceptive Methods Requiring Consultation with Physician		
Method	**What It Is, How It Works**	**Effectiveness and Acceptability**
		times more likely to develop in women over the age of 34. Women who have had blood clots in the legs, lungs, or brain should not use the pill. In addition, women who have cancer of the breast or uterus, serious liver conditions, or undiagnosed vaginal bleeding should see a physician for other methods of birth control. There is currently no proof that oral contraceptives can cause cancer in humans; however, that possibility continues to be studied. Women with other special health problems that could be aggravated by the use of the pill should see a physician for specific tests.
		The pill is by far the most acceptable method in terms of numbers because it is reliably effective and its non-messy, convenient use is unrelated to the timing of sexual play and coitus. It does not interfere with the spontaneity and passion of love-making.
Intrauterine Devices (IUD)	Objects of different shapes made of plastic or stainless steel are inserted into the uterus by a physician. They may be left in place indefinitely.	The protection afforded by the IUD is superseded only by the pill. Protection with the IUD is greater than with such "traditional" methods as the diaphragm or condom, even when these methods are used without any deviation in their regular use. Failures are about 2.7 per 100 women per year.
	How the devices prevent pregnancy is not completely understood. They do not prevent the ovary from releasing eggs. At the moment, the evidence suggests they probably speed descent of the egg, or the egg may reach the uterus at a time when it cannot nest there.	Some women cannot satisfactorily use the devices because of expulsion, bleeding or discomfort. Contraindications to insertion include pregnancy or suspected pregnancy, abnormalities which distort the uterine cavity, infection or inflammation of the uterus or adnexa, a history of postpartum endometritis, or of infection with abortion within the past three months, and endometrial disease (hyperplasia, carcinoma, polyps or suspected

TABLE 5-1 Birth Control Methods continued

	Contraceptive Methods Requiring Consultation with Physician	
Method	**What It Is, How It Works**	**Effectiveness and Acceptability**
		malignancy). Serious problems reported to be associated with the IUD are pelvic inflammatory disease and perforation of the uterus. Pregnancy can occur with the device in place. Insertion in nulliparous women is restricted because of their narrow cervical canals. Expulsions limit immediate postpartum insertions.
		IUDs are now inserted in about 7 percent of an obstetrician's contraceptive users. Few general practitioners insert them. IUDs are very acceptable when sustained motivation is lacking, when the user is fearful of using the pill or when other methods cannot be used successfully.
Diaphragms	Flexible hemispherical rubber domes, used in combination with cream or jelly which women insert into the vagina to cover the cervix, provide a barrier to sperm. They must be left in place for at least six hours after intercourse and may be left in place for as long as twenty-four hours. They must be fitted by a physician; refitted every two years and after each pregnancy.	Offers a high level of protection although occasional method failures may be expected because of improper insertion or displacement of the diaphragm during sex relations. A rate of 2 to 3 pregnancies per 100 women per year would seem to be a conservative estimate for meticulously consistent users. If motivation or self-control is weak much higher pregnancy rates must be expected. On the average, therefore, failures are about 17.5 per 100 women per year. Many women use the diaphragm successfully. Others have difficulty inserting it correctly, or dislike the procedure required.
Rhythm	This depends on abstinence from intercourse during the time of the month when a woman is fertile. Due to menstrual irregularity in many women and the inability to accurately determine the time of ovulation, success with this method may require abstinence for as long as half of	Self-taught "rhythm," haphazardly practiced, is one of the least effective methods of family planning. For most couples the "practice" of rhythm is a guessing game. Failures are to be expected in at least 24 per 100 women per year. However, the effectiveness of the rhythm

TABLE 5-1 Birth Control Methods continued

Contraceptive Methods Requiring Consultation with Physician		
Method	**What It Is, How It Works**	**Effectiveness and Acceptability**
	every month. While some couples have successfully worked out this system for themselves, most couples will require assistance from a doctor or rhythm clinic.	method may approach that of the diaphragm and condom when it is correctly taught, understood and religiously practiced.
		Rhythm is generally an unacceptable method, not only because it is unreliable but also because success requires that the woman have regular menstrual cycles (few have) and that both partners accept long periods of abstinence each month.
Surgery: Vasectomy	A vasectomy involves a relatively simple operation to prevent the sperm from entering the ejaculate through the tubes (vas deferens) leading from the testes to the urethra in the male. Cutting and tying or ligating of the vas deferens can be done under local anesthesia and performed usually in less than 30 minutes in the doctor's office or hospital. Ligation of the vas deferens should be considered a permanent procedure since there is no guarantee that fertility will be regained with the tubes reopened.	Once the sperm has been prevented from entering the ejaculate after a vasectomy, the male is considered sterile and his sperm can no longer fertilize the female egg. Many men find this method highly acceptable since it decreases neither the desire or the ability for sex nor the amount of ejaculate. Some men, however, experience psychological effects, a feeling of guilt or fear of lost manhood, after this surgical procedure.
Tubal Ligation	Tubal ligation involves blocking the Fallopian tubes through which the fertilized egg travels from the ovary to the uterus. This procedure, which involves cutting, separating and tying the tubes, can be done primarily through the abdominal wall or sometimes vaginally and is often performed just after childbirth. Reuniting the tubes is a major surgical procedure, and success may be defined by the fact that the tubes are reopened, but this does not necessarily mean that fertility is restored.	A tubal ligation is virtually 100 percent effective but failures with this method have been reported. While a tubal ligation is more involved than a vasectomy and must be performed in a hospital, it has become more acceptable to more women who desire permanent sterilization.

Contraceptive Methods Not Requiring Consultation with Physician		
Condom	This is a thin, strong sheath or cover, made of rubber or similar material, worn by the man to prevent sperm from entering the	A high degree of protection is offered if the man will use it correctly and consistently. Some couples find the use of con-

TABLE 5-1 Birth Control Methods continued

Contraceptive Methods Not Requiring Consultation with Physician

Method	What It Is, How It Works	Effectiveness and Acceptability
	vagina. (The woman may also use a vaginal foam, cream or jelly to provide added protection and lubrication.)	doms objectionable. Failures are due to tearing of the sheath or its slipping off after climax. The condom rates in effectiveness with the diaphragm. There are approximately 16 failures per 100 women (pregnancies) per year.
		The condom is universally accepted as the best preventive of venereal disease. A distinct advantage is that it can be purchased without a prescription.
Chemical Methods:	These products are inserted into the vagina. Their purpose is to coat vaginal surfaces and the cervical opening, and to destroy sperm cells; these products may act as mechanical barriers as well. They provide protection for about an hour.	The effectiveness of these vaginal chemical contraceptives used alone is lower than if they are used in combination with a diaphragm or a condom. Nevertheless, significant reductions in pregnancy rates may be obtained by the use of these simple methods.
Vaginal Foams	The foam is packed under pressure (like foaming shaving cream); it is inserted with an applicator.	Among these contraceptives the vaginal foams are the most effective, followed by the jellies and creams. Foaming tablets and suppositories are the least effective. Failures with the foam, the best of these methods, are about 28 per 100 women per year.
Vaginal Jellies and Creams	These are inserted into the vagina with an applicator.	Drainage of the chemical materials from the vagina is objectionable to some couples. Foaming tablets may cause a temporary burning sensation.
Vaginal Suppositories	These small cone-shaped objects melt in the vagina. They must be inserted in sufficient time to melt before the sex act.	The foam is acceptable to many women primarily because it is available to them without a prescription.
Vaginal Tablets	The tablets are moistened slightly and inserted into the vagina; foam is produced. They must be inserted in sufficient time for the tablets to disintegrate before the sex act.	

Source: Searle & Co., *Your Future Family* (1971), pp. 9–11, 12–17.

For purposes of this discussion, the kinds of birth control have been put into two broad categories—*natural* and *artificial*. The artificial methods are in turn put into subcategories labeled *mechanical, medicinal,* and *chemical*. The first involves use of devices such as the condom and the diaphragm, the second is concerned with oral contraceptives (the Pill), and the third with the use of nonprescriptive sperm-killing foams and creams.

Natural Methods

The one "natural" birth control practice that is fail-safe is, of course, total abstinence. But this discussion is concerned with kinds of birth control that are consistent with a normal sex life.

Rhythm   This system is one of the most widely practiced methods of birth control. It is commonly used by members of religions that contend that procreation is the sole purpose of sexual intercourse, and that the use of any artificial means to prevent conception is immoral. The rhythm system involves abstinence from intercourse at times when the woman is fertile. The problem, clearly, is determining just when those times occur.

Some women are able to predict their time of ovulation because they experience midcycle abdominal cramping called *mittelschmerz*. The discomfort is caused by irritation of the pelvic periteneum by fluid or blood escaping from the point of ovulation in the ovary. Women who have *mittelschmerz* are able to estimate with remarkable accuracy when their "safe days" will begin.

Some women rely on temperature measurements in an attempt to determine the onset of ovulation. The basal temperature drops, then takes a sharp upturn, at the onset of the fertile (unsafe) period. But doctors say the method is troublesome, and not too reliable, since the temperature changes involved are measured in fractions of degrees.

For most women, counting days after each menstrual period to decide when ovulation will start is guesswork. It's known that the period of fertility each month lasts about eight days (considering the time of ovulation and the life of the sperm and the mature ovum). But every woman has some variations in her menstrual cycle, and ovulation doesn't always begin on the same day of the cycle. As a consequence, many couples using the rhythm system abstain from sex for nearly half the month. Couples wanting to use the rhythm system are strongly advised to enlist the aid of a physician or a clinic.

Coitus Interruptus   This is another "natural" method of contraception that is considered quite risky. Its use is simple—at least in theory. When he feels his orgasm approaching, the man withdraws his penis from the woman's vagina, and ejaculates outside her body. The primary risks with this ancient method are two. It is sometimes difficult for the man to interrupt what he's doing at a time of intensifying pleasure and concentration. During intercourse and before ejaculation, the penis often releases a small amount of fluid, which may contain a small number of sperm, thus risking that the woman may become pregnant.

Some women still resort to postcoital douches in an attempt to prevent conception. This practice involves such a high risk of pregnancy that most doctors strongly recommend against it.

Medicinal Methods

Probably the most effective of all the birth control methods is the oral contraceptive, known popularly as "the Pill." Its development has been hailed as a revolutionary achievement in the field of contraception, and it is considered responsible for sweeping changes in the attitudes of many women toward sex and sexuality.

The pills now in common use are strictly for women, although research is going on to develop a pill for men. The pill is taken daily for 20 or 21 days, then discontinued for 7 or 8 to allow for menstruation. The oral contraceptive pills use synthetic versions of two female hormones, *progestin* and *estrogen,* to prevent ovulation. The synthetics inhibit the production of other hormones (called FSH and LH) that are needed to produce a mature egg.

The pills are of two kinds: combination and sequential. The combination type uses progestins and estrogens together (in amounts that vary with the brand). They are usually taken for 21 days (again, this may vary with the brand). Some manufacturers add placebos (sugar pills) for the remaining days of the month so that the women will develop the habit of taking a pill every day, without interruption.

The sequential method employs two different pills: the kind used for the first 14 to 15 days contain only the estrogens; the last five to seven pills contain combinations of estrogens and progestins. They are packaged in the proper order to achieve the desired sequence.

Oral contraceptives must be prescribed by a physician. The doctor will decide on the type and brand to be taken. Oral contraceptives are highly effective and they don't inhibit spontaneity or interrupt continuity of foreplay and coitus.

Hazards of the Pill But use of the Pill is not without its risks for women. Some of the hazards associated with the use of the Pill are the possible development of blood clots within the deep vein structure, and the increased chance of *pulmonary embolism* (blockage of one of the arteries carrying blood to the lungs) or *cerebral thrombosis* (stroke). But doctors, while warning of these potential hazards, are quick to note that statistically the risk is small: the incidence of such serious side-effects, including fatalities, is tiny when considered in relation to the number of pills taken yearly in the United States.

Physicians insist on thorough physical examinations and laboratory tests before they will prescribe—or refuse to prescribe—the Pill. Patients who have high blood pressure, diabetes, heart disease, or any of a number of other serious ailments, may be refused the Pill. Those who do take it are urged to have regular checkups, including the

Papanicolauo (Pap) test, which can detect cervical cancer in its earliest stages. The Pap test involves microscopic laboratory examination of cervical cells obtained in a vaginal smear.

Other side-effects of oral contraceptives may include depression, heavy menstrual flows or persistent bleeding between periods, headaches, water retention, and swollen, tender breasts. To counteract the possible side-effects, particularly clotting, many physicians try to select and prescribe the kind of pill which contains the least amount of hormone compatible with safe contraceptive use.

Mechanical Methods

The commonly used devices in this category include the condom, the diaphragm, and the interuterine device (IUD).

Diaphragm   This is a circular rubber dome, which is inserted into the vagina and forms a tight shield or cover over the cervix, thus blocking the path of the sperm. It is used in combination with a contraceptive jelly or cream, and it must be left in place for at least six hours after intercourse. It should be fitted by a physician and checked at regular intervals. A new one must be fitted following childbirth.

The diaphragm is considered about as effective as the condom, but not nearly as effective as the IUD. Pregnancy can occur if the device is improperly inserted, or dislodged by the penis during intercourse. Many women dislike inserting the diaphragm, while others find insertion difficult.

Condom   The condom is a sheath made of very thin rubber or latex which is pulled over the erect penis before intercourse, and which catches and retains the semen within its tip, keeping it from the vagina. Condoms are also useful for prevention of venereal disease. They are widely used because they are easily available. Although effective for both contraception and disease control, they can fail either when they split open during the activity of intercourse, or slip off after ejaculation. They are safer when used in combination with a spermicidal cream or jelly in the vagina.

Two complaints about the condom recur: the foreplay-intercourse rapport must be interrupted while it is put on, and its presence reduces the man's enjoyment by reducing the sensitivity of his penis.

IUD   The IUD is a tiny object that is placed in the uterus, where it prevents pregnancy even though it doesn't stop egg production. Doctors are not sure just how the device works, although it is possible that it creates an unreceptive environment for the implantation of a fertilized egg.

The IUD has become quite popular, and it is considered second only to the Pill in the degree of protection provided. IUDs are made in a wide variety of shapes and sizes and from a number of different materials. They are inserted by a physician and, unless complications develop, they can remain in place indefinitely and can be removed

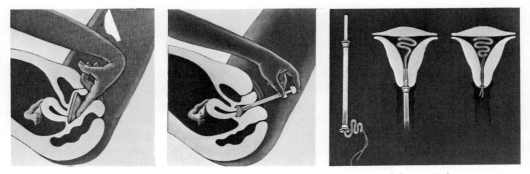

Some examples of contraceptive methods. Left: Diaphragm; Center: Vaginal foam; Right: Intrauterine device (IUD).

without difficulty if pregnancy is desired. A properly inserted IUD once in place should not be felt by its wearer, and it should in no way diminish the pleasure of sex for either partner. However, some women are unable to contain the IUD: they suffer severe bleeding, cramping, or abdominal discomfort. In some cases, the uterus stubbornly expels the device. There have been cases of perforation of the uterus by the IUD.

Many doctors, however, see the evolving IUD as the contraceptive wave of the future because it lacks the side-effects of the Pill. A recently developed version of the IUD that may hold high promise is a plastic device impregnated with progesteronelike particles that are slowly released into the wall of the uterus. Thus it combines the effectiveness of the basic IUD with that of the Pill, and without the blood-clotting potentials of the Pill.

Chemical Methods

The vaginal spermicides, such as jellies, foams, creams, and suppositories, are placed in the vagina before intercourse to provide short-term contraceptive protection. Their primary function is to kill the spermatozoa on contact. Some of them are used with a diaphragm, or in combination with the condom. They are generally considered far less effective than most other contraceptive methods.

The aerosol foams are considered the safest method. The foam is applied with a special applicator, as are the spermicidal creams and jellies. Suppositories are little cones that melt in the vagina to provide protection.

Surgical Methods

There are two kinds of surgery used by couples who want to be absolutely sure they can't conceive: the *vasectomy* in the male and *tubal ligation* in the female.

In vasectomy, the *vas deferens,* the tubes that carry the sperm from the testes to the urethra are cut and tied. The operation effectively blocks the passage of sperm, but it does not interfere with semen production, ejaculation, or orgasm. Nor does it inhibit desire.

But some men who have obtained vasectomies reportedly have had adverse psychological reactions afterwards, such as a feeling of lost manhood.

Tubal ligation consists of cutting the Fallopian tubes and tying off the cut ends. This prevents the eggs from reaching the uterus. It does not prevent sexual desire, or orgasm.

The major drawback to this surgery is that it is regarded as almost certainly permanent. Corrective surgery is possible, but so far the success rate for restoration of fertility has been low, although it is substantially higher in the female.

Abortion

Abortion is a medical term referring to the premature removal of the developing embryo or fetus from the uterus, terminating pregnancy.

Abortion is also a fighting word. "Right-to-Life" organizations say any kind of induced (medical) abortion should be equated with murder. Proponents of "therapeutic" abortion say it is often necessary to save the life of the expectant mother, for instance, or to prevent the birth of a deformed child; some argue the issue as a matter of women's rights. The partisans on both sides of the controversy are vocal, sincere, persuasive, and often emotional.

This discussion of abortion will concern itself mostly with what abortion is and how it is performed, rather than with whether it might be right or wrong.

There are two basic kinds of abortion: *natural* and *induced.*

Natural Abortion

Natural abortion, which occurs in perhaps 10 to 15 percent of pregnancies, is the spontaneous expulsion of the embryo or fetus from the uterus. This is commonly called *miscarriage,* and usually happens during the first three months of pregnancy. It can be caused by a number of things—including genetic abnormality or malformation of the fetus, or maternal diseases.

Induced Abortion

Induced abortion involves the use of artificial means to expel the embryo or fetus, usually during the first six months of pregnancy when the embryo or fetus is commonly described as "nonviable"—meaning it is incapable of sustaining life outside the uterus. The principal techniques used are:

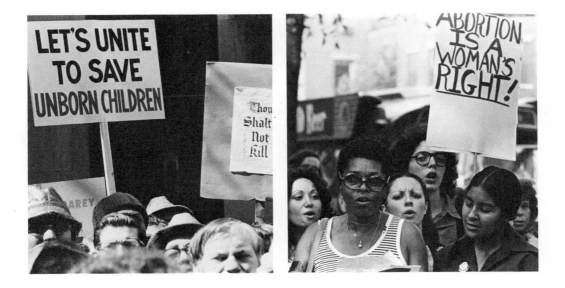

Vacuum Aspiration In this procedure a small tube is inserted through the cervix into the uterus and employed with a vacuum device to suck the embryonic tissue from the uterus wall. Properly used, this technique should have no deleterious effect on the woman.

Dilation and Curettage (D and C) The cervical opening is dilated to allow for the entry of a larger instrument called a curette or scraper, which is used to gently scrape the embryonic tissue from the surface wall of the uterus.

Aspiration and D and C are most commonly and effectively employed in pregnancies of under 12 weeks. A combination of the two methods is often used between the 12th and 20th weeks.

Saline Injection Using a long hypodermic needle, the surgeon penetrates the uterine wall and the *amniotic sac* (the membrane bag surrounding and protecting the embryo). A strong saline solution is injected, and usually causes expulsion of the embryo within 6 to 12 hours.

Summary

Unlike all other species, humans mate not only because they want to reproduce, but because they enjoy sex for its own sake. Men and women can be aroused to peaks of desire during foreplay, which involves manual or oral stimulation of erotically sensitive body areas. Sexual intercourse occurs when the male thrusts his erect penis into the woman's vagina. Orgasm, which produces intense genital pleasure in both male and female, also involves the male's ejaculation of sperm-carrying semen. If the woman is in her fertile period, a sperm or seed penetrating the ovum or egg in her Fallopian tubes will cause pregnancy.

Childbirth takes place after the embryo or fetus has grown and developed within the mother's uterus or womb for approximately nine months. Couples who don't wish to conceive practice various kinds of birth control—ranging from abstinence to "natural," chemical, and medical methods. Sometimes an unwanted birth is terminated in early pregnancy by abortion.

References

p. 58   Alex Comfort, ed., *The Joy of Sex* (New York, 1974).

p. 59   William H. Masters and Virginia E. Johnson, *Human Sexual Response* (Boston, 1966), pp. 191–93.

p. 60   Ibid., p. 66.

p. 61   Ibid., pp. 127–40.

p. 62   Ibid., pp. 66–67.

p. 62   Comfort, *The Joy of Sex,* pp. 61–63.

p. 67   W. M. Court-Brown, in *Journal of Medical Genetics* (1968); National Institute of Mental Health, *Report of the XYY Chromosomal Abnormality* (Washington, D.C., 1970).

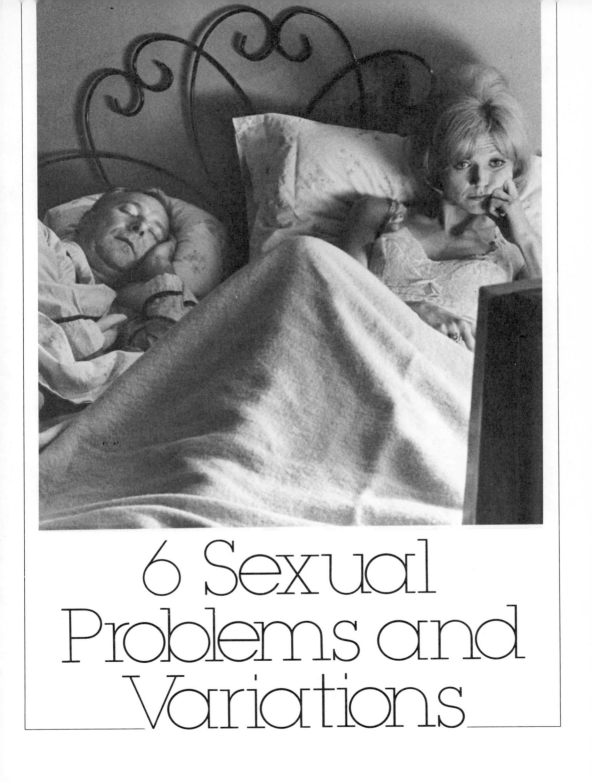

6 Sexual Problems and Variations

The researchers Masters and Johnson think contemporary society should forget the word *frigidity*, the term used for years to describe "inadequate sexual response" in women.

The way the word *frigidity* was used, inadequate sexual response could mean failure to achieve orgasm, fear or active dislike of intercourse, or physical pain, among other things. Masters and Johnson believe the catch-all word is imprecise, obsolete and meaningless. They have substituted their own lexicon. Their principal terms on the subject of female dysfunctions are discussed here.

Female Dysfunctions

Orgasmic Dysfunction

A woman who is unable to achieve orgasm is a victim of *female orgasmic dysfunction*. Masters and Johnson believe she falls into one of two subcategories. If she has never attained orgasm, by any kind of sexual stimulation, her affliction is called *primary orgasmic dysfunction*. If she has achieved orgasm in the past (at least once) but can no longer do so, her problem is called *situational orgasmic dysfunction*.

A number of things can cause, or contribute to, these dysfunctions. Most of the causes are emotional. They include fear, hostility, revulsion. Many of the causitive conflicts stem from childhood experiences that produced a negative view of sex.

Dyspareunia

Intercourse that is physically painful for the woman is called *dyspareunia*. It is usually marked by inadequate lubrication within the vagina—but the causes of that condition may be either physical or emotional, the researchers believe.

Vaginismus

Painful, involuntary spasms in the vagina are a response known as *vaginismus*. Masters and Johnson say the spasms may reflect a subconscious wish to avoid penetration—a wish that could be rooted in a temporary emotional conflict, or anchored in some deep-seated hostility stemming from childhood, or from the marriage itself.

Male Dysfunctions

The male is subject to two afflictions in terms of sexual dysfunction.

The inability to achieve or sustain an erection is called *impotence.* Failure to achieve an erection can be attributed to various things. Too much alcohol or guilt feelings can cause impotence. Impotence may be triggered by anxiety (including a sudden fear of failure). Or it might be caused by indifference. On the other hand, impotence might stem from fatigue, aging, or even medicine. Some of the drugs that lower blood pressure can also cause impotence.

All the conditions mentioned so far come under the heading of *transient impotence,* or *secondary impotence.*

Primary impotence, comparatively rare, is what bedevils the man who has *never* had erection. It sometimes has a physical cause, such as childhood injury—but it may stem from deep-seated psychoses.

Premature Ejaculation

When a man achieves orgasm (and ejaculation) before he wants to, he experiences *premature ejaculation.* Prolonged anticipation of intercourse, genital stroking in fore-play to the point of no return can cause a man to ejaculate almost immediately on insertion of the penis into the vagina.

Psychologists have found that most causes of premature ejaculation are emotional rather than physical. Some of the same psychological problems that induce impotence—fear, hate, revulsion, guilt, feelings of sexual inadequacy—contribute to the mutually dissatisfying occurrence of premature ejaculation.

Dyspareunia, or painful intercourse, also occurs in the male. So does the comparatively rare condition called *ejaculatory incompetence* (inability to ejaculate).

Sexually Transmitted Disease

Contagious diseases spread through various kinds of sexual contact are called *venereal diseases.* The word *venereal* derives from Venus, the Roman goddess of love. Among the most prevalant venereal diseases, the two most serious are syphilis and gonorrhea.

Syphilis

Syphilis begins in a small way. Its cause is a tiny micro-organism called a *spirochete,* which usually exists and grows within the human body for about three weeks—that's the average incubation period. The first manifestation of syphilis usually is a small (and, at first, painless) sore (a *primary chancre*) on the penis or within the vulva. The sore may go away in about two weeks, but its disappearance usually signals the onset of *secondary syphilis.* In this stage, the affliction has invaded the entire body. If unchecked, the disease may progress to heart disease, blindness, paralysis, insanity— even death.

Significant signals may include widespread skin rashes, moderate fevers, and (sometimes) a painless swelling of the lymph glands.

The spirochete, scientists have found, is readily killed by penicillin, and by a broad assortment of antibiotics. Both those infected and their sexual partners require competent medical treatment.

Gonorrhea

After the common cold, gonorrhea is probably the most widely circulated disease in the world. Medical science can cure gonorrhea, *if* the afflicted person seeks medical treatment. Unfortunately, too many sufferers don't take the problem to physicians.

The disease's statistics are staggering: It's estimated that two million people currently are afflicted by gonorrhea. Unlike syphilis, which can affect all parts of the body, gonorrhea has its main impact on the sex organs.

Its earliest signs, in man or woman, usually are a burn-like sensation in urination and a discharge of pus from the urethra. The discomfort is much more pronounced in the male—which explains why men seek and obtain medical cures in the early stages of the disease. Women, however, can harbor the disease for long periods of time without experiencing any physical signs of its presence. Thus the woman with gonorrhea often is unaware of its presence—and doesn't seek medical care—until the disease has progressed and spread into the Fallopian tubes, the ovaries, and other organs. The disease can even cause sterility in the woman through its scarring action in the Fallopian tubes.

Syphilis infections in a woman can cause congenital (birth) defects in her children, including heart malformations, bone deformities, and insanity. Both syphilis and gonorrhea can be passed to a newborn if an infection exists in the vagina or birth passage. While treatment is painless and easy, all sexual contacts must receive treatment to prevent spread of the disease.

Some Other Venereal Diseases

Other venereal diseases which frequently occur include:

Trichomoniasis   A common affliction of the vaginal area, trichomoniasis is the product of a small protozoan *(Trichomonas vaginalis)*. The infection incubates in the vulval area, and causes a burning and itching sensation. There is a profuse vaginal discharge. Trichomoniasis is easily transmitted to the male during sexual intercourse, and signals its presence by a burning and itching sensation in the urethra. Several rather new drugs are used in the treatment of this disease.

Moniliasis   *Monilia albicans* is a vaginal fungus that invades and infects any area of mucous membrane. This disease lives most often in the vagina or the mouth. The fungus multiplies and becomes highly infective when the woman starts taking antibiotics or birth control pills. Symptoms include a burning sensation during intercourse or urination. There are several drugs that attack monilia with great success.

Genital Warts and Herpes   Small sores in the genital area are the outward signs of these viral infections, which may or may not be transmitted by sexual contact. Other symptoms include discharge, painful urination, bad odors. Electrocautery (burning off the warts) is employed by many physicians treating genital warts.

Crabs and Scabies   There are three kinds of lice that infest the human body, usually due to unsanitary conditions. *Head lice* invade the scalp area. The other two—called *body lice* and *genital* lice—are active in the pubic regions.

Typically, the female lice burrows into soft layers of flesh and lays her eggs. In the pubic region, the eggs usually are laid near the base of a hair follicle. The lice multiply rapidly. Special medications are available by prescription.

Sexual Variations

All human institutions and practices have their norms or standards—definable as the way most people do whatever it is. Just as certainly, every norm or standard has its deviations. And deviates, in this sense, are simply people who do things differently. This is as true in sex as it is in any activity.

Homosexuality is the most widely known and practiced kind of sexual variation, but there are others: More and more has been heard in recent years about the *bisexual,* the *transsexual,* the *transvestite,* the *voyeur,* and the *exhibitionist.* And much has been written about those who practice *group sex.*

The general sexual liberation that has evolved in recent years has done much to increase public understanding and tolerance of some forms of sexual variation.

Homosexuality

Homosexuality is the attraction, psychological, emotional, and physical, to a person of one's own sex. The "why" of homosexuality isn't fully understood, although the causes appear to be emotional and are probably rooted in childhood. Role-playing in our society starts early in life. Boys are supposed to be like their fathers, girls like their mothers. But sometimes the person from whom the role should be learned is dead, absent, or doesn't play his or her own role. In these situations many children become "fixed," as Freud described it, in an early stage of emotional development, such as the oral or anal.

Studies show that children, particularly in early adolescence, do a lot of mutual exploring: they talk about sex, they compare their organs, and they engage at least tentatively in sexual acts. This is customarily done with others of the same sex. The figures vary, but studies have shown that perhaps half of today's adult males, perhaps more, have indulged in some sort of homosexual conduct. But in most cases it was exploratory and did not recur in adulthood. The same studies indicate that the number of persons actively and exclusively practicing homosexuality may amount to only three percent of the adult population.

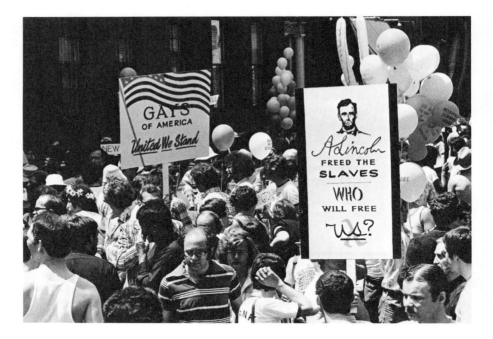

The ultimate physical expression of homosexuality is intercourse—oral-genital contact in male and female homosexuals *(lesbians)* and anal intercourse in males.

The Homosexual and Society   Homosexuality knows no social, educational, economic, or occupational barriers. Yet societal pressures can make life unpleasant for many homosexuals—and the pattern starts early: the little boy who is a loner, who isn't good at sports or simply shuns them, who shows even the tiniest hint of effeminacy, is likely to be hounded from the playground by taunting cries of "Sissy! Sissy!" During adolescence and later stages of youth, somebody even suspected of being a homosexual may be physically assaulted, humiliated, or silently shunned by contemporaries.

Treatment of Homosexuality   If a homosexual truly wants to change his or her sexual orientation, psychotherapy is recommended as the only logical treatment. It has met with some success, in a degree which varies with the experience of the psychotherapist and the desire of the patient to change.

Bisexuality

Bisexuals have been described as persons capable of having sexual relationships with the opposite sex—and with their own. Some recent psychoanalytic studies of the subject suggest that the typical bisexual is a homosexual who can perform adequately as a heterosexual, but some other studies suggest the opposite. It seems agreed that bisexuals have probably been around for a long time, but have been getting increased public attention in recent years. This is perhaps in part due to the number of celebrities who have openly proclaimed themselves as bisexuals.

Transsexuality

The most common description of a transsexual is that of a person of one sex trapped in the body of another, and wanting desperately to get out. And—knowing such escape is impossible—wanting to change the body to adapt to the misplaced sex.

There is scientific evidence that the preponderance of transsexuals strongly believe that they *are,* in fact, women in men's bodies or the reverse. On the basis of known cases, the transsexual trait occurs far more often in men than in women. Psychologists generally agree that the transsexual secretly "lives" as a person of the opposite sex, in terms of thoughts almost all of the time, and in actions when alone.

The possible cause of transsexualism cited most often is the not unusual case of the parents who wanted a child of one sex but had a child of the opposite sex and didn't adjust to the situation. Instead, they made their resentment clear, and at the same time treated their small child as if it were the sex they had wanted.

Sex-change operations have grown more common in recent years although surgery is just part of the sex change. The patient also receives intensive psychotherapy, hormonal treatments, hair removal, and wardrobe counseling.

The surgery itself serves two purposes: First, it removes the exterior signs of the unwanted sex. Second, it (sometimes) attempts artificial creation of the external signs of the new and desired sex.

Transvestism

Transvestites derive sexual gratification from posing as members of the opposite sex. This form of sexual expression shows itself far more often in men than in women, and generally resists psychiatric treatment because it's a source of such intense pleasure to the individual transvestite.

The typical transvestite probably is a man who has some deep-seated doubts about his own maleness—even though his basic orientation may be heterosexual. He may be married, but he's terribly unsure of himself with women, even his wife. He creates a fantasy life in which he plays two roles—his own and that of a woman he can possess almost at will with absolutely no fear of failure. Playing both—the ardent man and the sensual, willing woman—the transvestite draws sexual gratification from masturbating.

Fetishism, the use of an object as a source of erotic stimulation, often is associated with transvestism. It's believed to be an outgrowth of an adolescent use of such stimuli while masturbating.

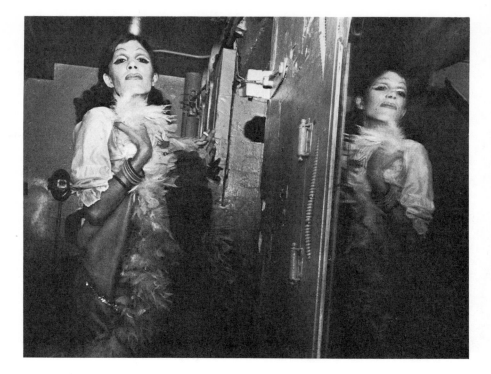

Voyeurism

Voyeurism is the attainment of sexual gratification through watching others have sex. The classic "Peeping Tom" stands in the darkness outside and peers in a bedroom window to get furtive glimpses of the naked female body. A more advanced stage of voyeurism involves the person who sits by the bed and watches as two other people (or sometimes more) engage in sexual intercourse, homosexual or heterosexual.

Some psychologists say the average male has a certain degree of built-in voyeurism, which is shown in the way he can be turned on by the mere sight of a naked woman. This theory is supported by the high popularity—mainly among men—of pornographic literature and movies.

Exhibitionism

Men alone seem to be cast in the role of the exhibitionist—one who gets sexual gratification by deliberately exposing his genitals to unsuspecting women. The standard cliché is the "flasher"—who stands in a conspicuous place and abruptly exposes his sex organs. The exhibitionist isn't intent on rape. His pleasure comes from showing his penis, whether it's limp or erect. The act of exposure may or may not include masturbation.

Psychological studies indicate the typical exhibitionist is a man with strong feelings of sexual inadequacy, even though a high percentage of exhibitionists are married.

Sado-Masochism

The sadist likes to inflict pain. The masochist likes to be physically punished. Frequently they team up to produce what might be called voluntary violence in sex: together, they dovetail their violent needs—and achieve sexual gratification.

Sado-masochism is commonly associated, in the public mind, with whips, chains, and leather. Many masochists like to be chained while their sadistic partners whip them savagely. Unfortunately, the sadist doesn't always get sexual pleasure by punishing somebody who *wants* to suffer. Sadism in its extreme forms has been responsible for many brutal rapes, beatings, and murders of innocent people.

Other Sexual Variations

There are other kinds of deviant sexual behavior which are generally as serious as those already discussed, but which occur less commonly. They include:

Pedophilia, or Child-Molestation   Almost all pedophiliacs are men, most are hetero-sexual, and all are believed to suffer from a fixation which has kept them from growing, psychologically, beyond an early childhood phase.

Bestiality, or Sexual Contact with an Animal   Most frequently it is performed by a boy or young man who is using the animal as an outlet for basically heterosexual urges. It isn't regarded as a lasting or harmful affliction.

Summary

The various sexual failures that sometimes plague men and women are called dysfunctions. In the woman, they include orgasmic dysfunctions (failure to achieve orgasm), painful intercourse, and spasms; in the man, they are impotence (failure to erect), premature ejaculation, and inability to ejaculate.

Venereal disease is a problem that concerns society at large, not just the individual. Public health officials are concerned that venereal diseases are so prevalent even when the most common of them—syphilis, gonnorhea, and some others—can be cured if treatment starts soon enough. All can be prevented—with a little common sense—but if not treated can have serious results.

In our society there are many people whose habitual sexual activities vary from our heterosexual "norm." Homosexuality is the best known and most widely practiced kind of deviant sex; homosexual alliances may involve men or women, and their relationships vary from the one-night pickup to enduring, live-together approximations of marriage. Other forms of variant sexual behavior include bisexuality, transsexuality, transvestism, voyeurism, and exhibitionism. A violent form of sexual deviation is sadomasochism, involving a person who likes to inflict pain and a person who likes to be punished. Some practices that go against accepted theories in our culture are pedophilia and bestiality.

References

p. 88   William H. Masters and Virginia E. Johnson, *Human Sexual Inadequacy* (Boston, 1970), pp. 266–88.

p. 88   Ibid., pp. 260–65.

p. 88   Ibid., pp. 137–56, 157–92, 193–213.

p. 89   Ibid., pp. 92–115.

p. 89   Ibid., pp. 116–36.

p. 90   John W. Grover, *VD: The ABCs* (Englewood Cliffs, N.J., 1971).

p. 91   Alfred C. Kinsey et al., *Sexual Behavior in the Human Male* (Philadelphia, 1948).

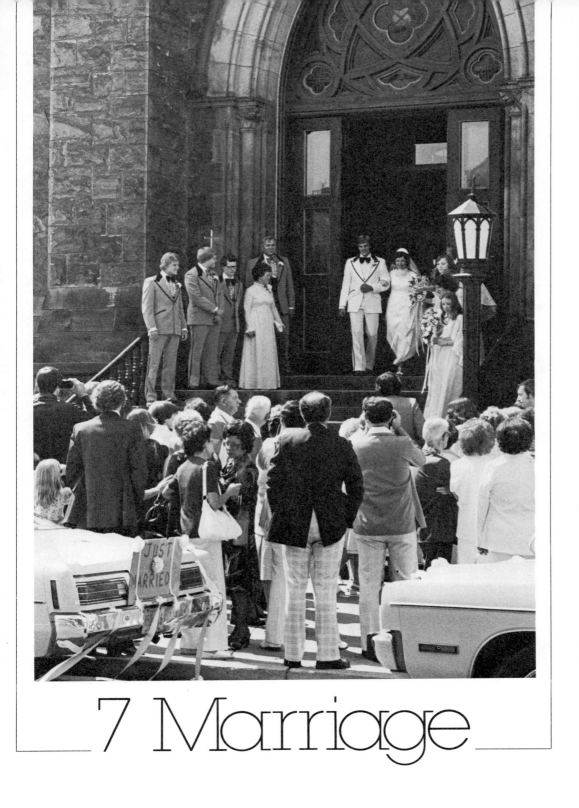

7 Marriage

Joe and Irma are young, happy, and in love. They want to be together always, so they decide to get married. They may not realize its full import at the time, but that decision is almost certainly the most serious and consequential of their lifetimes. By marrying, Irma and Joe are embracing an ancient institution which is the creator, protector, and perpetuator of the family and is considered central to most societies and civilizations. Marriage customs may differ in many ways from country to country, but there are two particular distinctions that should be noted: Marriage is either *monogamous* or *polygamous*. In the United States, our laws and established culture insist on monogamy— that is to say you may have only one mate at one time. The people of some nations are essentially polygamous, and a person may have more than one mate at the same time.

The Marriage Process

Joe and Irma could have simply decided to live together without marriage. Many people do that today because contemporary society is more accepting of the practice than it once was. Yet it's estimated that the vast majority of men and women in the United States still marry at some time in their lives. So despite sporadic, and sometimes perplexing, shifts in public attitudes toward marriage, the institution seems destined to survive.

In this chapter, we'll discuss the aspects of the institution beginning with courtship. Some of the many responsibilities of marriage will also be touched on, as the possible consequences that must be faced if a marriage fails.

Courtship

The chain of events leading to a wedding may have begun on a college campus, in an office, at a concert, or in a bar. The possibilities are as infinite as human personality is diverse. A man and a woman—perhaps they just met, perhaps they've been casual acquaintances for some time—decide a strong attraction is building between them emotionally, intellectually, physically. They begin to see much more of each other. They start doing things they mutually enjoy. They have begun the historic ritual of courtship.

As the relationship deepens, some couples engage in *premarital sex*. Liberalized attitudes about sex before marriage make its practice much more commonplace than it was two decades ago. But many couples—reflecting society's older attitudes toward the subject—avoid premarital sex. Their reluctance to practice it may stem from religious beliefs, and/or family teachings.

Length of Courtship Ideally, a couple should continue their courtship until they are confident they can live together with love; too short a courtship will not give them time to discover what they should know about each other. They must be able to accept the fact that every marriage has its inevitable conflicts and irritations. Things that happen in courtship should act as warning signals: If, for instance, the man has a quick temper, this must be considered by his partner in the light of spending the rest of her life with him.

Decision-Making During Courtship   Once the decision to wed has been made, the couple must make a number of other decisions—some important, some less so. They must set a date for the wedding, and decide whether it will be large or small, religious or civil. These are socially important decisions, but should not be allowed to take precedence over the decisions that will affect their lives together. They should decide where to live, and make arrangements to move in. They'll want to talk, seriously, about whether they want children and, if so, whether they want to start a family right away or defer it for a few years. Birth control, obviously, should be discussed. Religious beliefs are also critical: Differences, if any, must be aired and resolved before marriage; religious beliefs can be a major influence on attitudes about birth control, raising and educating children.

Decisions about work will also have long-range effects. One or both may be working away from the home after the marriage, and the couple should weigh this in deciding who will be responsible for what household tasks: cooking, housecleaning, laundry, ironing, shopping.

Finances must be discussed. Studies show that one of the major irritants in a marital relationship is money. If one partner is a spendthrift and the other is cautious about money, they must resolve their differences before marriage. To wait until after the wedding will only lead to conflict.

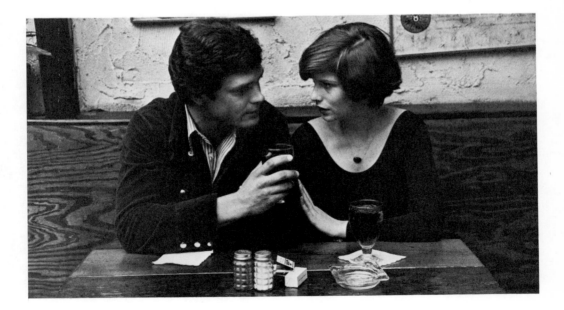

The License

All states have some kind of marriage licensing laws. In this country, these laws are administered at the local level. A license usually can be obtained for a small fee at a courthouse, city hall, or county seat. In many states, the couple must have medical examinations and blood tests before their license may be issued. Normally, they obtain these from their private physicians. The physical exam usually is a routine checkup. A few states also want to look for potentially serious psychological problems. The blood test is to detect venereal disease.

Some states impose a "cooling-off" period—a mandatory waiting time of several days—on the theory that some couples might be rushing into marriage and may need a little extra time to reconsider. Minimum age laws affect marriage almost everywhere but, as with many of these requirements, there is considerable variation.

When the legal requirements of licensing are satisfied, the couple may proceed to the ceremony itself.

The Wedding

People have been wed on television shows, on roller skates, or in their favorite bars. Our recent history even records one case where the couple and the person who wed them were skydivers. The ceremony took place as the three locked hands during a free fall from an airplane high in the sky. By the time their parachutes opened, the bride and groom were man and wife.

This sort of wedding is unusual, of course. Most ceremonies are either religious (performed by a minister, priest, or rabbi) or civil (performed by some authorized person such as a judge).

The kind of wedding ceremony the couple has is most often just a matter of the kind they want. But there's also the matter of what they (and their families) can afford. A large wedding, with a big wedding party, can be very expensive. Today, many couples seem to prefer quieter, less expensive weddings. Some couples decide to skip the ceremonial rituals altogether and *elope*—steal away someplace to wed privately, without fuss. The wedding ceremony almost universally ends with the ritual of the ring: The groom slips a wedding band on his bride's finger. If it's a double-ring ceremony, she reciprocates.

The Honeymoon

Another ancient wedding practice is the honeymoon, which is based on the plausible theory that the newly married couple need to get away for a while and begin their adjustment to marriage. For the wealthy, a honeymoon might be a long ocean cruise to some exotic place. For most, it's more likely to be a week or long weekend in pleasant, scenic, but not-too-expensive seclusion. Some couples have to settle for a night or two away somewhere because one or both are unable to get away from the job for a longer time.

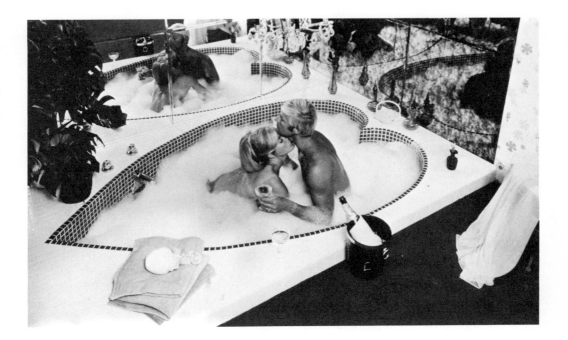

According to legend, the wedding night is supposed to be the time when the virginal bride is deflowered by her new husband—who has spirited her to a secret hideaway for the purpose. Many psychologists feel the newlyweds might be well advised to wait until the next day, say, for their first marital sex. The reasoning is that both will probably be physically and emotionally exhausted after the wedding and the days of hectic planning which preceded it.

Marriage: The Institution

Marriage traces its origins to primitive peoples who knew that the survival of their tribes depended on the propagation of the species. Early civilizations were constantly menaced by a hostile environment and enemy tribes. Death rates were high, and the basic procreative urge became a weapon for survival: the larger their family, the better their chances.

Monogamy became one of the earliest social customs of the human race—imposed by the tribe to prevent jealousy and fighting. Romantic concepts of love and marriage didn't emerge until the Renaissance, when men extolled the physical beauty of the women they loved. Love and beauty have been inextricably linked ever since, but procreation and the perpetuation of the family remain the strong subconscious motivations for marriage.

The Family

The structure of the family in the United States has undergone significant change in the country's relatively short lifespan. In colonial times, the common grouping was the *joint family,* which included all living descendants in either the male or female line. These families pretty well provided for all their own needs: The men furnished food (tending stock, fishing and hunting), the women cared for home and children, made clothing, and cooked the meals. But with the Industrial Revolution, cities began to grow around factories, men left their no longer self-sufficient farms to seek jobs, and the joint family began to be replaced by what is called the *nuclear family*—consisting of parents and their children. The nuclear organization of the monogamous family is credited with preserving and stabilizing the organization of society and providing a continuity from one generation to the next.

Why People Marry

The most common reasons why people marry and establish families— love and the procreative urge—have already been discussed. But there are other reasons.

Loneliness   There are many people who are desperately lonely. They suffer from feelings of isolation, anxiety, and low self-esteem; they often seize on marriage for companionship.

Money   Some people marry strictly for economic advantage—the boss's daughter isn't just a myth. Sometimes love will grow in such a marriage, sometimes it won't.

Social Advantage   There are often motives other than money behind a social-climbing marriage. It isn't too rare for the "climber" to have plenty of money, and to pick a marriage partner who'll provide entree to "high society."

Conformity   There are men and women who marry because it's socially acceptable or because all their friends are married. This attitude is far less common today than it was some years ago.

Idealized Love   Some people seem to approach marriage with a romanticized story-book notion that it will produce "eternal love." This could be inspired by the part of the wedding vows where the officiant commands bride and groom to love each other "until death do you part." Psychologists say the exhortation is foolish because it's so unrealistic. It tells people to love each other for all their lives when they can't say with certainty that they'll even *like* each other in two years.

Pregnancy   Marriages that take place because the woman is pregnant are comparatively unusual in these days of liberalized abortion laws and comparatively relaxed attitudes toward illegitimacy.

Children in Marriage

Parenthood can be one of the most perplexing, demanding, frustrating—yet one of the most richly rewarding—facets of marriage. The arrival of children creates new dimensions in the marriage and— as infant grows into toddler, toddler to preschooler—gives the parents new perspectives on themselves as man and wife, father and mother and, indeed, as lovers.

Today's society has been gnawing away at some long-held concepts of parental roles—particularly those which place all responsibility for child care on the mother. Increasingly, fathers are assuming part of the child-care responsibility in order to take some of the burden off the mother and, particularly, to establish a strong relationship with the child. Increasingly, mothers are getting out of the house—for shopping, recreational or cultural pursuits, for full-time or part-time jobs—especially after the child is old enough to attend preschool.

Mother, father, and child—collectively they are a unit, the family. But, psychologists say, the family collective must recognize that each of its components is an individual who must be encouraged to assert and develop that individuality.

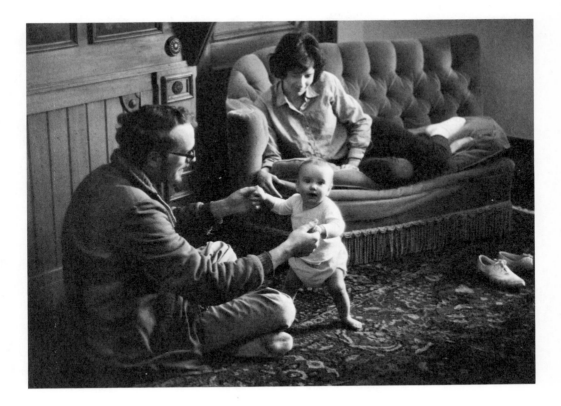

The Parents' Roles

The parents are the providers, the teachers. But there must be love, too. Shared experiences—shared with joy by parents and child alike. Birthday anniversaries and special days such as Christmas are obvious examples. But a stroll through the park or a picnic on the beach can mean as much. Sharing should be an everyday thing, not a special occasion.

However well-meaning, however effective the parental influences might be, the child will learn many things in a different perspective when he or she ventures out into the world. The parents must learn that they can't protect the child from the realities of life. They'll do better preparing him or her to learn these realities— including, of course, sex—in the proper perspective.

The parents, of however many children, must take care not to lose sight of their husband-wife relationship. Not just in terms of sexuality, but in other shared activities. They, and their marriage, need to be separated from their children occasionally.

Marital Problems

Any human institution involving the complex responsibilities of marriage can develop problems—sometimes easily resolved, sometimes not. Most marital crises are relatively minor, and based on misunderstandings that can be worked out between the partners. Others may require the aid of a marriage counselor, psychologist, or minister, if the marriage is to survive.

Some of the major and most common problems are:

Money   Or, perhaps, the lack of it. A spendthrift husband or wife can upset the most well-planned family budget. Management of the family finances should, ideally, be a team effort; major or unusual expenditures should be discussed. A sudden reduction in income (the husband or wife either loses or quits his or her job) can precipitate a crisis, particularly if the couple is already overextended on time-payments for that new clothes dryer or that two-year-old car.

Sex   The husband feels his wife is unresponsive, unloving—that she goes out of her way to think up reasons for not having sex. Or the wife makes similar complaints about the husband—who's so often "too tired." If the couple can't work out their problems— which can be difficult if they're shouting at each other—professional help may be the only answer.

Infidelity   Sometimes, but not always, the husband or wife is unresponsive at home because he or she is having a sexual liaison with someone else. Sexual infidelity by a married person is called *adultery*. Historically it has been regarded by society with outrage and contempt. It has long been considered an almost automatic ground for divorce. Many marital crises involving infidelity have been worked out by couples who consulted a marriage counselor instead of a lawyer.

Drunkenness Many marriages are seriously threatened when one of the partners develops a serious and continuing drinking problem. Typically, this might be the husband who has a few too many with his coworkers after work and develops a serious problem of drunkenness that might cost him his job. Or, it might be the bored housewife who starts buoying her spirits with a few nips in the morning—and ends up with a quart-a-day habit. Again, consultation with a marriage counselor, and the enlisting of various agencies specializing in drinking problems, may save the marriage.

Gambling In some people, gambling is an obsession every bit as compulsive—and potentially destructive of marriage—as alcoholism. There are organizations that cope with the problems of the compulsive gambler very much like the groups that deal with the problems of uncontrolled drinking.

The Trapped Housewife Many women feel, with great justification, that they are profoundly oppressed by the old convention that the woman's place is in the home with the children. This feeling of isolation ("I never see anybody over three feet tall") has contributed to marital unhappiness and sometimes to solitary drinking. Attitudes about the wife's role seem to be changing, however.

Children The emotional problems of growing children can range from throwing rocks on the playground to setting off fire alarms to experimenting with drugs. These problems, often occurring during adolescence, can cause considerable anguish to the parents—and sometimes parental hostility over how to cope with things.

Breaking Up

Many of the problems mentioned can cause the end of a marriage, which may not mean the end of the problems. The breakup, if legal and permanent, will mean working out agreements for division of property as well as child custody. Sometimes these things are worked out amicably but often they involve bitter disputes.

Many couples decide these matters while their marriage is still intact. Signed, legally binding agreements may specify exactly who gets what in terms of real estate or personal property should the marriage fail. Other kinds of agreements sometimes specify that the wife will receive a particular share of the combined assets on the basis of her work in the home as mother, housekeeper, cook, or whatever. In other words, what amounts to a cash value is placed on her services during the marriage even though her husband may be the sole wage-earner.

Divorce is the legal method of terminating a marriage. The legal grounds which must be proved before a court will grant a divorce vary from state to state, but usually include adultery, habitual drunkenness, and some of the other problems discussed earlier. Some states have liberalized their divorce laws. Recently some states have provided for *dissolution* of a marriage instead of divorce. This means that a couple can end the marriage by a showing of *irreconcilable differences* without one party formally

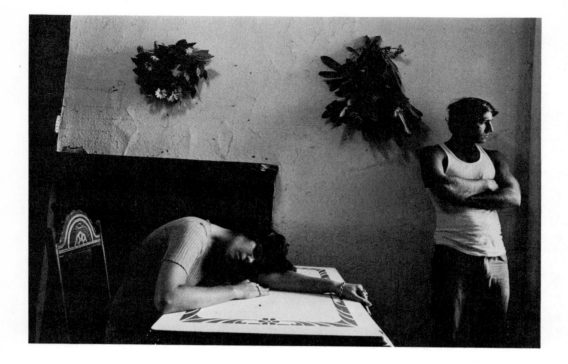

accusing the other on certain specified grounds and then proving these contentions in court. Dissolution has eliminated much of the acrimony from the ending of a marriage although not necessarily from property division and child custody.

Some states provide for *legal separation* through court procedures, but this does not end the marriage. It usually involves a decree that the couple shall live apart and that, in some cases, the husband will pay *separate maintenance*. One of the partners, customarily the husband, must in all cases make *child support* payments. In some cases, *alimony* must be paid to the former wife, usually until she remarries.

Annulment is a legal device for ending a marriage on grounds that it never legally existed as a marriage. The grounds may include bigamy, fraud, and failure to consummate (have sexual intercourse).

Alternatives to Marriage

Many people today—particularly younger ones—are rejecting conventional marriage and exploring alternatives.

Living Together   In most cases, this amounts to married life without benefit of the government sanction given by a license. The practice seems widespread although it has no real legal status. Its big advantage is that disengaging is in most cases simple—if things ever come to that. But studies indicate that most couples are in love and want to establish a long-term, sharing relationship involving more than just sex. In many cases, couples living together have children— but often the couples then legalize the relationship by wedding. Curiously, many couples in such liaisons sign agreements concerning what will belong to whom if they ever should part company.

Living together in this sense is also widely practiced by homosexuals. But homosexuals can't legally marry, although some of them go through various kinds of "wedding" ceremonies.

Living Apart   For whatever personal reasons, many people simply choose to live by themselves. Sometimes these "loners" satisfy their needs for sexual release and other emotional fulfillment through sporadic relations with other live-alone persons.

Communes   The exact nature of these experiments in group living seems to vary widely. So do the names by which they are called, and the number of people involved. Communal ownership of land, shelter, and material goods is practiced. Work is divided much as it was by the "extended family" in colonial days. Marriage is often polygamous, which has historically caused trouble in such communes. But sometimes the residents of the collectives practice a strict sort of monogamy-out-of-wedlock.

Our Liberated Sexuality

A growing number of Americans today seem to be approaching sex with greater knowledge, fewer inhibitions, and far more enjoyment. This liberated sexuality is the product of a number of factors, but the major contributors would seem to be the Pill, the feminist movement, and a continuing erosion of the stern Victorian attitudes so commonplace twenty years ago.

The main beneficiary of all this would seem to be the woman. The very nature of marriage as we have so long practiced it has kept the woman in her historic role: the wife, mother, cook, housekeeper, and laundress. And during most of this time, man has continued his dominant role: not just the husband and provider, but virtually the only living contact his wife has with the adult world. Both the husband and wife learned their roles from their parents.

The New Generation

Today there is a new generation of parents, and the differences are manifesting themselves: in parent, in child, and in attitudes. Consider, for a moment, a fairly typical mother of, say, twenty years ago. On the subject of sex, she told her daughters some of the things her own mother had instilled in her when *she* was a girl. For instance, this hypothetical mother (let's call her Mrs. Smith) was taught as a girl that sex before marriage was wrong. She was popular in high school and college, dated a lot, even went steady for a while. She did her share of kissing, occasionally even some moderately heavy necking, as it was called in those days. But through it all she remembered her mother's admonitions: Sex was for marriage. A *nice* girl went to the marriage bed a virgin. When she became Mrs. Smith, she had obeyed her mother's teachings. She was still a virgin.

She found on her wedding night that she wasn't at all repelled by sexual intercourse. She enjoyed being so close to her new husband, whom she loved. But she was something less than wanton and didn't experience orgasm until she'd been married ten years.

Neither of her daughters reached seventeen a virgin. Both had been told repeatedly the same things Mrs. Smith heard as a girl. But this new generation of women heard different stories from members of their peer group. They'd experienced a bit of peer-pressure, but had chosen to ignore it until, in each case, the boy and the chemistry were right.

Each daughter, in her own turn, confessed to Mrs. Smith, who reacted with shock in the first case and, several years later, with something close to resignation in the second. Mr. Smith's reactions were stormy, but he agreed that each of his daughters should go on the Pill. It may or may not have occurred to him that they were good examples of what we've chosen to call our liberated sexuality. But they were. Mrs. Smith was rather emancipated, not trapped in her kitchen. Among other things, she had a part-time job she liked—for the work and for the fact it paid her enough to buy some of those nice "extras" somewhat beyond the family budget.

Her relative emancipation reflected some of the ideas of the feminist movement, and probably took some of the sting out of her admonitions to her daughters. And the comforting knowledge that the Pill was there gave the girls a more relaxed attitude. The erosion of Victorian mores is more widespread than many people think. Our generally relaxed attitudes about sex include a more tolerant view—at least a live-and-let-live approach—to homosexuals. Many people are far less inclined to condemn unmarried couples who live together, who have children. Our society today is more tolerant of abortions.

There are many people, of course, who angrily condemn these trends as a slackening of our moral standards, an unconscionable slide into sin. Many of them blame pornographic books and films. Whatever the merits of the arguments, the trends are there.

The main contribution of the Pill to our society is, of course, its role as an effective and safe (for most women) oral contraceptive. But its very effectiveness reportedly has caused a new, relaxed sexual response in many users. Studies show that many women who rarely experienced orgasm started doing so regularly when they began taking the Pill. Similar responses have been reported in women who had passed menopause, and found they were no longer inhibited by the fear of an unwanted pregnancy.

The insistent drive for equality by the feminist movement clearly has spread into the area of sex—with, perhaps, mixed results. Women are, in many cases, asserting themselves vigorously in more than one aspect of sexuality—often as the aggressor in initiating liaisons. And they are demanding performance from their male partners. The performance demands, some researchers report, tend to bruise the psyches of some men to the degree that they suffer from temporary impotence.

Summary

Although it isn't as universal as it once was, marriage and the family remain the cornerstones of our society. Many couples still practice the rituals of courtship before deciding to wed. They then obtain a license and are wed in whatever kind of ceremony suits them and is within their means. The honeymoon, a time of seclusion after the wedding, is an ancient ritual still widely practiced. People marry for many reasons. Love is the most common but there are others, including money, security, and conformity.

The institution of marriage has primitive origins. In some societies it is polygamous, but in ours it is monogamous. People today are veering away from the old concepts that cast the husband as sole breadwinner and his wife as mother and housekeeper. Children can be at once a delight and a sometimes vexing challenge. Problems in marriage range from sexuality to infidelity to alcoholism. A failed marriage is ended through divorce, which sometimes involves knotty problems about property division and child custody. Alimony and child-support payments may be involved.

Many people today choose not to marry, though they live together as man and wife. If such a relationship fails, there are fewer complications involved in ending it. Some people simply choose to live alone, and still others group together in different kinds of communes.

People today, by and large, have a different perspective on sex than their parents did. They tend to be more relaxed about it, more open and tolerant. These changes in attitudes and reactions stem from a number of possible factors including an erosion of the prim Victorian standards of two decades ago; the Pill (oral contraceptive), so easy to take and so relatively fail-safe; the sexual self-assertion of many women, engendered at least in part by the feminist movement.

References

p. 98   Theodore Lidz, *The Person* (New York, 1968), pp. 386–409, 410–39, 440–56.

p. 98   Eleanor Hamilton, *Sex Before Marriage* (New York, 1970).

PART IV
The Mind-Altering Drugs

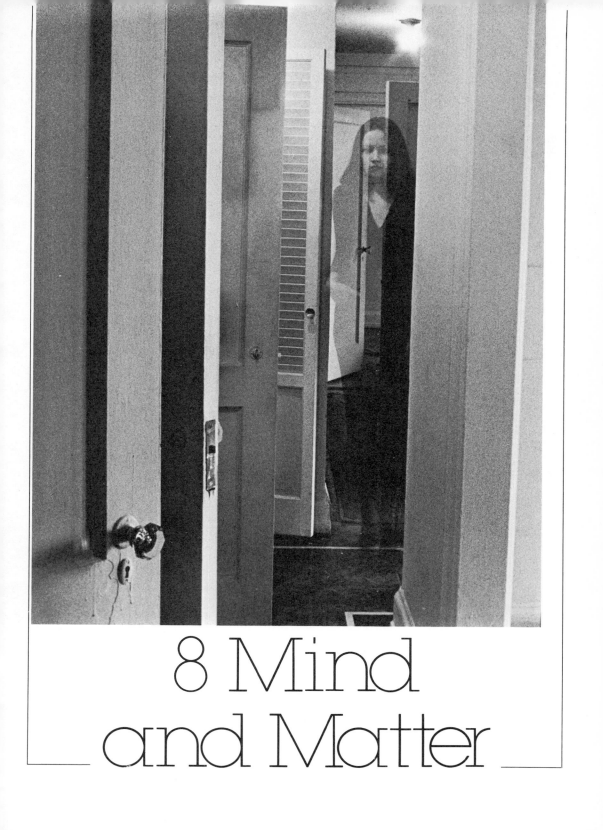

8 Mind and Matter

My father is a drunk, my mom is a speed freak (been using diet pills for over 10 years). One day my mother found a lid of weed in my room. When I told them I had been smoking weed for over 4 years they freaked—my father called me a hippie-fagot and said he would send me to a boys home. My mother flushed the lid down the toilet and cried for 2 days. Things have never been the same— I still live at home cause I have no place else to go. My father is still drunk and my mother is still wired and I'm still stoned.

Long before they started writing histories, people had discovered that swallowing the leaves or fruit or juices of certain plants had strange effects on their minds, as well as their bodies. The early discoveries were made by accident. Someone foraging for food sampled some unfamiliar vegetation and soon his heart was pounding and he felt unaccountably stronger; his mind raced, taking everything in with astonishing clarity. Someone else nibbled at another unfamiliar plant and the world began to look very strange. He experienced visions and heard voices. The risky business of finding food in those times must have had some terrifying results. No doubt many people died, became paralyzed, or went mad after eating poisonous leaves, roots, or berries. But in some cases the experiences must have seemed rewarding, because people went on eating some of those magical plants, and urging others to do likewise. To primitive minds, such substances were gifts from gods, or possibly snares set by less benign forces.

Psychoactive Drugs

Psychoactive substances are those that affect thoughts, moods, and sensory perceptions. Throughout history, in every culture, people have used psychoactive drugs, sometimes as medicines, often for other purposes—to escape anxiety, hunger, or boredom, or to relax, to "feel good," to have new experiences, or just because "everyone else does it."

In America in the late twentieth century almost everyone uses psychoactive drugs, including some that most people don't think of as drugs at all. Coffee and cocoa, for example, are psychoactive, as are tobacco and alcohol. Besides substances that occur in nature, there are a wide range of laboratory-created compounds that have psychoactive effects. Some—a variety of sedatives, stimulants, and tranquilizers—are legally available only when prescribed by a physician, but are often easily obtainable on the black market. Others may be purchased, without prescriptions, at drugstores and supermarkets and are intensively advertised on television. Still other natural and man-made psychoactive drugs—the ones most people think of when the drug problem is mentioned—are illegal but nonetheless used by millions of people.

Public policy toward psychoactive drugs has been a matter of recurring controversy that has been particularly intense in recent years. Before considering this controversy, however, we will consider the most commonly used psychoactive drugs the way a scientist does, without particular regard to their legality or illegality, but as chemicals that have certain effects or potential effects on individual organisms, in this case human bodies. The following is a brief discussion of some facts that apply to psychoactive drugs in general.

A Matter of Chemistry

A moment ago we said we would discuss the effects of certain chemicals on human *bodies,* even though our subject is *mind*-affecting drugs. It was no mistake. We often think of the mind as something mysterious, even supernatural. You can't see it or touch it. It seems to have a life of its own. The fact that we use the Greek word for soul, *psyche* (as in psychology or psychoactive), when we mean the mind, shows how people have thought of it in the past. And the workings of the mind—how it stores and processes information, registers pain or pleasure, creates dreams—are still not well understood even by the scientists. But it is clear that the mind is not something separate from the body. Surgical removal of parts of the brain or electrical stimulation of certain brain segments can affect thinking, emotions, and perceptions in ways that prove the mind is solidly rooted in physical matter. The mind is a function of the body, the process through which the organism controls itself and interacts with its environment. And the effects of psychoactive drugs are, initially, *physical* effects.

The human body is much more than a collection of limbs and organs. Researchers have spent many years synthesizing single enzymes or hormones that our bodies routinely manufacture in seconds. The amount of chemical and electrical activity going on in the body at any given time is bewildering, and science is still a long way from understanding all or even most of it. Basically, however, the body is an aggregate of chemicals reacting with other chemicals as a delicately self-regulated system. When someone takes a drug, he or she is introducing foreign chemicals into this delicate system. The chemicals in the drug react with some of those in the body. Some of the body's compounds may be destroyed, or their production may be stimulated or inhibited. The chemistry of the brain or other parts of the central nervous system may be affected directly, or nerve impulses from elsewhere in the body may be altered. These *physical* changes affect thoughts, feelings, and perceptions by altering, temporarily or permanently, the physical structure that underlies the mind.

Composition of Drugs

The drugs themselves possess no mystical properties. They are composed of some of the most common elements. Two parts of carbon, six of hydrogen, and one of oxygen, combined in a certain way, give you 190 proof ethyl alcohol. The very same elements, in different proportions and in a different molecular arrangement, form cocaine. And still another combination of the same elements produces tetrahydrocannabinol, the key ingredient of marijuana. The three drugs, as a rule, have very different effects on the user, but the differences are results of their dissimilar molecular structures, which affect the way they react with body chemicals.

The subjective experience of the drug taker—what *seems* to him or her to be happening—may convince that person the world "out there" has changed. But the illusions, delusions, and hallucinations of a drug taker are built, like dreams, out of information stored in his or her brain, or from everyday sights and sounds that are distorted because the nervous system has been, in effect, short-circuited or otherwise deranged.

Trips Without Maps

One person swallows a little pill and drifts off into a happy dreamland. Another takes the same kind of pill and shortly thereafter is shrieking in terror. The kind of "trip" a given individual will have as a result of taking a particular drug is unpredictable. It depends in part on the purity of the drug and the size of the dose. It also depends on a number of other factors, including the physical makeup of the individual, his past experience, his mood, his expectations, and the circumstances under which the drug is taken. With some drugs, especially the so-called psychedelics, conditions described as "set" and "setting" may have more to do with the nature of the experience than does the direct chemical effect of the drug. "Set" means the set of the mind—the drug taker's mood, his or her conscious or unconscious anxieties, what he or she desires and what he or she expects from the experience. "Setting" is the environment in which the drug effects are experienced. A person who takes LSD, for example, in a pleasant place where he or she feels secure, and under the supervision of a trusted and experienced "guide," is much less likely to have a bad trip than someone who takes it in the middle of a party, or on the street, where strange faces may turn into fearsome enemies or an automobile into a rampaging monster.

Even Safe Drugs Can Be Dangerous

Even a doctor's prescription does not insure that a normally safe drug will not have unwelcome effects on some individuals. Consider, for example, the following information, supplied to physicians by the manufacturer of a certain psychoactive drug:

> WARNINGS: . . . As is true of most preparations containing central nervous system-acting drugs, patients receiving . . . [this drug] should be cautioned against engaging in hazardous occupations requiring complete mental alertness such as operating machinery or driving a motor vehicle. . . .
>
> Since [the drug] has a central nervous system depressant effect, patients should be advised against the simultaneous ingestion of alcohol or other central nervous system depressant drugs. . . .
>
> *Physical and Psychological Dependence:* Withdrawal symptoms (similar in character to those noted with barbiturates and alcohol) have occurred following abrupt discontinuance of [this drug] (convulsions, tremor, abdominal and muscle cramps, vomiting and sweating). These were usually limited to patients who had received excessive doses over an extended period of time. Particularly addiction-

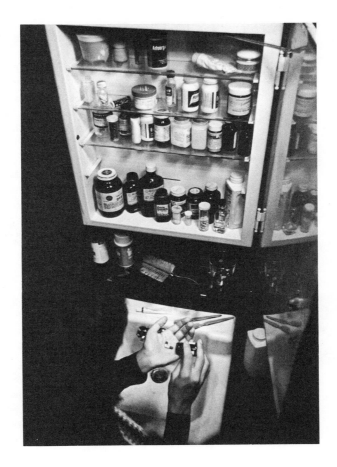

prone individuals (such as drug addicts or alcoholics) should be under careful
surveillance when receiving. . . .

ADVERSE REACTIONS: . . . Side effects most commonly reported were
drowsiness, fatigue and ataxia. Infrequently encountered were confusion, constipation, depression, diplopia [double vision], dysarthria [difficulty in articulation],
headache, hypotension [low blood pressure], incontinence [inability to control
urine or feces], jaundice, changes in libido, nausea . . . slurred speech, tremor . . .
vertigo and blurred vision. . . .

The drug to which those warnings apply is diazepam, a tranquilizer marketed
under the trade name of Valium, the most widely prescribed drug in the United States.
Valium is used as an example here because it is familiar to so many people; it is not
unusually hazardous. Similar warnings accompany most legally manufactured drugs.
Unfortunately, the same service is not provided for users of "street" drugs. The point is
that no drug, not even one manufactured under government-regulated conditions and
prescribed by a physician, is absolutely predictable as to its effects on every individual.

Some Definitions of Drug Use

The manufacturer's warnings to physicians, cited in the preceding paragraphs referred to *physical* and *psychological dependence* and to *addiction*. These are much-used terms, but what exactly do they mean? Even established authorities don't always agree.

Psychological dependence is also called *habituation*. A person gets into a habit of using a particular drug and feels deprived if, for one reason or another, he or she has to do without the drug. Some people become psychologically dependent on things other than drugs, such as television or food. Physical dependence is recognized by the *withdrawal syndrome*. The drug user suffers physical distress, sometimes terrible agony, if he stops taking the drug, voluntarily or otherwise. *Addiction* (from the Latin *addictere*, to consent, to give up) is a word whose usage in the drug context is derived from ancient Roman law; to be addicted meant to be bound to another person by judicial order—in other words, to be enslaved. Some authorities apply the term *addiction* only to cases in which three factors are present: physical dependence, psychological dependence, and *tolerance*, which is a condition in which the body learns to tolerate more and more of a given drug, so that the user has to take larger and larger doses to achieve the desired effect. On the other hand, there are authorities who feel that psychological dependence alone should be described as addiction.

Drug Dependence

Disagreement about the precise meaning of addiction has led to complete abandonment of the term by major national and international health organizations. Rather, they have agreed to apply the term *drug dependence* to any case in which a user feels a strong need for a drug and has difficulty giving it up. As defined by the World Health Organization Expert Committee on Addiction-Producing Drugs, "Drug dependence is a state of psychic or physical dependence, or both, on a drug, arising in a person following administration of that drug on a periodic or continuous basis."

Another imprecise term is *drug abuse*. The National Commission on Marihuana and Drug Abuse, established by Congress and the president at the beginning of the 1970s to investigate the use of psychoactive drugs in the United States and to recommend drug policies, concluded after a two-year study:

> Drug abuse is another way of saying drug problem. Now immortalized in the titles of federal and state government agencies (and we might add, in our own), this term has the virtue of rallying all parties to a common cause: No one could possibly be *for* abuse of drugs any more than they could be *for* abuse of minorities, power or children. By the same token, the term also obscures the fact that "abuse" is undefined where drugs are concerned. Neither the public, its policy makers nor the expert community share a common understanding of its meaning or the nature of the phenomenon to which it refers.
>
> The Commission has noted over the last two years that the public and press often employ drug *abuse* interchangeably with drug *use*. Indeed, many "drug abuse experts," including government officials, do so as well. . . .

The Commission believes that the term drug abuse must be deleted from official pronouncements and public policy dialogue. The term has no functional utility and has become no more than an arbitrary codeword for that drug use which is presently considered wrong. . . .

The commission's conclusion notwithstanding, drug abuse remains a frequently used term, and a definition is required. As it relates to health, the subject with which this book is concerned, a good definition is the one adopted by the World Health Organization's Expert Committee: "persistent or sporadic excessive drug use inconsistent with or unrelated to acceptable medical practice."

Classifying Drugs

Many people think of alcohol as a stimulant because they feel "high" after a couple of drinks; a wallflower becomes the life of the party—temporarily. Actually, alcohol is a powerful depressant. By "turning off" some of the brain's functions, it can suppress inhibitions, giving the drinker a sense of freedom that sometimes turns into acute embarrassment the morning after.

All psychoactive drugs have multiple effects, some of them much more subtle than the deceptive alcohol "high." The subtleties sometimes make it difficult for scientists to agree when they try to classify certain drugs according to their principal effects. For example, nicotine, the psychoactive ingredient in tobacco, seems to act sometimes as a stimulant and other times as a depressant. As a result of such inconsistencies, drugs may be placed in different categories by different scientific investigators. And drug users may find that their subjective experiences do not tally with scientific descriptions of the effects of some drugs. What the drug taker thinks is happening, however, often has little to do with objective reality. Many drug users believe that certain drugs enhance their creativity, but peer review of such creations does not substantiate their fantasy.

In general, psychoactive drugs can be grouped into three broad categories: stimulants, or "uppers"; depressants, or "downers"; and that group sometimes called "turn-arounds," of which LSD is the classic example. The drugs are so categorized in the following chapters. One or two of the drugs might be placed in different categories by some investigators; those are identified in the text.

Buyer Beware

A final comment before going on to specific drugs: Impure drugs, or drugs that aren't what they've been represented to be, are a major risk for people who buy "street" drugs—those sold illegally on the black market. Pills sold as mescaline or LSD or THC (tetrahydrocannabinol) have often turned out to be PCP (phenylcyclidine), a potentially dangerous animal tranquilizer. Marijuana is sometimes laced with PCP—a combination

TABLE 8-1 Drugs and Their Medical Uses, Symptoms, and Dependence Potentials

Name	Slang Name	Chemical or Trade Name	Source	Classification	Medical Use	How Taken
Heroin	H., Horse, Scat, Junk, Smack, Scag, Stuff, Harry	Diacetyl-morphine	Semi-Synthetic (from Morphine)	Narcotic	Pain relief	Injected or Sniffed
Morphine	White stuff, M.	Morphine sulphate	Natural (from Opium)	Narcotic	Pain relief	Swallowed or Injected
Codeine	Schoolboy	Methylmorphine	Natural (from Opium), Semi-Synthetic (from Morphine)	Narcotic	Ease Pain and coughing	Swallowed
Methadone	Dolly	Dolophine Amidone	Synthetic	Narcotic	Pain relief	Swallowed or Injected
Cocaine	Corrine, Gold Dust, Coke, Bernice, Flake, Star Dust, Snow	Methylester of benzoylecgonine	Natural (from coca, NOT cacao)	Stimulant, Local Anesthesia	Local Anesthesia	Sniffed, Injected, or Swallowed
Marijuana	Pot, Grass, Hashish, Tea, Gage, Reefers	Cannabis sativa	Natural	Relaxant, Euphoriant, In high doses Hallucinogen	None in U.S.	Smoked, Swallowed, or Sniffed
Barbiturates	Barbs, Blue Devils, Candy, Yellow Jackets, Phennies, Peanuts, Blue Heavens	Phenobarbital, Nembutal, Seconal, Amytal	Synthetic	Sedative-hypnotic	Sedation, Relieve high blood pressure, epilepsy, hyper-thyroidism	Swallowed or Injected
Amphetamines	Bennies, Dexies, Speed, Wake-Ups, Lid Prop-pers, Hearts, Pep Pills	Benzedrine, Dexedrine, Desoxyn, Meth-amphetamine, Methedrine	Synthetic	Sympatho-mimetic	Relieve mild depression, con-trol appetite and narcolepsy	Swallowed or Injected
LSD	Acid, Sugar, Big D, Cubes, Trips	d-lysergic acid diethylamide	Semi-Synthetic (from ergot alkaloids)	Hallucinogen	Experimental study of mental function, alcoholism	Swallowed
DMT	AMT, Businessman's High	Dimethyl-triptamine	Synthetic	Hallucinogen	None	Injected

Usual Dose	Duration of Effect	Effects Sought	Long-Term Symptoms	Physical Dependence Potential	Mental Dependence Potential	Organic Damage Potential
Varies	4 hrs.	Euphoria, Prevent withdrawal discomfort	Addiction Constipation Loss of Appetite	Yes	Yes	No
15 Milligrams	6 hrs.	Euphoria, Prevent withdrawal discomfort	Addiction Constipation Loss of Appetite	Yes	Yes	No
30 Milligrams	4 hrs.	Euphoria, Prevent withdrawal discomfort	Addiction Constipation Loss of Appetite	Yes	Yes	No
10 Milligrams	4–6 hrs.	Prevent withdrawal discomfort	Addiction Constipation Loss of Appetite	Yes	Yes	No
Varies	Varies, Short	Excitation, Talkativeness	Depression Convulsions	No	Yes	Yes?*
1–2 Cigarettes	4 hrs.	Relaxation, increased euphoria, Perceptions, Sociability	Usually None	No	Yes?	No
50–100 Milligrams	4 hrs.	Anxiety reduction, Euphoria	Addiction w/ severe withdrawal symptoms, Possible convulsions, toxic psychosis	Yes	Yes	Yes
2.5–5 Milligrams	4 hrs.	Alertness Activeness	Loss of Appetite Delusions Hallucinations Toxic psychosis	No?	Yes	Yes?
100–500 Micrograms	10 hrs.	Insightful experiences, exhilaration, Distortion of senses	May intensify existing psychosis, panic reactions	No	No?	No?
1–3 Milligrams	Less than 1 hr.	Insightful experiences, exhilaration, Distortion of senses	?	No	No?	No?

TABLE 8-1 Drugs and Their Medical Uses, Symptoms, and Dependence Potentials continued

Name	Slang Name	Chemical or Trade Name	Source	Classification	Medical Use	How Taken
Mescaline	Mesc.	3,4,5-trimeth-oxyphenethyl-amine	Natural (from Peyote)	Hallucinogen	None	Swallowed
Psilocybin		3 (2-dimethyl-amino) ethylin-dol-4-oldihydro-gen phosphate	Natural (from Psilocybe)	Hallucinogen	None	Swallowed
Alcohol	Booze, Juice, etc.	Ethanol ethyl alcohol	Natural (from grapes, grains, etc. via fermentation)	Sedative hypnotic	Solvent, Antiseptic	Swallowed
Tobacco	Fag, Coffin nail, etc.	Nicotinia tabacum	Natural	Stimulant-sedative	Sedative, Emetic (nicotine)	Smoked, Sniffed, Chewed

*? denotes areas of disagreement by some experts.

Source: U.S. Department of Health, Education and Welfare, Resource Book for Drug Abuse Education.

known as "angel dust"—to give the impression that the weed is particularly potent. Strychnine, arsenic, insecticides, and detergents are among the adulterants sometimes found in street drugs. Buying drugs from a trusted acquaintance—the usual case in small-quantity black market transactions—is no guarantee of purity. However well-meaning he may be, the small-time dealer may have no way of knowing that his source told, or knew, the truth.

Summary

Prehistoric man, foraging for food, discovered that his mind and body reacted differently—he *felt* differently—when he ingested certain leaves, fruits, and juices. Throughout recorded history, humans have used psychoactive substances to alter their moods, thoughts, perceptions.

Some of these substances, such as coffee, alcohol, tobacco, are in wide use. Others are laboratory-made drugs—sedatives, stimulants, and tranquilizers—obtained legally

Usual Dose	Duration of Effect	Effects Sought	Long-Term Symptoms	Physical Dependence Potential	Mental Dependence Potential	Organic Damage Potential
350 Micrograms	12 hrs.	Insightful experiences, exhilaration, Distortion of senses	?	No	No?	No?
25 Milligrams	6–8 hrs.	Insightful experiences, exhilaration, Distortion of senses	?	No	No?	No?
Varies	1–4 hrs.	Sense alteration Anxiety reduction, Sociability	Cirrhosis Toxic psychosis Neurologic damage, Addiction	Yes	Yes	Yes
Varies	Varies	Calmness Sociability	Emphysema, Lung cancer, mouth & throat cancer, Cardiovascular damage, loss of appetite	Yes?	Yes	Yes

by prescription or illegally on the black market. Still others are the substances, mostly illegal, regarded by the public as components of "the drug problem."

Each substance affects the user in different ways geared to the chemical nature of the substance, the strength of the dosage, and the physical and mental state of the user. Some are addictive, others aren't. The reactions produced range from mild euphoria to hallucination. Excessive doses of some drugs can be serious, even fatal. So-called street drugs may be adulterated and impure— and thus doubly dangerous.

References

p. 114   San Francisco Opportunity High School II, *Dope Notes, A Project of the Drugs and Society Class* (1972). This booklet contains unedited statements by thirty-five students about drug experiences. Errors in spelling, grammar, and punctuation in quotations from *Dope Notes* are the students'.

p. 117   Roche Laboratories, Valium package insert (Nutley, N.J., September, 1971).

p. 118   Nathan B. Eddy et al., "Drug Dependence: Its Significance and Characteristics," *Bulletin of the World Health Organization,* Vol. 32, No. 5 (May 1965), p. 722.

p. 119   *Drug Use in America: Problem and Perspective, Second Report of the National Commission on Marihuana and Drug Abuse* (Washington, D.C., 1973), pp. 11–13.

p. 119   *WHO Expert Committee on Drug Dependence, Sixteenth Report,* World Health Organization Technical Report Series, No. 407 (Geneva, 1969), p. 6.

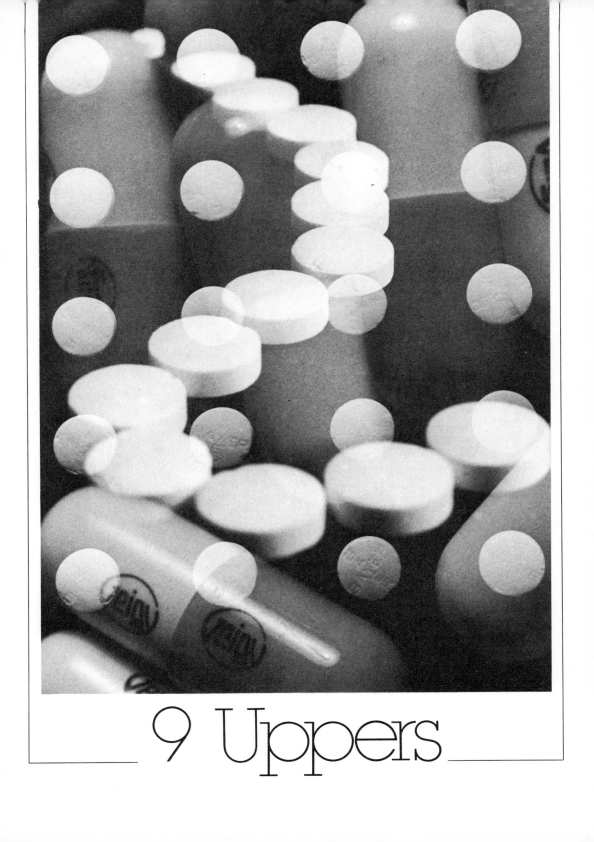

9 Uppers

In the course of evolution, survival frequently depended on an ability to respond quickly to danger, to fight hard, or to run fast. Humankind inherited from their ancestors a built-in emergency response system. In moments of stress, the adrenal glands, located at the top of each of the kidneys, release hormones that trigger a series of instant reactions. The liver releases stored sugar into the bloodstream—extra fuel to enable the brain and muscles to work harder and faster. The lungs pull in more oxygen, and the heart beats faster, pumping blood laden with fuel and oxygen throughout the body. The pupils of the eyes dilate, widening the field of vision. Hair sometimes "stands on end," a reaction probably inherited from some shaggy ancestor who, like a combative cat, could thus puff itself up so as to look bigger and more ferocious.

This "fight or flight" response is useful, sometimes vital, when we have to cope with sudden emergencies. But if our adrenal glands should malfunction and produce too many hormones, or produce them at the wrong time, the results could be very unpleasant, even seriously damaging to the body. There are certain drugs whose effects, in many ways, mimic those of the adrenal hormones. Some are closely related to these hormones in their molecular structure. Some actually stimulate production of the hormones by the adrenal glands. Such drugs are called stimulants or excitants or "uppers." We will discuss the ones most commonly used in this country.

The Xanthines

A fatal dose of caffeine given to an animal produces convulsions because of the central stimulating effect. Early in the poisoning, these are epileptiform [spasmodic convulsion followed by relaxation] in nature; as the action of the drug on the spinal cord becomes manifest, strychnine-like convulsions [unremitting spasms of most muscle groups] may appear. Death results from respiratory failure.

An unpleasant picture, but could that really be caffeine, the very same caffeine we consume in our morning coffee? It is, but there is little cause to become alarmed; no one is likely to drink the seventy to one-hundred cups of coffee at a sitting that, it has been estimated, would be necessary to provide an adult human with a fatal dose of caffeine. The gruesome description is used to emphasize a fact that never occurs to many people; caffeine *is* a drug. It is one of a group of drugs called the *xanthines,* a group that also includes theophylline (an alkaloid obtained from tea leaves) and theobromine (an alkaloid from cacao beans and kola nuts). Caffeine is found in tea, cocoa, and cola drinks, as well as in coffee. In moderate amounts, none of these beverages is likely to be harmful to a healthy person. As with all drugs, however, the effects vary from individual to individual, and what is moderate for one person may be immoderate for another.

The xanthines are an example of what might be called a "tamed" drug. While they are potentially as dangerous as some of the more notorious chemicals that are usually associated with the drug problem, they are customarily used in ways that are accepted

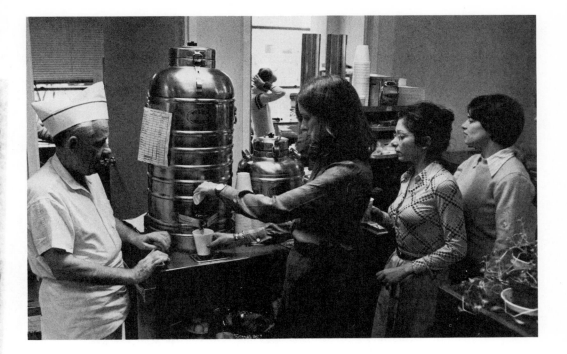

and even encouraged by society. An ordinary cup of coffee is a highly diluted solution containing a very small quantity of caffeine. Yet the effects of even that small amount can be remarkable.

Why Coffee Breaks?

The usual effects of small doses of caffeine help to account for the fact that many employers as well as employees find coffee breaks during working hours beneficial:

> Caffeine stimulates all portions of the (cerebral) cortex. Its main action is to produce a more rapid and clearer flow of thought, and to allay drowsiness and fatigue. After taking caffeine one is capable of a greater sustained intellectual effort and a more perfect association of ideas. There is also a keener appreciation of sensory stimuli, and reaction time to them is appreciably diminished. This accounts for the hyperesthesia [overstimulation of the senses], sometimes unpleasant, which some people experience after drinking too much coffee. In addition, motor activity is increased; typists, for example, work faster and with fewer errors. However, recently acquired skill in a task involving delicate muscular coordination and accurate timing may . . . be adversely affected. These effects may be brought on by the administration of 150 to 200 milligrams of caffeine, the amount contained in one or two cups of coffee or tea.

The Coffee Abusers

Everyone is familiar with the term *coffee nerves,* and with the fact that many people have trouble going to sleep after drinking coffee. And most of us have heard people say that they "need" their morning coffee to wake up, or to "get going." Not everyone, however, realizes that many people become dependent on the xanthine drugs, even to the point of suffering physical withdrawal symptoms if they have to do without. One team of researchers reported the following results of a study involving a group of housewives:

> . . . Eighteen non-coffee drinkers and 38 drinkers of five or more cups a day were each supplied with nine coded vials containing specially compounded instant coffee. They were told to use one vial each morning in preparing their morning cup. The coffee prepared with the various vials could not be distinguished either by appearance or by taste; but three of the vials contained 300 milligrams of caffeine (the equivalent of two or three cups of brewed coffee), three contained 150 milligrams, and three contained no caffeine at all. The subjects were asked to score their moods in various respects before drinking the morning cup and again at half-hour intervals for the subsequent two hours. The 9,240 mood scores thus secured were analyzed with the aid of a computer.
>
> . . . The five-cups-or-more-a-day users felt less alert, less active, less content, more sleepy, and more irritable before their morning coffee. On days when they drank caffeine-free coffee, they continued to feel that way throughout the next two hours; and they felt increasingly jittery, nervous, and shaky as the caffeineless hours dragged by. On days when their morning cups contained caffeine, however, these withdrawal symptoms were dramatically relieved. They also reported fewer headaches on caffeine mornings. The favorable effects were more marked with the 300 milligram dose than when the morning cup contained only 150 milligrams of caffeine.
>
> The effects were reversed among the participants who did not ordinarily drink coffee. These housewives reported an increase in *unpleasant* stimulant effects such as jitteriness and nervousness, plus more gastrointestinal complaints on caffeine mornings. . . .

In addition to their direct effects on the nervous system, the xanthine drugs—like the adrenal hormones—increase the heartbeat rate, blood pressure, and circulation. They also act as diuretics, stimulating urination. Secretion of gastric acids, too, is stimulated by these drugs, and some investigators have suggested that they may contribute to the development of stomach ulcers in some heavy users. Besides nervousness and inability to sleep, heavy users of the xanthines may experience rapid or irregular heartbeats, sensory disturbances, such as ringing in the ears, and other unpleasant symptoms. Because of the effects of the xanthines on the circulatory system, people with heart trouble or high blood pressure are encouraged by doctors to use coffee and tea from which the caffeine has been removed.

Caffeine Pills

Many students, cramming for exams, have kept themselves awake with the help of caffeine tablets that are sold without prescription in drugstores and supermarkets under various trade names. A one-hundred-milligram tablet contains roughly the amount of caffeine found in an average cup of coffee. Because it is easier to swallow a lot of little pills than to drink great amounts of coffee or cola beverages, the tablets lend themselves to excessive use. In large doses they can produce confusion, disorientation, and irrational behavior, among other unwelcome symptoms.

Cocaine

Dr. Sigmund Freud, a disciple of his wrote later, "was rapidly becoming a public menace." The year was 1884, and the young Viennese neurologist, destined for immortality as the father of psychoanalysis, had found what seemed to be a remedy for his chronic exhaustion and depression. To his fiancée, Martha Bernays, Freud wrote:

> Woe to you, my Princess, when I come. I will kiss you quite red and feed you till you are plump. And if you are forward you shall see who is the stronger, a gentle little girl who doesn't eat enough or a big wild man *who has cocaine in his body* [Freud's italics]. In my last severe depression I took coca again and a small dose lifted me to the heights in a wonderful fashion. I am just now busy collecting the literature for a song of praise to this magical substance.

Not content with publishing his "song of praise" in a medical journal, in language sometimes more poetic than scientific, Freud eagerly urged cocaine on his fiancée, his sisters, his friends, his colleagues, and his patients. One of the friends he introduced to cocaine was Ernst von Fleischl-Marxow, who had become dependent on the morphine he took for a painful nervous system disease.

Within a short time medical investigators began publishing reports that cocaine not only produced a strong dependence in regular users, but caused serious mental disturbances in some of them. Freud, an occasional user who escaped dependence, eventually gave up the drug altogether. His friend Fleischl-Marxow, however, was less fortunate. Fleischl found that cocaine enabled him to give up morphine—but he couldn't give up cocaine. By then he had discovered something else about cocaine; he rapidly developed a tolerance for the drug, and required ever-larger doses. And since cocaine was then, as now, the most expensive of drugs, Fleischl was soon impoverished. He also suffered from psychotic episodes in which he imagined white snakes creeping over his skin. Freud sometimes helped nurse his friend through such wide-awake nightmares during the final years before Fleischl-Marxow died of the disease that had first driven him to drugs.

Chewing and Snorting

Decades before Freud and his colleagues began experimenting with cocaine, the drug had been isolated from the leaves of *erythroxylon coca,* a shrub that grows in the mountains of South America. Coca leaves have been used as a stimulant for centuries by Andean Indians, who chewed the leaves as they worked. Coca makes them feel stronger, helps them endure long periods of hardship—and to do so with little food, since cocaine also acts as an appetite suppressant. Probably because the leaves contain only small quantities of cocaine, the Andean Indians, who still chew coca leaves, do not seem to become dependent on the drug. When they leave the mountains and give up coca, they suffer no apparent ill effects. In a sense, their use of the drug can be compared to the use of coffee in the United States—although there is a danger in such comparisons: someone always jumps to the erroneous conclusion that "cocaine is no worse than coffee." Comparing coca leaves to coffee is not the same as comparing cocaine to caffeine. In similar quantities, cocaine—even diluted with various adulterants as it almost always is when sold on the street—is much more powerful than caffeine. It can also be much more seductive.

Cocaine usually comes in the form of a very fine, white powder. It is sometimes dissolved and injected into a vein or under the skin, but most users sniff it into their nostrils—"snort," in the vernacular. It is then absorbed through the mucus membrane. Some experimenters find the results disappointing:

> Coke to me, baby, is definitely a rich man's high. Although I'm not rich, I've gotten down a few times, and this is what it is to me . . . nothing, not a damn thing but a waste of money. During my short relationship with coke I felt my nose getting stiff (called froze), I felt high but it was a far away high and for about 45 minutes it was so far away it was gone. How much coke did I snort? . . . I spent twenty dollars for an hour's high.

The drug's effects on other users are more pronounced: "The subjective effects of cocaine include an elevation of mood that often reaches proportions of euphoric excitement. It produces a marked decrease in hunger, an indifference to pain, and is reputed to be the most potent antifatigue agent known. The user enjoys a feeling of great muscular strength and increased mental capacity and greatly overestimates his capabilities. . . ."

Drips and Crawly Things

Like Freud's friend Fleischl, frequent cocaine users are likely to find that their tolerance for the drug develops very rapidly, that acquiring enough cocaine to achieve the desired effect soon becomes extremely expensive. Nevertheless, they may feel by that time that they need the drug. While giving up a cocaine habit does not produce strong physical withdrawal symptoms, users who are deprived of the drug may plunge into a deep mental depression, which, it seems to them, can be relieved only by more cocaine. At the same time, the cocaine-induced euphoria (sense of well-being) that first captured the user's interest may be replaced by frightening hallucinations. Like Fleischl-Marxow, many cocaine users "see" and "feel" insects or snakes crawling over or under their skin. Unlike the alcoholic's pink elephants, cocaine hallucinations do not come after the drug use has been discontinued, but during the "high." Some heavy cocaine users become paranoid, plagued by irrational fears. Some start carrying guns or knives to protect themselves from imagined enemies.

Over a period of time, cocaine snorting causes some peculiar physical damage. When cocaine is sniffed into the nostrils, it anesthetizes, or deadens, the *cilia,* tiny hairs that line the walls of the nasal passages. The function of the cilia, which normally sway with a wave-like motion, is to brush mucus toward the outer openings of the nasal passages. This disposes of potentially infectious microbes trapped in the mucus. Anesthetized by cocaine, the cilia stop waving, and the microbes remain in the passages. Resulting infections sometimes eat holes through the nasal *septum,* the partition between the nostrils. Cocaine sniffers also develop a characteristic postnasal drip, which is a discharge of mucus from behind the nose onto the surface of the pharynx, which necessitates continual throat-clearing and swallowing.

Eventually, regular, heavy cocaine users are likely to suffer general deterioration, physically as well as mentally. Because the drug kills their appetites, they suffer from malnutrition, and because the drug keeps them awake, they suffer from a lack of sleep. They become slovenly in appearance. Neglect of personal hygiene and weakened resistance make them susceptible to infectious diseases. They are sometimes psychotic, and they may be easily moved to violence.

Cocaine and Sex

Some users claim that cocaine increases their enjoyment of sexual intercourse because it heightens awareness of sensory stimuli. Since cocaine causes a drying up of various body secretions, including vaginal fluids, women sometimes suffer vaginal tightness and rawness following prolonged coitus after taking cocaine. Sometimes men rub the powder on the tips of their penises in the belief that it will enable them to maintain an erection for a long time without ejaculation. Since locally applied cocaine may anesthetize the sexual organs of both partners, any increased enjoyment in this case is probably more fancied than physical.

The Amphetamines

In the late nineteenth century a doctor in the German Army injected cocaine into some soldiers on maneuvers and reported that it greatly reduced their fatigue. In the Second World War many servicemen on both sides of the battle lines, including Americans, were issued *amphetamines.* These synthetic drugs had much the same effects as cocaine, plus some added advantages; unlike cocaine, which is poorly absorbed by the body when swallowed, the amphetamines could be taken orally in tablets or capsules. And whereas the effects of a dose of cocaine wore off rather quickly, amphetamines kept the troops stimulated for hours. After the war amphetamines became fashionable. Pharmaceutical manufacturers, who turned them out in enormous quantities, advertised them intensively in medical journals as effective agents against a variety of complaints, and drug salespeople pressed samples on physicians, along with literature extolling their

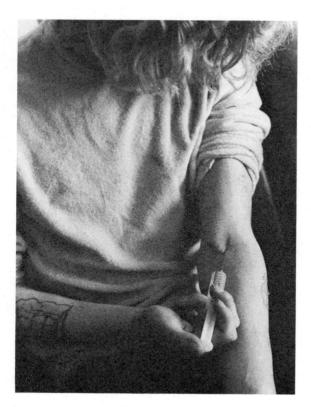

virtues. Soon amphetamines were among the most widely prescribed drugs. And for those who didn't have prescriptions, there was a thriving black market in amphetamines that had somehow been diverted from legal channels.

> . . . Early black-market patrons included in particular truck drivers trying to maintain schedules which called for long over-the-road hauls without adequate rest periods. Soon truck stops along the main transcontinental routes dispensed amphetamines as well as coffee and caffeine tablets . . . to help the drivers stay awake. Students, who had long used caffeine tablets, now turned instead to these new amphetamine ''pep pills'' when cramming for exams. . . .

Amphetamines were compounded in a variety of ways and marketed under numerous trade names. There were, for example, amphetamine sulfate (marketed as Benzedrine), dextroamphetamine sulfate (Dexedrine), and methamphetamine hydrochloride (Methedrine and Desoxyn). There were also some amphetaminelike drugs with much the same effects, methylphenidate (Ritalin) and phenmetrazine (Preludin). The amphetamines are medically useful in treating victims of narcolepsy, a rare condition in which the victim continually falls asleep. Students unable to stay awake in class were not infrequently diagnosed as having narcolepsy. However, the students' problem was most often boredom, not narcolepsy. Children with a certain kind of brain damage that makes them *hyperkinetic* (overactive) are found to benefit from amphetamines and amphetaminelike drugs through one of those paradoxes that always crops up in the study of psychoactive chemicals. When taken by such children, the drugs had a calming instead of a stimulating effect.

By far the greatest number of amphetamine prescriptions, however, were issued for other purposes. Because of their mood-elevating and fatigue-suppressing effects, the drugs were widely prescribed for people suffering from mild depressions or from general tiredness. And because, like cocaine, they suppress the appetite, amphetamines were perhaps even more widely prescribed for people who needed or wanted to lose weight. All over America bored and frustrated housewives found that these "diet" pills brightened their dreary days, and many became more or less permanent dieters. "Mother's little helpers," some called the pills. By the 1960s millions of people of every age and social condition were using amphetamines—and more and more of them were learning, often painfully, that along with cocaine's benefits these synthetic drugs could bring all of cocaine's grief.

Ups—and Downs

Highballing down a superhighway, a big-rig driver peers through sunken, dark-ringed eyes at the ribbon of concrete streaming up into the glare of his headlights. Jacked up on "pep pills," he is streaking closer to the bonus at the end of a tightly scheduled transcontinental run that has been broken only by fuel stops and catnaps. But things are getting . . . weird. Snatches of sound from nowhere. Menacing shapes popping up and . . . what's that? Air brakes scream and the rig careens crazily. . . .

Mrs. Prentiss is being firm. No more diet pills. No more jittery days and sleepless nights and pounding heart, lying there listening to Frank snore, wondering if she's having an attack. No more . . . but right now everything is so depressing; just a couple of pills to get through today and then no more. . . .

Little bits of fiction, but not very different from countless real-life experiences of amphetamine takers. Many people started taking small doses to stay awake or to relieve depression or to lose weight and then increased the doses as they developed tolerance until they became habituated. They found themselves on a roller coaster of drug-induced euphoria followed by depression, and so on.

. . . even low-dose amphetamine consumption can cause tremulousness, anxiety, drying of the mouth, alteration of sleep habits and other unpleasant effects. It may also lead to an increased awareness of heart function, which can be compounded by tachycardia, a rapid, forceful pounding that stems from extreme cardiovascular stimulation.

Tachycardia also shows up in cases of acute amphetamine toxicity due to intentional or accidental overdosage. Although no fatalities have been recorded as a direct result of high-dose consumption, it commonly produces restlessness, hypertension, . . . impaired judgment, hyperventilation (a state of excessively rapid breathing), hallucinations and possible psychosis. . . . patients may require isolation and reassurance that they are not suffering heart attacks or losing their sanity.

More serious, and increasingly common in this country, is chronic amphetamine toxicity. The chemicals are not addictive in small doses, but people who take larger amounts do experience extreme psychological dependence and may even suffer mild physical withdrawal symptoms when deprived of the drugs. Such dependence is complicated by the fact that as the body develops a tolerance to amphetamines, increasingly higher doses are required to maintain their effects. Prolonged high-dose amphetamine consumption often results in physical deterioration and in a toxic psychosis characterized by perceptual alterations, visual and auditory hallucinations, severe depression and a state that resembles paranoid schizophrenia. It may also lead to organic brain damage and personality change. . . .

The "Speed Freaks"

In the 1960s Methedrine and Desoxyn could be purchased in liquid form in ampuls (glass containers holding small quantities of the material). Injected directly into the bloodstream, these short-acting varieties of amphetamine produce a "flash" that some users liken to a "full-body orgasm." The drug in this form was known on the streets by a number of names, including "meth" and "crank," and, especially, "speed," the latter a name that was eventually applied to all of the amphetamines. Someone who had injected speed was "wired" or "cranked up."

Amphetamines could also be taken by injecting dissolved tablets, but the ampul form was particularly convenient. Methedrine and Desoxyn ampuls were available on the black market as a result of drugstore burglaries and, more often, as a result of shipment from Mexico, where "legitimate" dealers ordered huge quantities from phar-

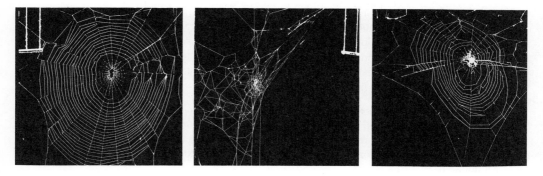

Left: A normal spider web. Center: The web spun by the spider twelve hours after receiving a dose of dextroamphetamine. Right: The web spun by the same spider twenty-four hours after receiving the dose.

maceutical manufacturers in the United States. Some users also obtained the drugs by prescriptions issued by doctors who believed the amphetamines provided a beneficial way to wean heroin dependents off their habit—as Freud's friend Fleischl used cocaine to end his dependence on morphine. And there were a few physicians, some of whom later went to prison, who prescribed "meth" to almost anyone who had the price of an office call. Eventually, the Methedrine and Desoxyn ampuls were to be forced off the market by concerned authorities, but the public demand for the drugs was quickly met by amateur "cooks" who turned out methamphetamine in home laboratories. For someone who knew a little chemistry, methamphetamine was easy to make and highly profitable to market. It was also frequently contaminated by adulterants that sometimes made its undesirable effects even worse.

The beginning amphetamine "mainliner" may give him- or herself injections "once or a very few times over a day or two," one researcher reported. Days or weeks may intervene between sprees. Gradually the sprees become longer and the intervening periods shorter; doses become higher and injections more frequent. After a period of several months, the final pattern is reached in which the user (now called a "speed freak") injects his drug many times a day . . . and remains awake continuously for three to six days, getting gradually more tense, tremulous and paranoid as the "run" progresses. The runs are interrupted by bouts of very profound sleep (called "crashing") which last a day or two. Shortly after waking . . . the drug is again injected and a new run starts. . . .

Like the habitual cocaine user, the speed freak deteriorates mentally and physically. Many become dirty, diseased, and violent. Roger C. Smith, a criminologist and drug researcher who worked with San Francisco's Haight-Ashbury Free Medical Clinic and studied the speed epidemic of the 1960s at close range, reported: "It is common to see speed freaks with open running sores or scabs on their faces or arms as a result of picking or cutting out . . . hallucinated crank bugs." Explaining what "crank bugs" are, Smith quoted one speed freak:

> It's just that when you're shooting speed constantly you start to feel like there's bugs going around under your skin and you know they're not there, but you pick at them anyway. . . . Once in a while you'll see a little black spot and you'll watch it for ten minutes to see if it moves. If it doesn't move it isn't alive. You can feel them on your skin. I'm always trying to pick them out of my eyebrows.

The speed freaks in the Haight-Ashbury neighborhood "frequently substituted drugs for interpersonal relations and experienced a complete isolation reinforced by their paranoia and psychotic behavior. They sometimes had sex, but their lives were ego trips dominated by speed."

A Slowdown on Speed

By the mid-1970s mounting evidence of the dangers of amphetamines had led to considerable tightening of laws governing their manufacture and distribution by phar-

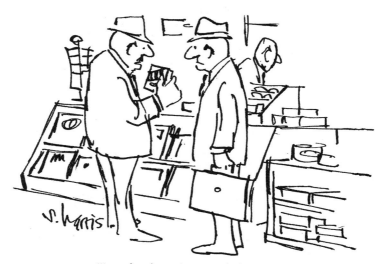

*"I prefer these imported cigarettes.
They don't have a health warning."*

maceutical companies, and the medical profession had greatly reduced the numbers of prescriptions issued for their use. The only remaining legitimate uses are in the occasional case of narcolepsy and for brain-damaged hyperkinetic children. Even the latter use has become controversial because of claims that many children were improperly diagnosed as brain damaged, and given the drugs simply because their overactiveness caused problems for parents and teachers. Such claims have been challenged, and the controversy continues.

Tobacco

It was an exquisitely tender moment. As the lovers gazed soulfully into each other's eyes, Paul Henreid placed two cigarettes between his lips, lighted both, and wordlessly presented one of them to Bette Davis, as he might have presented a bouquet, the keys to paradise, his heart on a silver platter.

In the darkened movie house, your grandmother sighed; your grandfather squeezed her hand. It was so touching, so elegant, and—in an era of chaste romance—so erotic. The scene in *Now Voyager* (made in 1942), became an instant classic. A generation of teen-agers, the parents of today's college students, reenacted the moment in thousands of parked cars, incurring immeasurable disillusionment when sacramental cigarettes stuck stubbornly and debasingly to the lower lips of adolescent Paul Henreids.

Psychologists and other researchers have devoted countless hours in efforts to determine why people begin using various drugs. The reasons are numerous. Peer pressure is a well-known one, the desire to be like everybody else. Parental example is another. Relief of boredom, "kicks," the search for a mystical experience, the hope of improving one's self-image are others. The reasons are often complex—and seldom are they more complex than in the case of tobacco.

Tobacco—or nicotine, its main psychoactive ingredient—no longer has any recognized medical use. It does not provide users with very far-out trips. Everyone knows, as stated in the warning printed on every package of cigarettes made in the United States: "The Surgeon General Has Determined That Cigarette Smoking Is Dangerous to Your Health." To the beginner, at least, tobacco smoke doesn't usually taste good. Initial experiences with tobacco are likely to be unpleasant, producing dizziness, coughing fits, and, not infrequently, a frantic dash for some receptacle to throw up into. Yet almost everyone at least experiments with cigarettes, and millions of Americans have taken up smoking as a regular habit, consuming billions of cigarettes a year, not to mention large quantities of cigars, pipe and chewing tobacco, and snuff.

For the adolescent, the inducements seem almost irresistible. Chances are that one or both parents smoke. Everywhere he or she goes, other adults are smoking. Friends smoke. Favorite movie stars smoke in glorious, wide-screen color. Although cigarette advertising was banned from television about ten years ago, magazines, newspapers, and billboards blossom with a profusion of alluring come-ons provided from the enormous advertising budgets of a multibillion-dollar tobacco industry. Handsome, virile men and beautiful women in enticing settings—the South Seas, "Marlboro Country," ski lodges, expensive sports cars, intimate boudoirs—inhale as though tobacco smoke were a gaseous form of nectar. The models glow with health. The subliminal message is that smoking Brand X will assure adventure, romance, success, sex. Besides offering all that happiness, the ads often emphasize the manliness of smoking at the same time other ads are implying that smoking is womanly. "You've come a long way, baby" the increasing numbers of female smokers are flatteringly assured by copywriters with an eye on the women's liberation movement and an ear apparently deaf to the chauvinism implicit in that "baby."

In impressionable minds, smoking is associated with all the things the young yearn for. Learning to smoke becomes a rite of passage into the real or imagined delights of the adult world.

Tobacco's Effects

Tobacco is one of those substances whose subtle psychoactive effects are difficult to classify. The first act of many inveterate smokers after opening their eyes in the morning is to light a cigarette to help them wake up. On the other hand, people in tense situations light a cigarette (a standard movie scene) in order to calm themselves down.

The drug is placed among the "uppers" in this book partly because the initial effect of nicotine is excitation, or stimulation, of the nervous system, although that effect is transient and is followed by depression of the nervous system. Nicotine causes the adrenal glands to release epinephrine, one of those "fight or flight" hormones (see p.

268), with resulting increases in respiration, heart rate, and blood pressure. Nicotine also affects other body functions in ways that are not completely understood.

Nicotine is only one of several hundred chemical compounds that are inhaled in tobacco smoke. The others range from twenty-five different acids to the 126 aromatic hydrocarbons and phenols that have been identified as carcinogens (cancer causers) or possible carcinogens. Cigarette smoking is the leading cause of lung cancer, chronic bronchitis, and emphysema, and, because of its effects on the heart and blood pressure, it is a contributing factor in heart disease and strokes. Smoking cigars or pipes is less likely to cause those diseases, but may result in cancers of the mouth or bladder, as may the use of chewing tobacco and snuff.

Many cigarette ads emphasize the effectiveness of the filter tips on their brands, with the implication that the filters make smoking less hazardous. Some researchers have concluded, however, that "cigarette filters did not offer protection against the health hazards of smoking." But the fact that today's young people smoke more filter-tipped cigarettes than their parents did may have at least one minor benefit; since the filters stick to lips less readily than does cigarette paper, it's probably easier to play Paul Henreid than it used to be.

Nicotine Dependence

Sigmund Freud, whose infatuation and disillusionment with cocaine were described earlier, found tobacco harder to give up than cocaine. Despite a lifelong struggle, he was never able to escape from his twenty-cigars-a-day habit for more than a short time. It finally killed him.

"Soon after giving up smoking," Freud wrote during one of his brief attempts to abandon cigars, "there were tolerable days. . . . Then there came suddenly a severe affection of the heart, worse than I ever had while smoking. . . . And with it an oppression of mood in which images of dying and farewell scenes replaced the more usual fantasies. . . . The organic disturbances have lessened in the last couple of days; the hypo-manic mood continues. . . ."

Freud complained that smoking interfered with his work, but he still smoked. He developed frightening pains and irregular rhythms in his heart, blamed by a physician on his smoking, but he kept smoking. Then came cancer of the mouth and throat. Somehow, the great psychoanalyst survived to the age of eighty-three, but only after many years of agony that included thirty-three operations for the cancer that eventually caused his death. He smoked cigars until the end. For Freud, an associate wrote, the "torture" of trying to quit smoking was "beyond human power to bear."

Not all smokers, of course, suffer so profoundly when they try to quit. A good many succeed in stopping, and some of them report only minor discomfort. But millions have found that trying to break the habit can bring on afflictions ranging from physical withdrawal symptoms such as shakiness, headaches, and constipation to persistent anxiety and—in rare cases—paranoid psychosis and violence. And dependence, while not inevitable, can be acquired quickly. One researcher concluded:

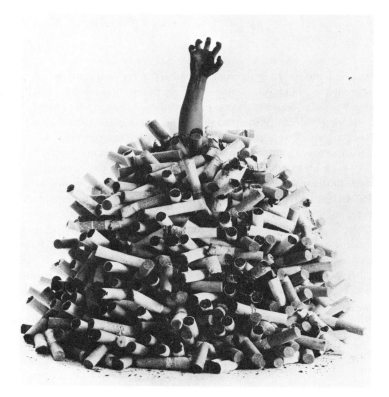

It requires no more than three or four casual cigarettes during adolescence virtually to ensure that a person will eventually become a regular dependent smoker. . . . If we bear in mind that only 15 percent of adolescents who smoke more than one cigarette avoid becoming regular smokers and that only about 15 percent of smokers stop before the age of 60, it becomes apparent that of those who smoke more than one cigarette during adolescence, some 70 percent continue smoking for the next 40 years.

The researcher does not claim, of course, that a single cigarette addicts a person for life. Many experimenters dislike the first cigarette so much that they never try another one. Among those who, despite the initial unpleasantness, keep on trying,

tolerance soon develops to the unpleasant side-effects and skill is quickly acquired to limit the intake of smoke to a comfortable level, thus lowering the threshold for further attempts. Herein lies a possible cause of the virtual inevitability of escalation after only a few cigarettes. With curiosity satisfied by the first cigarette, the act is likely to be repeated only if the physical discomfort is outweighed by the psychological or social rewards. If these motives are sufficient to cause smoking to be repeated in the face of unpleasant side-effects, there is little chance that smoking will not continue as these side-effects rapidly disappear.

Synanon, the therapeutic community for heroin dependents, decided in 1970 to ban cigarette smoking among its members. A reporter for the *New York Times* wrote a year later: "About 100 people left during the six-month period following the ban and chose possible readdiction to drugs outside Synanon to life without cigarettes." Said one Synanon resident: "With most drugs, you get over the [withdrawal] symptoms in a few days, a week at most. But with tobacco, we've noticed them for at least six months." Said another: "It was much easier to quit heroin than cigarettes."

Even knowledge of the strong possibility that the habit will prove fatal does not deter most cigarette smokers for very long. Immediately following the highly publicized 1964 report of an advisory committee to the surgeon general of the United States detailing the strong evidence that cigarette smoking caused cancer and other diseases, cigarette sales in this country dropped by fifteen to twenty percent. But within a few months the sales were back up almost to the previous levels. Public attitude surveys have shown that a majority of smokers believe that cigarettes cause cancer and are otherwise harmful to health. But most smokers continue to brave those perils, along with bad breath, yellow teeth, stained and burned fingers, smelly clothes, hair, and living quarters, hacking coughs, the irritation of nonsmokers, occasional accidental fires, and other concomitants of the tobacco habit. In the middle of the 1970s, Americans are smoking more than ever.

Summary

Some drugs are called "uppers" because they excite and stimulate the senses. One group, xanthines, includes the caffeine in our coffee and tea as well as the more potent cocaine, which, when chewed or sniffed, can produce feelings ranging from intense euphoria to frightening hallucinations.

The amphetamines are synthetic drugs that have about the same effects as cocaine but are better absorbed by the body and don't wear off as quickly. They are widely prescribed for people who want to stay awake and alert; they elevate moods and suppress fatigue. They also suppress appetite, and are sometimes used by those on diets. But as tolerance increases, so, often, does dosage. Habituation increases as does a cycle of artificial "highs" followed by depression. Amphetamines are known on the street as "meth," "crank," and "speed."

Tobacco has no known medical value and is, according to the Surgeon General, hazardous to your health. The nicotine in tobacco is one of the most addictive substances known to mankind. Its initial effect on the nervous system is that of an "upper," but depression follows. Trying to quit smoking can produce all kinds of physical withdrawal symptoms, and many people can kick the habit only through expensive group therapy sessions.

References

p. 126   J. Murdoch Ritchie, *The Pharmacological Basis of Therapeutics,* 4th ed., ed. Louis S. Goodman and Alfred Gilman (New York, 1970), p. 365.

p. 127   Ibid., p. 359.

p. 128   Edward M. Brecher and *Consumer Reports* Editors, *Licit and Illicit Drugs: The Consumers Union Report on Narcotics, Stimulants, Depressants, Inhalants, Hallucinogens, and Marijuana—Including Caffeine, Nicotine, and Alcohol* (Boston, 1972), p. 202.

p. 129   Ernest Jones, ed., *The Life and Work of Sigmund Freud, Vol. I (1856–1900)* (New York, 1953), p. 81.

p. 129   Ibid., p. 84.

p. 130   San Francisco Opportunity High School II, *Dope Notes, A Project of the Drugs and Society Class* (1972).

p. 130   Jerome H. Jaffe, *The Pharmacological Basis of Therapeutics.* 3rd ed., ed. Louis S. Goodman and Alfred Gilman (New York, 1965), pp. 298–99.

p. 132   Brecher and *Consumer Reports* Editors, *Licit and Illicit Drugs,* p. 280.

p. 134   David E. Smith and John Luce, *Love Needs Care, A History of San Francisco's Haight-Ashbury Free Medical Clinic* (Boston, 1971), pp. 15–16.

p. 135   John C. Kramer, "Introduction to Amphetamine Abuse," *Journal of Psychedelic Drugs,* Vol. II, No. 2 (1969), pp. 2–3.

p. 135   Brecher and *Consumer Reports* Editors, *Licit and Illicit Drugs,* p. 285.

p. 137   *Smoking and Health, Report of the Advisory Committee to the Surgeon General* (Washington, D.C., 1964), p. 69.

p. 138   Ibid., p. 51.

p.138   Alfred Kershbaum et al., "Regular, Filter Tip and Modified Cigarettes," *Journal of the American Medical Association,* Vol. 201, No. 7 (August 14, 1967), pp. 545–46.

p. 138   Jones, *The Life and Work of Sigmund Freud, Vol. I,* pp. 309–10.

p. 138   Ibid., p. 311.

p. 138   John S. Tamerin and Charles P. Neumann, "Casualties of the Anti-Smoking Campaign" (Paper delivered at the annual meeting of the American Psychiatric Association, Washington, D.C., May, 1971).

p. 139   M. A. Hamilton Russell, "Cigarette Smoking: Natural History of a Dependence Disorder," *British Journal of Medical Psychology,* 44 (1971), pp. 12–13.

p. 140   Ibid., pp. 8–9.

p. 140   *New York Times* (May 23, 1971).

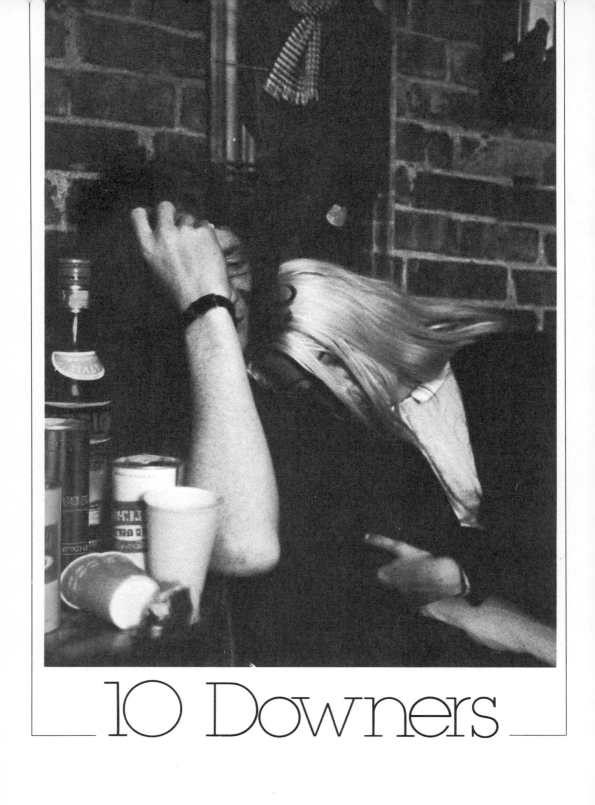

10 Downers

Hundreds of those long-haired young people they used to call hippies are lining up six to eight deep these nights at the big, bustling Catalyst bar in Santa Cruz.

Many of them are buying up and swilling down far-freaking-out quantities of hard liquor—straight shots of tequila and whiskey, in particular.

The scene, on a smaller scale, perhaps, is occurring in countless other Northern California bars.

On Berkeley's Telegraph Avenue, it is not uncommon to see some of the strange-looking denizens they call street people taking swigs of port wine from bottles thinly hidden in paper bags.

Going barefoot at rock concerts has now become hazardous. Some promoters have complained that broken bottles are a major clean-up problem.

Beer busts are once again a staple of college life in the Bay Area, and not just among the fraternity crowd.

In short, booze is definitely back. . . .

It was front-page news in the *San Francisco Chronicle*. For close to two decades, that newspaper had been covering in colorful detail the succeeding waves of counterculture movements—and attendant drug use—that seemed always to find their extremes, if not their origins, in San Francisco.

Youth Revolutions

In the late 1950s it was the beat generation who turned a once-quiet Italian neighborhood into a bizarre bohemia built largely around avant-garde art forms, restless nomadism, and existential philosophy. Some of the "beats" dabbled in drugs, but wine was their staple. Around the beginning of the 1960s, rising rents, run-ins with the police, and other problems drove most of them out of North Beach. Many faded into another quiet neighborhood, a low-rent residential district called the Haight-Ashbury. And many began to turn from alcohol to marijuana, LSD, and other psychedelic drugs.

The beats were the precursors of the "psychedelic revolution" that in the mid-1960s drew tens of thousands of young people to the Haight-Ashbury, which was the prototype of similar communities that sprang up all over the country. The newcomers were the "flower children," the "hippies," who came with flowers in their hair and utopian dreams in their heads seeking cosmic consciousness and love in a pill or in a puff of smoke. Crowded into communes and "crash pads," they found, in thousands of cases, poverty, disease, and bad drug experiences. By the end of the sixties the flower children had largely abandoned Haight-Ashbury. Crime and drug addiction increased, and the neighborhood became a violent slum.

In the mid-1970s, rehabilitation of Haight-Ashbury was begun. Boarded-up storefronts were refurbished and new boutiques and antique shops emerged. The various upheavals of the sixties became, for most people, strange memories. There was more talk about the state of the economy and the energy crisis than about countercultures. Across the bay in Berkeley students at the University of California were studying hard, more interested in careers and security than in revolution. And the bars around the campus were doing a booming business. While there was still a lot of traffic in drugs of all kinds, and while the drinking habits of some Northern California young people may have represented another of those San Francisco extremes, the *Chronicle* had put its finger on a trend that had been under observation for some time by scientific investigators. Next to tobacco, alcohol had become the most favored drug among young people—as well as their elders—throughout the country, with marijuana running a poor third in popularity among the young. Alcohol is the most widely used of the depressants, or "downers," which are described in this chapter.

Alcohol

In nature ethyl alcohol is created without human intervention as a result of a collaboration between bacteria, fungi (yeasts), and any of a large array of fruits, grains, and vegetables. The bacteria and yeasts break down sucrose, a natural sugar, into alcohol, water, and carbon dioxide. Escaping carbon dioxide accounts for the bubbles that rise from fermenting brews. The alcohol content of naturally fermented beverages never rises above about 13 percent, because at that point the alcohol kills the bacteria. As we know from evidence found among the relics of prehistoric cultures, stone-age people discovered by accident the peculiar qualities of natural fermentations, and they learned how to put the necessary ingredients together to brew their own alcoholic drinks. Ever since, alcoholic beverages have been a part of almost every culture. Eventually people found methods of distilling those beverages to increase the alcohol content, or to produce pure alcohol, greatly increasing the effect of their drinks. Today, beer and wine begin as products of natural fermentation, although chemists often turn the drinks into something only vaguely resembling the originals, and many wines are fortified with extra alcohol. Whiskey, gin, vodka, brandy and other "hard" liquors are products of distillation.

Alcohol, a form of carbohydrate, provides the body with calories, which supply energy but no other nutrients or vitamins. The notion that alcohol is fattening is only indirectly accurate. People who drink a lot of alcohol and eat regularly tend to gain weight because the body metabolizes alcohol easily and stores much of the remaining food intake as fat. Skid row alcoholics, who don't eat much, are usually emaciated and almost always suffer from malnutrition. The body absorbs alcohol rapidly through the walls of the stomach and the small intestine. Carbonation increases the rate of absorption, which accounts for the fact that people seem to get drunk faster when they mix their liquor with bubbly beverages, such as club soda or ginger ale. The alcohol is carried by the bloodstream from the stomach and the intestine to the liver, but the liver is capable of processing only a small quantity of alcohol at a time. As a result, most of the alcohol returns to the bloodstream and thence throughout the body, including the lungs, heart, and brain. Alcohol itself exerts a toxic (poisonous) effect on nerve tissue when consumed in large quantities.

Only a small fraction of the alcohol is exhaled by the lungs. Most of it returns to the liver over and over again, while the processing in that organ slowly proceeds. Small amounts of alcohol are changed into a poisonous substance called acetaldehyde. Fortunately for the drinker, the toxic acetaldehyde quickly undergoes another transformation, both in the liver and in other body cells, into acetic acid. The acetic acid in turn is broken down into energy, water, and carbon dioxide. The water is excreted and the carbon dioxide is exhaled. But all that takes time. Meanwhile, the drinker, to a greater or lesser extent depending on his or her consumption, is *intoxicated*. That word is most familiarly applied to the effects of alcohol, although it is equally applicable to the effects of other drugs. Its root is the Latin word *intoxicare,* to smear with poison, which is what the ancient warriors did to their arrows. Intoxicated means, literally, poisoned.

Alcohol's Effects

Under the laws of most states, an alcohol content of more than one-tenth of one percent in a blood sample is regarded as evidence of intoxication—evidence enough, in many cases, to secure a conviction of drunken driving. The content of alcohol in the blood reaches that percentage, as a rule, shortly after the consumption of two or three average-sized drinks. Even one drink, tests have shown, increases the amount of time it takes the average person to react to stimuli, such as another driver suddenly pulling in front of the drinker's car. But the effects of small quantities of alcohol can be so subtle that drinkers are often unaware that they are affected at all. Alcohol's first effect is irritation of the stomach lining, which accounts for the nausea often experienced by inexperienced drinkers. Once into the bloodstream, alcohol quickly exerts a sedative (quieting) effect. Heartbeat and respiration are slowed, and blood pressure is reduced. The drinker feels relaxed, especially as the drug goes to work on certain parts of the brain.

Among other things, alcohol impairs the functioning of the cerebral cortex, the most highly evolved part of the brain, the reasoning and thinking part. Inhibitions and judgment are affected. People "loosen up," the effect that makes alcohol such a popular icebreaker at social gatherings. To social imbibers who limit their intake to a drink or two, this effect may be a welcome anxiety reducer and social lubricant. But as the party continues, and alcohol intake escalates, less welcome effects may appear. The workings of the brain's motor centers are impaired; speech thickens, drinks are spilled, people stagger. Social judgment becomes poor. Deep secrets slip out. Dignified men don lampshades. People feel free to make sexual advances. Pacifists pick fights. And these people are not necessarily among those regarded in this society as "problem drinkers."

The Hangover

Before going on to the effects of prolonged, heavy consumption of alcohol, some attention should be given to a somewhat mysterious affliction that is familiar even to moderate social drinkers who have occasionally gone overboard in their drinking. The morning after such excess often brings a combination of symptoms including headache, nausea, shakiness, dizziness, clouded thinking, and a consuming thirst, compounded by mental depression—commonly referred to as "hangover."

The exact causes of hangovers are poorly understood. Since alcohol is a diuretic, dehydration accounts for the thirst, and dehydration of the brain combined with the toxic effects of alcohol may produce the other symptoms. Home remedies for hangovers include thousands of concoctions featuring such ingredients as Worcestershire sauce, raw eggs, and oysters, but aside from their food value such "medications" are generally ineffective. Rest, aspirin, fluids, and nourishing food may be helpful. The classic resort to more alcohol often leads to renewed intoxication and a worse hangover the next day.

Alcohol and Sex

Alcohol has long had a reputation as an *aphrodisiac* (from Aphrodite, the Greek goddess of love), a stimulater of sexual passion. The drug's undeserved reputation in this regard is based not on any magical property of the chemical, but on the fact that it suppresses inhibitions. In reality, immoderate quantities often render the male impotent. If his inability to perform sexually after imbibing occurs repeatedly, the man may become convinced that he is permanently impotent. This conviction may have the psychosomatic effect of making him unable to perform even when he is sober. So common is this problem that it has become one of the major causes of male impotence.

The Heavy Drinker

Every time a human being consumes a large quantity of alcohol, some brain cells are destroyed by the poisoning. Unlike most other body cells, those that make up the brain and the rest of the central nervous system do not replace themselves; once lost, they are gone forever. Since we have billions of brain cells, the work of those that are lost is normally taken over by others, and occasional intoxication has no serious long-term effects on the functioning of the body. But heavy drinking over a long period can destroy so many nerve cells that functioning becomes permanently impaired. Memory and the ability to think clearly may be affected. The personality may change. Portions of the brain that may be damaged by alcohol include the cerebellum, which controls physical coordination. Alcohol may also break down the fatty *myelin* sheath that covers and protects the nerves, with resulting *neuritis,* an often painful inflammation of peripheral nerves. Eventually the heavy drinker may have difficulty coordinating movements, may walk with the rolling "drunken sailor" gait characteristic of many alcohol-damaged bodies.

Not only the nervous system is damaged. Organs including the heart, the kidneys, and, especially, the liver may suffer. The liver sometimes swells and fills with fat, and a condition called *cirrhosis* sets in. Impaired liver function causes jaundice (increased yellow pigment in body tissues), a protuberant abdomen, and swollen legs and feet.

Once the process becomes well established, cirrhosis is progressive, irreversible, and, finally, fatal. The precise cause of cirrhosis has not been established. One theory is that the condition results from a vitamin deficiency brought on by failure to eat properly. Consequently, many people believe that as long as they eat, they are safe from cirrhosis of the liver no matter how much they drink. Studies have shown, however, that even some well-fed drinkers develop cirrhosis. Nondrinkers, on the other hand, may develop cirrhosis only as an occasional outgrowth of some other condition affecting the liver, such as hepatitis, but the most common cause of cirrhosis of the liver remains chronic excessive alcohol consumption.

Alcoholism

Alcoholics are drug addicts, or, in the currently favored terminology, drug dependents. More than nine million Americans are dependent on alcohol, more than are dependent on any other drug except nicotine. Only a small percentage of alcoholics end up on skid row. The ranks of alcoholics include businessmen and women, homemakers, members of the clergy, teachers, students, police officers, politicians, butchers, bakers, candlestick makers, doctors, lawyers, and Indian chiefs. Some people can consume large amounts of alcohol daily for many years before their alcoholism begins to have serious effects on their functioning. Others succumb rapidly. In France, where many families customarily drink wine at home with most meals, adolescent alcoholism has become a matter of concern. And in America the incidence of teen-age alcoholism has risen in the 1970s.

There are many definitions of alcoholism. Basically, an alcoholic is anyone who "needs" to drink and who has trouble controlling the amount he or she drinks. Typically, budding alcoholics develop *tolerance* for alcohol; they can pour down drink after drink for hours, tipple throughout the day and never seem to be terribly drunk. They may even boast about their capacity to drink. And if they "black out" from time to time—suffer temporary amnesia that erases from their memories part of an evening during which they may have "lost" their cars—it's good for a laugh with their drinking companions the next day. The social acceptance of alcohol renders hilarious effects that would be serious cause for alarm if produced by another drug.

Blackouts are one of the most common early symptoms of alcoholism. Sooner or later, alcoholics—who consider themselves merely "heavy drinkers" and would deny even to themselves that they have "problems"—find that some of their friends aren't laughing anymore. They have committed too many social blunders, made a nuisance of themselves too often. Their self-images suffer—and, as a consequence, they drink to drown their troubles. Drunk, they feel sure of themselves; they feel clever, charming. Sober, they are defensive and depressed. Drunk is better. Their lives begin to revolve around alcohol. Their family lives deteriorate. Financial problems develop. There may be trouble on their jobs. Every difficulty becomes an occasion for more drinking (and every triumph an excuse for celebration). More drinking brings more problems, thus creating a vicious circle.

There comes a time when drinkers' vaunted capacities diminish, their tolerances reverse. They get drunker and drunker on less and less booze. They find this hard to accept, but eventually they begin to worry. They go on the wagon, then fall off. They may become binge drinkers, interspersing periods of abstinence with debilitating sprees. The end of a spree leaves them sick, weak, shaky, and abysmally depressed. Detoxification can take days, even if they enter a hospital where they will be treated with vitamins, sedatives, and given diets that include lots of (nonalcoholic) fluids. In many cases sudden cessation of drinking, whether by a binge drinker or a daily drinker, is followed hours or even days later by an attack of *delirium tremens*—"DTs"—symptoms which include hallucinations, convulsions, paranoia, and tremor. Occasionally people die during such attacks. Exactly what brings on such a withdrawal syndrome is unclear. It is believed to be a result of the body's constant efforts to achieve *homeostasis,* a comfortable state of balance among the myriad chemical reactions taking place in the body. When large amounts of a foreign chemical are introduced the system is unbalanced; the pendulum swings too far in one direction. The body then produces counteragents in an attempt to restore balance. When the foreign chemical is suddenly stopped the body takes a while to catch up. It continues to produce the counteragents, swinging the pendulum too far in the other direction. The effects are opposite to those produced by the drug. Formerly relaxed drunks become shaky and jumpy; their once-slow heartbeats and respirations speed up alarmingly; their brains, no longer sedated, race out of control. This theory could explain the effects of withdrawal from other drugs, as well as from alcohol.

There is no certain cure for alcoholism. Organizations, such as Alcoholics Anonymous and some religious groups, provide a supportive function and strong psychological motivation and have succeeded in keeping many alcoholics sober. Therapy with psychiatrists or other doctors who specialize in treatment of alcoholics has helped many others. More drastic treatments include *aversion* therapies, electric shock treatments and administration of drugs such as Antabuse, which is an alcohol antagonist that makes patients very ill if they take a drink. Some alcoholics, but relatively few, manage to kick their habits without help. But millions go on drinking.

Why Alcoholics?

A majority of people who enjoy a cocktail or two, or wine with dinner, or even a one-night spree on special occasions, do not become alcoholics. Their moderate drinking, unless they have an accident while under the influence, rarely gets them into trouble. They do not feel a need to drink. Why, then, does one out of every dozen or so drinkers become dependent on the drug?

The question could be asked of drug dependence in general. How can some people take frequent small doses of amphetamines or even cocaine without becoming dependent, while others escalate their intake until they are speed freaks or cocaine slaves? Researchers are still looking for answers, and there is evidence that both psychological and biological factors may be involved. Some authorities have identified what they call "addictive personalities," people who have a tendency to become dependent on *some* drug, and if one isn't available another will do. Alcoholics sometimes maintain sobriety by switching to other drugs. And heroin dependents who kick that habit often do so only at the expense of becoming alcoholics. Psychologically, all kinds of factors may contribute to making individuals dependence-prone. Because of various childhood experiences they may suffer from lack of self-esteem, from difficulty in relating to other people, from inability to cope with problems. Then, when intoxicated by one drug or another, their problems seem to disappear for a while. Not only do they feel good, but they are members of a drug-using group. When they sober up or come down from their high, everyday life seems bleaker than ever. Consequently, they can't wait to get intoxicated again.

There are some obvious reasons for alcohol attracting more dependents than other drugs. It is legal; it is intensively and attractively advertised. Alcohol is, within rather loose bounds, not only socially approved, but often pressed on reluctant drinkers, who in certain groups may be treated with contempt if they refuse to drink with the rest. Until their behavior becomes too unacceptable, alcohol dependents are socially rewarded for their drug use. "Peer pressure," it is called.

For some people, there are other pressures. Heavy drinking is much more common among certain national and ethnic groups than among others. It has been observed that those of Chinese or Jewish extraction have a lower incidence of alcoholism, while alcoholism is a national problem in Sweden, Ireland, and France. Alcoholism is nonexistent among Moslems and Hindus while American Indians appear to have low tolerance to alcohol's effects. That fact may involve not only cultural but biological influences. In one investigation of such influences in alcoholism, a number of sets of identical twins in Sweden and Denmark, who had been separated at birth and placed in foster homes, were studied over a period of years. Those who were the natural children of alcoholics proved to have a much higher incidence of alcoholism than the general population, even in cases in which the foster parents did not drink. And when one twin became an alcoholic, the other was likely to follow the same path, even though they lived in different surroundings. The results of the study indicate that the subjects had a *hereditary*—biological—predisposition to become alcoholics. Presumably, biological factors could contribute to dependence on other drugs too.

Alcohol's Toll

"In nine states, alcoholic disorders lead all other diagnoses in mental hospital admissions. Maryland, for example, reports that 40 percent of all male admissions are for alcoholism." "In 1965, out of close to five million arrests in the United States for all offenses, over 1,535,000 were for public drunkenness (31 percent). In addition, there were over 250,000 arrests for driving while intoxicated. Another 490,000 individuals were charged with disorderly conduct, which some communities use in lieu of the public drunkenness charge. Thus at least 40 percent of all arrests are for being drunk in a public place or being under the influence [of alcohol] while driving. . . ."

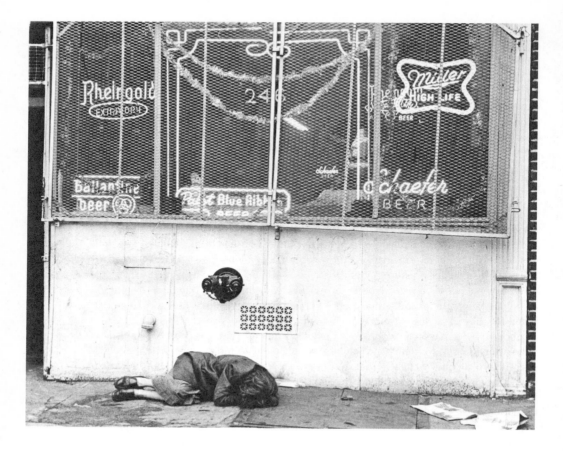

"Coroner's reports on levels of blood alcohol found in autopsies reveal high concentrations . . . in fatal accident victims. Among drivers rated as probably responsible for their accidents, 73 percent had been drinking to some extent. . . ."

"A 1954 Ohio study revealed that 43 percent of those who committed homicide had been drinking. . . ."

"A 1962 Washington state study . . . showed that 23 percent of suicide attempts were made by persons who were known to be alcoholics and 31 percent of the successful suicides were known to be committed by alcoholics. . . ."

"Dr. Karl Menninger and other psychiatrists have suggested . . . that alcoholism is itself a form of 'chronic suicide.' . . ."

While alcohol consumption in the United States continues to rise, more and more people will suffer the ravages of excessive alcohol intake. Alcohol, along with tobacco, remains the most popular drug consumed in the world. In moderation it adds enjoyment to life; in excess it may terminate life.

> Reds have a lot of facts about them. There only good to have because they are cheaper than alcohol, and feel about the same. But they can easily be abused. Once you start to take them every day you want more! 3 a day can start you off, two week's later you're taking 15 or more a day if you can get them. After a while they make you feel ugly outside and in and your too stoned to tell. Some people most I know get very high tempered. They will turn around and want to fight about anything. So don't mess with a red freak.. . . .

Family medicine cabinets in American homes are more likely than not to contain psychoactive drugs. Many children have their first "trips" after sampling the contents of those fascinating little pill containers. Because they are prescribed by doctors, most people think of these chemicals only as medicines. Often, however, they are the very same substances that, when sold on the street, are legally classified as dangerous drugs, and criminal penalties are prescribed for both seller and user in black market transactions. The amphetamines, described in the last chapter, are among these medicine-chest drugs. More common are the *barbiturates,* prescribed by the millions as sleeping pills and for the relief of anxiety and tension. And most common of all are the minor tranquilizers, which are very much like the barbiturates in their effects.

The barbiturates—all of which are laboratory-created synthetics—are valuable as medicines, since insomnia and anxiety are endemic in modern society. Used according to the physician's directions, barbiturates are not usually harmful. Patients are expected to report any untoward effects to their doctors, who sometimes deem it advisable to discontinue the medication. Properly used, barbiturates can be taken by most people in small quantities over considerable periods of time without undesirable results, just as most people can drink a cocktail or two each evening without becoming alcoholics. But many people take the pills whenever and in whatever quantity they feel like. This is "drug abuse" in the medical sense. Spouses, roommates, guests, and children, for whom no medication has been prescribed, help themselves to bathroom supplies. Pills are shared over back fences and office water coolers. And immense quantities are diverted into the black market.

There are long-acting barbiturates, such as phenobarbital, and short-acting varieties, such as pentobarbital (marketed as Nembutal) and secobarbital (marketed as Seconal). A major peculiarity of barbiturates is that the shorter the duration of biological activity, the greater the psychoactive effects. "Reds," a common favorite among high school students, are in reality a short acting but highly potent and dangerous barbiturate.

The Effects of "Barbs"

Barbiturates are cheaper than alcohol, and feel about the same. They can simulate alcohol's effects, from staggering drunkenness to hangovers and even mimic delirium tremens during withdrawal. Like an alcohol nightcap, a barbiturate sleeping pill provides sedation that can help bring sleep. For someone not seeking sleep, barbiturates in small doses suppress inhibitions. The user feels "high" and may become giddy and show signs of *ataxia* (loss of coordination). The results of taking larger doses were clearly demonstrated in a study conducted at the U.S. Public Health Service Hospital in Lexington, Kentucky, by a team of researchers headed by Dr. Harris Isbell. The study involved five prisoner-patients, serving time for violations of drug laws, who volunteered to be subjects. At the beginning, each patient was given a large dose of a barbiturate. Like alcohol users, they reacted differently. One seemed outwardly to be little affected, but the other four showed "a marked degree of intoxication," and all five "had difficulty in thinking and deterioration in their ability in performing the psychologic tests." The next morning, the patients "were nervous and tremulous and complained of anorexia [loss of appetite] and headache. They compared these symptoms to a 'hangover' after an alcoholic debauch."

The subjects were then placed on a schedule that for more than three months included a small dose of barbiturate on waking in the morning, and larger doses at intervals throughout the day, duplicating the drug-taking pattern of many alcoholics. And like alcoholics, the barbiturate takers became "drunker" as the day progressed. They also "neglected their appearance, became unkempt and dirty, did not shave, bathed infrequently, and allowed their living quarters to become filthy. They were content to wear clothes soiled with food which they had spilled. All patients were confused and had difficulty in performing simple tasks or in playing cards or dominoes." Some of the subjects, who got along well together before the experiment began, became "irritable and quarrelsome. They cursed one another, and at times even fought." Like drunks pleading with a bartender for "just one more," some of the subjects kept asking for more barbiturates, even when they were already thoroughly intoxicated. And like an alcoholic "swearing off," one of the subjects "frequently asked to be released from the experiment, but would always change his mind within thirty minutes after missing a dose." The subjects had developed tolerance and had become dependent on barbiturates. Their moods swung from elation to depression. One talked of "the joys of death." Another became paranoid. Of the five subjects, two "showed less pronounced changes in behavior. They continued to maintain good relationships with the other patients and with the attendants, and their personal appearance deteriorated less. . . . The general picture in both these men was that of a person who was drunk and enjoyed it."

By eleven o'clock at night, "all the patients would be staggering and unable to walk except by sliding along the walls. In spite of close supervision, they occasionally fell and were injured. The patients also tended to become more boisterous and quarrelsome at night, and most fights occurred at that time. . . . Great care had to be exercised to prevent patients from smoking in bed and setting fires. . . ."

At the end of the experiment, when their barbiturate dosages were cut off, the subjects went through agonizing withdrawal symptoms like those suffered by alcoholics. "The similarity of the barbiturate withdrawal syndrome to alcoholic delirium tremens is striking," the researchers concluded. The effects of barbiturates, another authority noted, "vary considerably with the dose, the situation and the personality of the user. . . . The patterns of abuse are as varied as those for alcohol and range from infrequent sprees of gross intoxication, lasting a few days, to the prolonged, compulsive, daily use of huge quantities and a preoccupation with securing and maintaining adequate supplies."

Barbiturates and Alcohol

It has been suggested that the two drugs, barbiturates and alcohol, are so similar in their effects that "barbiturates might be labeled a 'solid alcohol' and alcohol classed as a 'liquid barbiturate.'"

> . . . A man who drinks increasing quantities of alcohol, for example, becomes tolerant to alcohol effects—but he simultaneously develops cross-tolerance for barbiturate effects as well, and can tolerate an enormous dose of a barbiturate the very first time he tries the drug. The same is true in reverse; as the barbiturate addict increases his dose, he simultaneously achieves cross-tolerance for the alcohol as well as barbiturates, and can take enormous doses. Some alcoholics under pressure to give up alcohol do give it up completely, without any of the usual suffering, "shakes," "rum fits," and delirium tremens—by substituting barbiturates for alcohol. (Some who make the changeover report that they prefer the barbiturates.) Many addicts use alcohol and barbiturates interchangeably, depending on which is cheaper or more conveniently available at the moment. Many use the two drugs at the same time. Simultaneous use is dangerous, however; for with either drug, there is only a narrow margin between the maximum dose that an addict can manage and the lethal dose—and it is harder to gauge the dose when both drugs are taken together.

Barbiturates and alcohol, in fact, *potentiate* each other's effects, so that each seems to become more powerful when mixed with the other; one and one, in effect, add up to more than two. Accidental overdoses resulting from taking barbiturates during or soon after drinking alcohol have caused many deaths.

> Finally, the similar effect of alcohol and barbiturates is demonstrated during delirium tremens; either drug can *relieve* delirium tremens. Indeed, one of the standard treatments for delirium tremens is to place the patient on large doses of a barbiturate, and then slowly to taper off the dosage. Drugs of another closely related group, the minor tranquilizers, are also now used for this purpose.
>
> There are also significant practical differences between alcohol and the barbiturates. The latter are less likely to lead to serious malnutrition and accompanying neurological damage, . . . and are less damaging to the gastrointestinal system [barbiturates can, however, hasten the degeneration of an already damaged liver]. Alcohol in the form of light wines and beer is less concentrated, so that the imbibing of a moderate series of doses can be spread over a period of time. An overdose of alcohol is toxic and sometimes lethal; but it is much easier to pop a whole handful of pills than to down a quart of whiskey. Hence, death from barbiturate overdose (or from a combination of alcohol and barbiturate), either accidental or with suicidal intent, is more common. . . .

Among women, who are less likely than men to kill themselves by violent means, such as gunshots, taking an overdose of barbiturates is the most frequently used method of suicide in this country.

Downers and Uppers

In their history of the Haight-Ashbury Free Medical Clinic, Drs. David E. Smith and John Luce reported that multiple drug abusers often "became inordinately disturbed and paranoid when they were strung-out on speed. If they then shot barbiturates to come down from extended runs, they were likely to become assaultive as well. When taken in combination, the drugs seem to produce a toxic state of confusion. . . . As one speed freak told criminologist Roger Smith, 'barbs make you want to get out on the street and start kicking ass. Speed gives you the energy to get up and do it.'" The same speed freak told of a friend who

> always freaks out on speed and barbs. He's a very nice person but when he gets all jacked up and he's also doing reds . . . then he's in trouble, because pretty soon he's got a shotgun and everybody else has got a shotgun, or so he thinks. I've seen him out, in front of the freeway entrance west of the Haight, herding the hitchhikers away because he's so paranoid on them. At four o'clock in the afternoon, with a full-length shotgun, he's screaming, "Move on—you can't stand there—move on!" That's the way he gets when he's mixing barbs and speed.

The Minor Tranquilizers

Earlier, we quoted from the manufacturer's warnings to physicians contained in a package of Valium, the most widely used of the minor tranquilizers and, in fact, the most prescribed drug in the United States. The doctors were warned that Valium, like the barbiturates, could affect physical functioning, could be dangerous if taken in combination with alcohol or other depressants, and could produce dependence, withdrawal symptoms, and a variety of unpleasant side effects. Indeed, there are great similarities between barbiturates and the minor tranquilizers, which include, in addition to Valium, *meprobamate* (marketed as Miltown and Equanil) and *chlordiazepoxide* (Librium). These tranquilizers, in small doses, tend to result in less sleepiness and loss of muscular coordination than the barbiturates, but in general what one authority said of meprobamate applies to all of the minor tranquilizers: "The pharmacological effects of meprobamate are very similar to those of the barbiturates. Indeed, in clinical usage it is difficult, if not impossible, to differentiate between the two drugs. . . . Like the barbiturates, the tranquilizers are valuable medicines and are usually harmless if taken according to doctors' directions. But, like the barbiturates, they are much abused."

Early in 1975 the federal government announced that prescriptions for Valium and Librium, which had often been open-ended, that is, refillable for indefinite periods, would no longer be valid for more than six months. The action was prompted, the *Washington Post* reported, by "hundreds of reports of . . . hospital emergency-room admissions, usually for attempted suicides. . . ."

Other Sedatives and Tranquilizers

There are a number of nonbarbiturate prescription sedatives, marketed under trade names including Placidyl, Doriden, and Noludar, that are basically indistinguishable

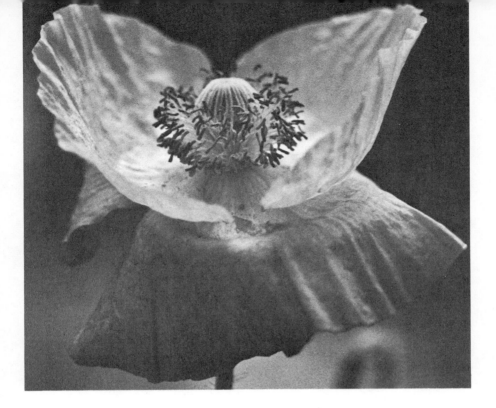

from the barbiturates in their effects and hazards, although their chemical content is different. Also widely used are over-the-counter sleeping pills, such as Sominex and Sleep-Eze, and tranquilizers, such as Compoz, which are heavily advertised on television and are available without prescriptions. While these compounds are usually harmless in small doses, they have been known to produce "a state of mental disturbance and physical agitation" and other unpleasant effects when taken in large quantities.

The Opiates

The flowers, delicate purple, red, and white petals flickering beguilingly in the sun, look good enough to eat. When the pods are cut open, a milky juice oozes out. No one knows just how many thousands of years ago someone first tasted this juice and found that it was no ordinary food. Its strange properties were already known in prebiblical times in Egypt, where mothers gave it to their babies to put them to sleep. The ancient Greeks called it *opion,* a diminutive of *opos,* their word for sap. We call it *opium.*

The flower is *Papaver somniferum* (from the Latin *papaver,* poppy; *somnus,* sleep, and *ferre,* to bring), "the poppy that brings sleep." It is cultivated in many regions, particularly in Asia, the Middle East, and Mexico. A century ago it was also widely cultivated in the United States. A Massachusetts official reported in 1871:

There are so many channels through which the drug may be brought into the State, that I suppose it would be impossible to determine how much foreign opium is used here; but it may easily be shown that the home production increases every year. Opium has recently been made from white poppies, cultivated for the purpose, in Vermont, New Hampshire, and Connecticut, the annual production being estimated by hundreds of pounds, and this has generally been absorbed in the communities where it is made. It has also been brought here from Florida and Louisiana, while comparatively large quantities are regularly sent east from California and Arizona, where its cultivation is becoming an important branch of industry, ten acres of poppies being said to yield, in Arizona, twelve hundred pounds of opium.

In those days opium and its derivatives (opiates), as well as numerous preparations containing opiates, could be purchased legally by anyone, without prescription, almost anywhere in America. Grocers as well as druggists sold these products over the counter, and they could be ordered by mail from patent medicine manufacturers who advertised in newspapers and magazines. Laudanum, a mixture of opium and alcohol, sold briskly. Opiates were used as home remedies for a great many ailments. People took them for pain, anxiety, and insomnia as casually as people today take aspirin, tranquilizers, and barbiturates. And many soon found that they had become dependent on their medicines. In 1914 Congress passed the Harrison Narcotic Act, outlawing sales of most opiates unless prescribed by doctors.

Opium Derivatives

Opium contains a number of psychoactive ingredients. The most important are morphine (from Morpheus, the Greek god of dreams) and *codeine* (from the Greek *kodeia,* poppy head). Heroin (diacetylmorphine) is manufactured by heating morphine in the presence of acetic acid. When taken into the human body, heroin turns back into morphine, but heroin is shorter-acting and more powerful than the unprocessed morphine. Pharmacologically, the opiates are *narcotics* (from the Greek *narkotikos,* numbness, torpor). Narcotic is a much misused word, both in law and in everyday conversation. It has a bad connotation and is often mistakenly applied to all illegal drugs. Legally, such drugs as cocaine and, formerly, marijuana were classified erroneously as narcotics. On the other hand, alcohol and barbiturates, which have narcotic effects, have rarely been thought of as narcotics. There are synthetic narcotics, such as methadone (marketed as Dolophine) and meperidine (Demerol), which have effects very similar to those produced by the opiates, but are not derived from opium.

Opiates as Medicine

In the nineteenth century, before most of the synthetic analgesics (pain relievers), sedatives, and tranquilizers now available had been created, morphine was known among doctors as G.O.M.—God's Own Medicine. Then as now, narcotics were indispensable in medical practice. Acting primarily on the central nervous system, narcotics provide profound relief from pain. They tranquilize anxious patients and put insomniacs to sleep. In many patients they produce euphoria and a general feeling of warmth and comfort. Narcotics are also useful for other medical purposes, such as relief from coughing (some cough medicines contain codeine) and diarrhea, which is sometimes treated with paregoric, also known as tincture of opium.

In earlier times, the doctor's prescription was the most common route to dependence on narcotics. Physicians prescribed morphine, patients got better—and then discovered that they were addicted. Nowadays, more careful and learned control of dosage and frequency of administration make dependence as a result of medical prescription relatively rare. As one authority wrote, "Considering the frequency with which opiate analgesics are used in clinical medicine, addiction as a complication of medical treatment is quite uncommon."

Nonmedical Use of Opiates

In the past, and at present in some parts of the world, opium itself, rather than its derivatives, was the choice drug of many who used drugs nonmedically. It was sometimes eaten, though more often it was smoked in tiny, long-stemmed pipes. It was heated rather than burned in these pipes, so that smokers inhaled the volatile gases without all of the solid particles found in tobacco and marijuana smoke. The opium used for smoking was ordinarily a weak preparation, containing small quantities of the psychoactive ingredients. Opium smoking produces a blissful, dreamy state of euphoria, from which comes the expression "pipedreams." Many, but not all, opium smokers became dependent:

> There is a pattern of self-limitation or restraint in opium smoking as practiced in countries where it is socially acceptable. It is common for natives of these countries to indulge in opium smoking one night a week, much as Americans may indulge in alcoholic beverages at a Saturday night party. . . .

Today in the United States opium smoking is not widespread, and heroin is the opiate most commonly used for nonmedical purposes. A fine, white powder, it is sometimes mixed with tobacco or marijuana and smoked, sometimes snorted like cocaine, but most often dissolved and injected under the skin (skin-popping) or into a vein (shooting up or mainlining). First-time or infrequent users often report that injecting heroin into a vein produces an initial "rush" that is described by some as an "abdominal orgasm" and by others as nauseating. Regular users experience this rush less frequently, if at all. The rush may be followed by profound relaxation and euphoria. The heartbeat and respiration become slower, and the user becomes drowsy, goes "on the nod." Not all users achieve those desired effects. Some become anxious, restless, or frightened; some vomit, become dizzy, suffer shortness of breath. Contraction of the pupils, which hampers night vision, is a common effect. Another effect is constipation.

The effects of heroin usually wear off in a few hours—unless the user has taken too much. Overdose victims die of respiratory failure; their breathing becomes slower and slower until it stops. It is believed that many of the deaths attributed to overdoses of heroin may actually result from adulterants or contaminants in the drug. The product sold on the street (called "smack," "horse," "H," "junk," or any of a dozen other names) contains only a small percentage of heroin "cut" with milk sugar or quinine and often containing various other adulterants, some of them toxic. In addition, many heroin users are multiple drug abusers. Alcohol or barbiturates increase the effects of opiates, as alcohol increases the effects of barbiturates.

Opiate Dependence

All of the opiates produce strong dependence, which develops rapidly in frequent users. People who become dependent on codeine go to great lengths to acquire large quantities of codeine-based cough medicine, which they consume like whiskey. Codeine dependence, however, is much less common than heroin dependence. There are some occasional, or "weekend," heroin users who do not become dependent, but most people who become dependent start by using it only occasionally. The popular idea of the professional dope pusher lurking around schoolyards ensnaring children is largely a myth; people are usually "turned on" for the first time by friends or acquaintances—peer pressure at work again. Experimenters begin "skin popping" occasionally, usually escalate the frequency of injections and the size of doses, and don't realize they are hooked until they start experiencing withdrawal symptoms. Before long, they may have a powerful and expensive habit.

Tolerance develops quickly; bigger doses are required to stave off the withdrawal symptoms. Users have to shoot up several times a day, and if they miss an injection they may face almost unendurable suffering. Some heroin dependents say that once they have acquired a high tolerance for the drug they no longer obtain any great pleasure from taking it, but keep shooting up only to avoid the agony of withdrawal. As one authority describes heroin withdrawal:

> . . . lacrimation [tears], rhinorrhea [runny nose], yawning, and perspiration appear . . . the addict may fall into a tossing, restless sleep known as the "yen," which may last several hours but from which he awakens more restless and miserable than before . . . additional signs and symptoms appear . . . dilated pupils, anorexia, violent yawning, severe sneezing . . . and coryza [coldlike nasal symptoms]. Weakness and depression . . . nausea and vomiting . . . intestinal spasm and diarrhea. Heart rate and blood pressure are elevated. Marked chilliness, alternating with flushing and excessive sweating . . . waves of gooseflesh . . . the skin resembling that of a plucked turkey . . . is the basis of the expression "cold turkey" to signify abrupt withdrawal without treatment. Abdominal cramps and pains in the bones and muscles of the back and extremities are also characteristic, as are the muscle spasms and kicking movements that may be the basis for the expression "kicking the habit." Other signs . . . the failure to take foods and fluids, combined with vomiting, sweating and diarrhea, results in marked weight loss, dehydration. . . . Occasionally there is cardiovascular collapse. At any point in the course of withdrawal, the administration of a suitable narcotic will completely and dramatically suppress the symptoms of withdrawal.

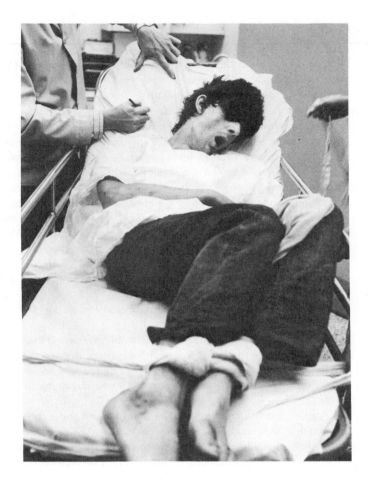

The preceding description of narcotics withdrawal occurs each time an addict kicks the habit. Long after an ex-addict has stopped using heroin, he may still crave the drug. The craving is not *continuous* but seems to come and go in waves of varying intensity, for months, even years, after withdrawal. It is particularly likely to return in moments of emotional stress. Following an intense wave of craving, drug-seeking behavior is likely to set in, and the ex-addict relapses. When asked how he feels following a return to heroin, he is likely to reply, "It makes me feel normal again"—that is, it relieves the ex-addict's chronic triad of anxiety, depression, and craving.

"It is this view—that an addict takes heroin in order to 'feel normal'—that is hardest for a nonaddict to understand and to believe. Yet it is consonant with everything else that is known about narcotics addiction. . . . The ex-addict who returns to heroin, if this view is accepted, is not a pleasure-craving hedonist but an anxious, depressed patient who desperately craves a return to a *normal* mood and state of mind."

Effects of Drug Use

Diminution of sexual desire in both males and females, and of potency in males, is common although not universal among regular heroin users. Some female users stop menstruating, or menstruate irregularly. Women are less likely to become pregnant while using heroin, although many users do become pregnant. When a pregnant woman takes heroin, the drug may pass through the placenta to the unborn child; the baby may suffer withdrawal symptoms after birth, such as convulsions, inability to feed properly, and hyperirritability. Because opiates make users less sensitive to pain, disease symptoms may go unnoticed or be ignored, and users may fail to seek medical help until they are seriously ill. Sweating, constipation, vision problems, difficulty urinating, runny noses, and a variety of other minor ailments are common among regular users.

Heroin and morphine do not, however, appear to produce the serious, long-term physical damage often caused by alcohol and tobacco, or the mental deterioration to which alcoholics are prone. Here are conclusions reached by some investigators:

"As to possible damage to the brain, the result of lengthy use of heroin, we can only say that neurologic and psychiatric examinations have not revealed evidence of brain damage. . . ."

"The incidence of insanity among addicts is the same as in the general population."

"It was shown that continued taking of opium or any of its derivatives resulted in no measurable organic damage. The addict when not deprived of his opium showed no abnormal behavior which distinguished him from a non-addict."

"Cigarette smoking is unquestionably more damaging to the human body than heroin."

Such *negative* findings, however, tell us more about the hazards of alcohol and tobacco than they do about heroin and morphine. The unwary might infer that heroin is better than alcohol, another of those dangerous comparisons so common in the emotionally charged atmosphere surrounding psychoactive drugs. Consider another comparison: While many people can drink cocktails every evening for years without becoming alcoholics, few if any can take heroin daily for more than a week or two without becoming dependent, with all of the dire consequences that implies.

Who Uses Heroin?

Opium-eating, unlike the use of alcoholic stimulants, is an aristocratic vice and prevails more extensively among the wealthy and educated classes than among those of inferior social position; but no class is exempt from its blighting influence. The merchant, lawyer, and physician are to be found among the host who sacrifice the choicest treasures of life at the shrine of Opium. The slaves of Alcohol may be clothed in rags, but vassals of the monarch who sits enthroned on the poppy are generally found dressed in purple and fine linen.

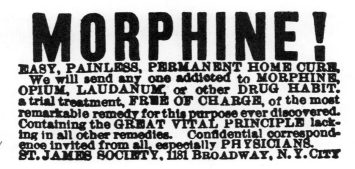

MORPHINE!

EASY, PAINLESS, PERMANENT HOME CURE.
We will send any one addicted to MORPHINE,
OPIUM, LAUDANUM, or other DRUG HABIT.
a trial treatment, FREE OF CHARGE, of the most
remarkable remedy for this purpose ever discovered.
Containing the GREAT VITAL PRINCIPLE lacking in all other remedies.   Confidential correspond-
ence invited from all, especially PHYSICIANS.
ST. JAMES SOCIETY, 1181 BROADWAY, N.Y. CITY

Nineteenth-century advertisement.

That florid bit of imagery was published in an 1881 edition of the *Catholic World*. Since then, opiates have been outlawed, alcohol has become respectable, and drug-taking patterns have changed in many ways. During most of this century, heroin users—the modern equivalent of the nineteenth century opium eaters—were widely believed to be found almost exclusively among poor ethnic minorities living in urban ghettos. There were many explanations for such a theory; narcotics seem to affect the primitive areas of the brain, including the hypothalamus, where powerful drives including hunger, thirst, sex, and aggression are controlled; heroin's effectiveness in suppressing hunger and rage, as well as anxiety, seemed to account at least in part for its use in the ghettos.

It came as a shock to many people when, in the 1960s, increasing numbers of white, middle-class young people were discovered to be using heroin. They simply didn't fit the popular "dope fiend" image—an image that was further damaged in 1969 when the House of Representatives' Select Committee on Crime heard testimony that, according to files of the Federal Bureau of Narcotics and the U.S. Public Health Service Hospital at Lexington, Kentucky, "roughly 30 percent of all the drug abusers actually are legitimate people, in the sense that they have a job which they keep. . . . They tend to be professional people, doctors and lawyers, quite a number of housewives, some musicians but not too many, people who appear to the outside world to be fairly normal, and people who do not seem to get in trouble with the law, except after long periods of use, when they get picked up through a contact, or in some cases when they turn themselves in for treatment. . . ."

Jerome H. Jaffe, who later became director of the Special Action Office for Drug Abuse Prevention, said in a textbook published in 1970:

> The addict who is able to obtain an adequate supply of drugs through legitimate channels and has adequate funds usually dresses properly, maintains his nutrition, and is able to discharge his social and occupational obligations with reasonable efficiency. He usually remains in good health, suffers little inconvenience, and is, in general, difficult to distinguish from other persons.

Of course, there are no legitimate channels through which Americans can obtain heroin, but that "fairly normal" 30 percent that the members of Congress heard about presumably had adequate funds and were able to obtain their supplies through other channels. But they represent a minority of heroin users. What about the rest?

Heroin and Crime

> . . . If you do get hooked into smack what can you expect? You can expect to do things unimaginable to you now in order to keep your body satisfied. If your habit costs $50 per day or more you would have to come up with $350 per week . . . just for the Heroin. What about food, rent, clothing, spending money.
>
> A hard core junkie . . . will do just about anything to get the bread for his junk—rip off his family, friends and strangers. When his family and friends can't tolerate him anymore, his only alternative is to turn to crime like stick-ups, burglaries, or, yes, even prostitution. You see a junkie gets sick when he's not getting a regular dose of smack, so sick, in fact, that he would sell out his grandmother to feel better. . . .

A fifty-dollar-a-day heroin habit is not uncommon, and yet most people don't have that much money to spend on drugs. Even if they are employed, heroin dependents often find they must quit their jobs so they can hustle more money. As the high school student observed in the preceding quotation, many turn to burglary, robbery, or prostitution.

Heroin users have often been stereotyped as "walking corpses" who spend most of their time in a dream world. Some are like that, but they are no more typical of the average user than is the skid row derelict of the average alcoholic. Here is quite another picture, sketched by an anthropologist and by an economist who studied hard-core heroin dependents in New York City's slums:

> [Typical users are] actively engaged in meaningful activities and relationships seven days a week. The brief moments of euphoria after each administration of a small amount of heroin constitute a small fraction of their daily lives. The rest of the time they are aggressively pursuing a career that is exacting, challenging, adventurous, and rewarding. They are always on the move and must be alert, flexible, and resourceful. The surest way to identify heroin users in a slum neighborhood is to observe the way people walk. The heroin user walks with a fast, purposeful stride, as if he is late for an important appointment—indeed, he is. He is hustling (robbing or stealing), trying to sell stolen goods, avoiding the police, looking for a heroin dealer with a good bag (the street retail unit of heroin), coming back from copping (buying heroin), looking for a safe place to take the drug, or looking for someone who beat (cheated) him—among other things. He is, in short, *taking care of business*. . . .

It sounds almost romantic—until still another side of the picture is examined. Even if the constant threat of withdrawal doesn't drive them to stealing or other crimes, heroin dependents are criminals by virtue of the fact that possession and use of the drug is against the law. They are ever in danger of arrest and imprisonment, of poisoned drugs and overdoses, of the violence inherent in daily association with heroin dealers and other criminals. The anxieties are extreme. Users are also susceptible to infectious diseases from contaminated drugs and needles; serum hepatitis, a serious liver disease, is endemic among people who share hypodermic needles. Most of whatever money users can lay their hands on goes for heroin. They live in poverty; their self-images are destroyed; society regards them as the lowest of the low.

Kicking the Habit

Very few heroin dependents are able to kick the habit without help, and relatively few succeed in staying away from heroin use even when they do get help. Whether their failure results from lack of will power, as many people believe, or from irresistible psychological or biological drives, the fact remains that users go on using, and ex-addicts become readdicted, despite every discouragement, including the very real threat of imprisonment.

Federal officials have claimed considerable success for the program of the U.S. Public Health Service Hospital at Lexington, Kentucky, where many thousands of heroin dependents have been incarcerated, or have surrendered voluntarily, and treated since the hospital opened in 1935. Follow-up studies have shown, however, that while the patients may have been ex-addicts when they left Lexington, few maintained that status. " . . . One study traced 1,912 Lexington alumni for periods of from one to four and a half years. Only 6.6 percent remained abstinent throughout the follow-up period.

"A second study checked on 453 Lexington alumni six months, two years, and five years after release. Only 12 of the 453 (less than 3 percent) were abstinent on all three follow-ups. The failure rate was thus in excess of 97 percent." Similar programs at other institutions run by federal, state, and local government agencies have not been notably more successful.

In recent years, much attention has been given to Synanon and other therapeutic communities in which many former heroin dependents have remained abstinent in an atmosphere of strict paternalism, family-style relationships, work schedules with opportunities for upward mobility, and regular encounter-group therapy. Such communities are, in effect, separate societies that require their residents to abandon their former life-styles. While therapeutic communities unquestionably have helped considerable numbers of people, controlled scientific studies of their cure rates are lacking, and their success is difficult to assess. According to one report:

> By the mid-1960s . . . even Synanon itself conceded that its program had with few exceptions failed to turn out abstinent alumni. Members apparently cured beyond any possibility of relapse promptly relapsed when they left the sheltering confines of Synanon or of other therapeutic communities to which they had been transferred. [Synanon founder Charles E.] Dederich himself estimated in 1971 that the relapse rate among Synanon graduates was in the neighborhood of 90 percent.
>
> "We once had the idea of 'graduates,'" he told a reporter. "This was a sop to social workers and professionals who wanted me to say that we were producing 'graduates.' I always wanted to say to them, 'A person with this fatal disease will have to live here all his life.'

"I know damn well if they go out of Synanon they are dead. A few, but very few, have gone out and made it. When they ask me, 'If an addict goes to Synanon, how long will it take?' my answer is, 'If he's lucky, it will take forever. . . .'"

Even this one-in-ten success rate, moreover, must be viewed with caution. For Synanon accepted in the first place only highly motivated addicts who were willing to go through the rigorous Synanon procedures, including "cold turkey" withdrawal. Many "split" within a few days or weeks after entering Synanon—*before* they were formally enrolled or included in the statistics. Synanon procedures applied to an unselected cross-section of addicts rather than this very select group would no doubt yield a far lower success rate.

Maintenance Programs

Since most efforts to cure heroin and morphine dependents have failed, authorities have looked for other ways to mitigate the consequences of such drug use. In Britain any physician legally may prescribe morphine or methadone, the synthetic narcotic, to people who are dependent on those drugs—and since cross-tolerance develops among the narcotics, morphine and methadone work for heroin dependents too. Heroin itself may be prescribed for dependents by approved clinics in Britain. The users are guaranteed, at little or no cost, a steady supply of pharmaceutically pure drugs in controlled doses, along with sterile, disposable injection equipment. The dangers of overdoses, of adulterated or contaminated drugs, and of infections are thus greatly reduced. The illegal black market (which still operates in Britain on a small scale) is deprived of customers, and users do not have to turn to stealing or prostitution to support their habits. Some other countries, including Sweden, Denmark, and the Netherlands, permit all physicians to prescribe heroin, as well as the other narcotics, to dependents.

In the United States, while doctors are permitted to prescribe narcotics for treatment of illnesses, the courts have not recognized opiate dependence as an illness; nonmedical users can obtain heroin or morphine only from illegal sources. In recent years, however, methadone maintenance clinics have been established in many American communities, and many authorities now see such clinics as the best hope for people addicted to narcotics until a cure is found.

Methadone's Effects

Methadone itself creates dependence in regular users. There is some black market traffic in methadone, and users say that when mainlined it produces subjective effects very similar to those produced by heroin. The use of street methadone carries with it all the hazards of illegality, adulteration, contamination, and lethal overdose associated with street heroin. In clinical use for treatment of narcotic dependence, however, methadone has a number of advantages over the opiates. It is effective when taken orally, which eliminates the need for injection equipment and the dangers of infection. As provided in clinics, the drug is pharmaceutically pure. Its cost is very low, so that methadone maintenance programs—like the British system—relieves users of the need to acquire large amounts of money to pay for their drugs.

Taken orally, methadone does not provide the user with any "kick." And it blocks the effects of other narcotics, so that a person who has taken methadone receives no enjoyment from taking heroin. However, methadone prevents the withdrawal symptoms that follow "cold turkey" abandonment of heroin. It also prevents the postwithdrawal syndrome, the depression and craving that otherwise follow withdrawal from heroin. The heroin dependent who switches to a clinical methadone maintenance program can thus feel "normal." Unlike heroin, methadone is a long-acting drug; an adequate dose will prevent withdrawal symptoms for twenty-four to thirty-six hours. Whereas the heroin user has to take heroin several times a day, a single dose of methadone in the morning keeps the patient well all day to hold a job and enjoy a normal family life.

Complete methadone maintenance programs involve not only controlled administration of the drug, but they also include employment and psychological counseling, diet supervision, and other rehabilitative services to help restore the dependents' self-image and enable them to resume normal positions in the community. Programs that include such services have reported that 50 to 75 percent of their patients have been rehabilitated. After three to five years on methadone maintenance, some patients are able to taper off and eventually give up methadone as well as the other drugs. Others must continue taking methadone, or their craving returns—and not for methadone but for heroin. These people must take methadone, as a diabetic must take insulin, as a lifetime medication.

In Britain many heroin dependents have shifted voluntarily to methadone maintenance. "The fact that more than half of all the addicts known to the United Kingdom Home Office are being maintained on methadone alone is of particular significance, for any one of those . . . methadone patients can at any time decide to go back to heroin and have a legal right to get it, free of charge. . . ."

In the United States the limited number of methadone maintenance clinics in operation in 1975 had long lists of heroin dependents waiting to enter their programs as soon as facilities and supplies became available.

Inhalants

Various volatile substances that can produce "highs" when inhaled have had limited popularity among drug abusers from time to time. Some have stimulant effects, but most are central nervous system depressants. They include nitrous oxide (laughing gas), ether, chloroform, organic solvents, such as toluene (found in model airplane glue) and benzene, and even gasoline. All of these substances are extremely toxic and can be lethal. Their effects range from euphoria to hyperstimulation and hallucinations to deep depression. They can cause severe liver and kidney damage, among other things.

In the nineteenth century, inhaling certain of the volatile gases was believed in some circles to produce consciousness expansion, as drugs like LSD were supposed to do in more recent history. One experimenter was Oliver Wendell Holmes of Harvard Medical School, who reported:

> I once inhaled a pretty full dose of ether, with the determination to put on record, at the earliest moment of regaining consciousness, the thought I should find uppermost in my mind. The mighty music of the triumphal march reverberated through my brain, and filled me with a sense of infinite possibilities, which made me an archangel for a moment. The veil of eternity was lifted. The one great truth which underlies all human experience and is the key to all the mysteries that philosophy has sought in vain to solve, flashed upon me in a sudden revelation. Henceforth all was clear: a few words had lifted my intelligence to the level of the knowledge of the cherubim. As my natural condition returned, I remembered my resolution; and, staggering to my desk, I wrote, in ill-shaped, straggling characters, the all-embracing truth still glimmering in my consciousness. The words were these (children may smile; the wise will ponder): "A strong smell of turpentine prevails throughout."

Summary

The most widely known and used of the "downers" is alcohol, which has begun to supplant drugs in the lifestyles of many younger people. Alcohol is an important factor in the social lives of many adults, too. In the bloodstream alcohol has a relaxing, quieting effect. It slows the heartbeat and respiration and lowers blood pressure. It eases inhibitions, too. But as intake increases, motor control diminishes and judgment slips away.

A bout of heavy drinking can produce the pain and anguish of a hangover. Heavy drinking also affects sexual performance and—if it becomes sustained and habitual—can cause brain and liver damage, can become addictive (alcoholism). These excesses are the exception, not the rule.

Barbiturates are prescribed to induce sleep, and tranquilizers to reduce stress and tension. They are used by many and are widely abused by those who get them illegally or ignore the limits on the labels. They can become addictive. Excessive dosages—or heavy use along with alcohol—can cause serious illness or death.

Opium and its derivatives (opiates) are the true narcotics, although the word has been widely and incorrectly applied to other substances. Two opiates—morphine and codeine—are indispensible in medical practice. Nonmedical use of opium is uncommon in the United States. Here, the opiate called heroin is the most widely used, and abused, narcotic. It can produce an intense "high" followed by profound euphoria—or it can cause fright and physical illness. Overdoses can kill. Heroin and other opiates are highly addictive. Tolerance increases with dependence, and increasingly heavy doses are needed to stave off withdrawal. Many addicts resort to crime for the money they need to support their habits. Few can end their addiction without medical and psychological help. In some countries, doctors legally prescribe morphine, or the synthetic methadone, for addicts. Many American cities have begun methadone maintenance programs.

References

p. 143 William Moore, "Youth Back on Booze," *San Francisco Chronicle* (November 11, 1974), p. 1.

p. 147 Thomas F. A. Plaut, Appendix I in *Task Force Report: Drunkenness,* President's Commission on Law Enforcement and Administraton of Justice (Washington, D.C., 1967), pp. 120–31.

p. 147 Ibid., p. 122.

p. 150 J. R. McCarroll and W. Haddon, Jr., cited by Richard H. Blum assisted by Laurain Braunstein, Appendix B in *Task Force Report: Drunkenness,* p. 38.

p. 150 L. M. Shupe, cited by Blum assisted by Braunstein, Appendix B in *Task Force Report: Drunkenness,* p. 41.

p. 150 E. G. Palola, T. L. Dorpat, and W. R. Larsen, cited by Blum assisted by Braunstein, Appendix B in *Task Force Report: Drunkenness,* p. 35.

p. 150 Edward M. Brecher and *Consumer Reports* Editors, *Licit and Illicit Drugs: The Consumers Union Report on Narcotics, Stimulants, Depressants, Inhalants, Hallucinogens, and Marijuana—Including Caffeine, Nicotine, and Alcohol* (Boston, 1972), p. 263.

p. 151 San Francisco Opportunity High School II, *Dope Notes, A Project of the Drugs and Society Class* (1972).

p. 152 Brecher and *Consumer Reports* Editors, *Licit and Illicit Drugs,* pp. 249–52.

p. 153 Jerome H. Jaffe, *The Pharmacological Basis of Therapeutics,* 4th ed., ed. Louis S. Goodman and Alfred Gilman (New York, 1970), p. 289.

p. 153 Brecher and *Consumer Reports* Editors, *Licit and Illicit Drugs,* pp. 252–53.

p. 153 Ibid.

p. 154 David E. Smith and John Luce, *Love Needs Care, A History of San Francisco's Haight-Ashbury Free Medical Clinic* (Boston, 1971), p. 20.

p. 154 Murray E. Jarvik, *The Pharmacological Basis of Therapeutics,* 4th ed., ed. Goodman and Gilman, p. 174.

p. 154 "Federal Curbs for Valium, Librium," reprinted in *San Francisco Chronicle* (January 31, 1975), p. 1.

p. 155 Smith and Luce, *Love Needs Care,* p. 242.

p. 156 S. Dana Hays, quoted in *Annual Report of the State Board of Health, Massachusetts* (1871). Cited in *The Opium Problem,* ed. Charles E. Terry and Mildred Pellens (New York, 1928), p. 7.

p. 156 Brecher and *Consumer Reports* Editors, *Licit and Illicit Drugs,* p. 8.

p. 157 Jaffe, *The Pharmacological Basis of Therapeutics,* 4th ed., ed. Goodman and Gilman, pp. 285–86.

p. 157 Marie Nyswander, cited by Jerome H. Jaffe, *The Pharmacological Basis of Therapeutics,* 3rd ed., ed. Lewis S. Goodman and Alfred Gilman (New York, 1965), p. 285.

p. 158   Jaffe, *The Pharmacological Basis of Therapeutics,* 4th ed., ed. Goodman and Gilman, pp. 287–88.

p. 159   Brecher and *Consumer Reports* Editors, *Licit and Illicit Drugs,* pp. 13–14.

p. 160   George H. Stevenson et al., "Drug Addiction in British Columbia: A Research Survey" (University of British Columbia, 1956), pp. 514–15.

p. 160   Marie Nyswander, *The Drug Addict as a Patient* (New York, 1956).

p. 160   George B. Wallace, "The Rehabilitation of the Drug Addict," *Journal of Educational Sociology,* No. 4 (1931), p. 347.

p. 160   Vincent P. Dole, quoted by Brecher and *Consumer Reports* Editors, *Licit and Illicit Drugs,* p. 25.

p. 160   "The Opium Habit," *Catholic World,* No. 33 (September 1881), p. 827.

p. 161   Stephen Waldron of Arthur D. Little, Inc., consultants to the President's Commission on Crime and to the National Institute of Mental Health, *Hearings Before the Select Committee on Crime,* House of Representatives, 91st Congress, 1st Session (1969), p. 291.

p. 161   Jaffe, *The Pharmacological Basis of Therapeutics,* 4th ed., ed. Goodman and Gilman, p. 286.

p. 162   San Francisco Opportunity High School II, *Dope Notes.*

p. 162   Edward A. Preble and John J. Casey, Jr., "Taking Care of Business—The Heroin User's Life on the Street," *International Journal of the Addictions,* No. 4 (March 1969), pp. 2–3.

p. 163   Brecher and *Consumer Reports* Editors, *Licit and Illicit Drugs,* p. 69.

p. 164   Ibid., pp. 78–79.

p. 165   Ibid., p. 177.

p. 166   Quoted by Brecher and *Consumer Reports* Editors, *Licit and Illicit Drugs,* p. 316.

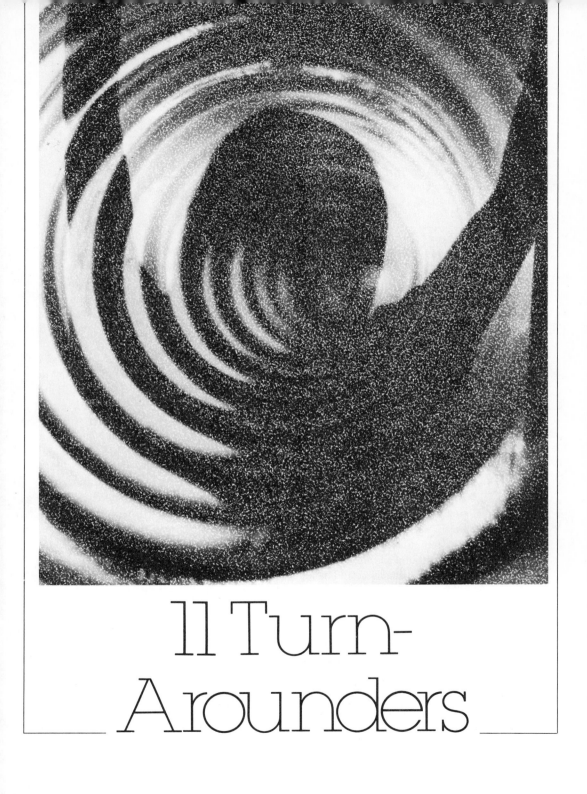

11 Turn-Arounders

. . . I saw a man sitting on the ground, his face turned almost in profile. I approached him until I was perhaps ten feet away; then he turned his head and looked at me. . . . His head was pointed like a strawberry; his skin was green, dotted with innumerable warts. Except for the pointed shape, his head was exactly like the surface of the peyote plant. . . . I heard him talking to me. At first his voice was like the soft rustle of a light breeze. Then I heard it as music—as a melody of voices—and I "knew" it was saying, "What do you want?"

In one of Scheherezade's tales from *A Thousand Nights and a Night,* Aladdin rubbed a lamp and a djinni appeared saying, "What do you want?" In the strange encounter described in the chapter opening, Carlos Castaneda met something very like a djinni in the form of Mescalito, a more or less anthropomorphic embodiment of the power of peyote. This happened, Castaneda wrote later, after he ritually consumed a number of peyote mushrooms under the guidance of a Yaqui Indian *brujo,* a twentieth century sorcerer called Don Juan.

Castaneda, an anthropology student who recounted his curious experiences in a series of best-selling books, met Mescalito during the 1960s, an era in which belief in the occult reached proportions probably unprecedented in the United States since the Salem witch trials. This outbreak of "magic" coincided with the widespread use of certain psychoactive substances that, to many users, sometimes seemed to possess the powers of all the elixirs, potions, and philters in the pages of *A Thousand Nights and a Night.*

Like all psychoactive drugs, these substances that were used widely in the 1960s worked their "magic" by chemically altering the functioning of the central nervous system—the physical structure of the mind. Because they worked in different ways on different parts of the nervous system, their effects were unlike those usually produced by "uppers" or "downers." We have categorized these drugs informally as "turn-arounders," a term that has no particular scientific basis, and that is used here only because no one has found a completely satisfactory name for this class of chemicals. They have been called psychedelics and hallucinogens, among other things, but none of the terms in use has won unanimous acceptance among scientific investigators, for reasons that will be explained in this chapter.

Some Hallucinogenic Drugs

Among the more widely known of the "turn-arounders" is mescaline, a derivative of the peyote cactus. Mescaline, which can also be synthesized in the laboratory, is said to have been named for the Mescalero Apaches, who, like many other Indians throughout North America, have used peyote for centuries as a part of religious rites. Psilucybin is

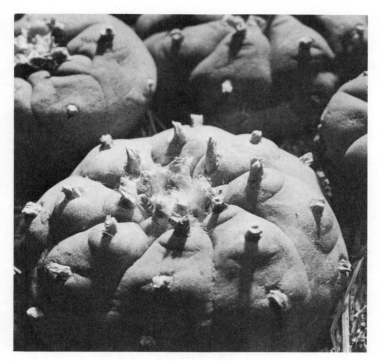

Peyote cactus.

another well-known "turn-arounder" that is found both in natural and synthetic forms. It occurs in a number of species of mushrooms, such as the celebrated "magic mushrooms" of Mexico. The roots of the small plant *Mimosa hostilis* yield N, N-dimethyltryptamine, or DMT. The seeds of certain kinds of morning glories, and even ordinary nutmeg, can produce some psychedelic, or hallucinogenic, effects when taken in large quantities; they can also cause severe stomach upsets.

LSD

The drug most people associate with the term psychedelic is a synthetic that was derived originally from ergot, a fungus that grows on rye. Scientifically, the drug is d-lysergic acid diethylamide; popularly, it is LSD, or "acid." LSD is colorless, odorless, tasteless—and almost unbelievably powerful. Effective doses of the other drugs are usually measured in milligrams, or thousandths of a gram; effective doses of LSD are measured in micrograms, or millionths of a gram. Some people can get intoxicated on as little as twenty-five micrograms of LSD; the usual dose taken by those experienced in using LSD is about 250 micrograms. "An amount of LSD weighing as little as the aspirin in a five-grain tablet is enough to produce effects in 3,000 people." In the 1960s LSD was often dripped onto sugar cubes or blotting paper or other easily swallowed substances.

Nowadays it is usually found in tablet form. The tablets consist mostly of inert materials (or various adulterants and contaminants) and contain tiny quantities of the drug.

The effects of LSD, as the classic example of drugs in this category, will be explored in the following pages. With some exceptions, particularly where the size of the dose is concerned, what is said about the effects of LSD is generally true of similarly classified drugs.

LSD's Effects

In Chapter 8, it was noted that *subjective* effects of psychoactive drugs—what the user thinks is happening—may be very different for different users, or for the same user on different occasions. This is particularly true of LSD and similar drugs. The effects described here are among the most common.

LSD usually begins to produce noticeable effects within a few minutes to half an hour after it is swallowed. The "trip" may last for eight hours or longer. Physical signs may include rapid breathing, flushing of the skin, reddening of the eyes, heart palpitations, and apparent fluctuations in body temperature. Nausea and vomiting are not unusual. The user commonly experiences euphoria, often accompanied by what seems to him or her to be a suspension or slowing down of time; minutes may seem like hours. Sensory perceptions seem to be greatly heightened. Colors become unusually intense. A person may think that music sounds better. Tactile sensations are exaggerated; some users say their skin creeps. Perceptions of all kinds may become wildly distorted; solid objects move about, colors run. Many users experience *synesthesia* (Greek *syn,* together, and *aisthesis,* sensation), a phenomenon caused by the drug's toxic effects on the reticular activating center, which plays a basic role in regulating the background activity of the central nervous system. LSD acts on this center, causing people to "see" sounds, to "hear" colors.

The peculiar visual and auditory effects often produced by LSD and like chemicals are largely responsible for the description of the drugs as hallucinogens, or generators of hallucinations. "Illusogens" might be a better description. A hallucination is something a person sees or hears when there is really nothing at all to be seen or heard; imagining something when it is not there. While users of LSD may sometimes hallucinate, their experiences are most often *illusions;* there really is something out there, but it is distorted by the intoxicated mind so that it appears to behave strangely, or to be something else altogether. A bush or a boulder, for example, might appear to the drug user to be a person with a strawberry-shaped head and warty green skin.

Mind Expansion

"If the doors of perception were cleansed, every thing would appear to man as it is, infinite." This quotation from William Blake, the eighteenth century poet, painter, and mystic, provided the title for a book that created a considerable stir when it was published in 1954. In *The Doors of Perception,* Aldous Huxley wrote glowingly and intriguingly of his experience with mescaline. Huxley, whose other writings revealed a broad streak of mysticism, theorized that mescaline "cleansed the doors of perception," opened up the individual mind to "Mind at Large," a universal consciousness that, he believed, linked all things. Consciousness, in other words, was expanded. After Huxley, many others who tried mescaline, LSD, and similar drugs reported almost identical experiences. They were convinced that the chemicals provided profound insights into cosmic truths hidden from ordinary consciousness. How did this happen?

In Chapter 10, we observed that alcohol, by suppressing certain functions of the brain, impairs judgment. LSD and other "illusogens" also affect judgment, in different ways. As Sidney Cohen, an authority on drugs, wrote: . . . the judgmental attitude . . . toward the experience itself is diminished. . . . Insights are accepted without reservation and seem much more valid than under nondrug conditions. In this state of diminution of "the judgmental attitude," the drug taker also may experience these effects: a "marked heightening of . . . suggestibility"; distortion of the sense of time, which may make a moment seem "eternal"; a feeling that has been called "portentousness," which one writer describes as "the sense that something—even a trivial platitude—is fraught with a cosmic significance too profound to be adequately communicated." This feeling of portentousness is probably connected with another effect of the drug's intoxication of the nervous system: the increased selectivity of the mind, or narrowing of awareness, that causes the drug user to focus on one bit of sensory input at a time, such as the shade of green of a particular leaf, or the notes of a single instrument in a symphony orchestra, to the exclusion of other stimuli. Such intense concentration gives its object an unusual vividness, and the leaf or the musical instrument takes on a great and mysterious importance.

The same kind of selectivity seems sometimes to affect thought processes; in drugged consciousness, the user focuses on a single strand of the web of thought, as a spotlight beams on a soloist in a choir; the other "voices," the interplay of positive and negative considerations that are the elements of reason, are muted; the single, shining, ill-considered fragment of an idea is accepted without reservation. In the intoxicated mind, it rings with the mighty resonance of Absolute Truth.

By now, most people have read or been told that LSD expands consciousness. With that thought in their drugged, suggestible, nonjudgmental minds, in an "eternal" moment fraught with portentousness, it is not surprising that LSD takers experience what seem to be cosmic truths. Such experiences account for the term *psychedelic,* which, in Greek, means mind-manifesting. It is a somewhat misleading term. Actually, it might be said that at least a considerable portion of the mind hides, rather than manifests itself, during LSD intoxication. In a sense, consciousness is contracted rather than expanded. The drug taker, to paraphrase William Blake, holds infinity in the palm of his hand and eternity in an hour. The drug taker's world, in short, is a small one.

Bad Trips The perceptual distortions and other strange effects of LSD are as frightening to some people as they are fascinating to others. Some users become convinced that they are going insane, that their bodies are dissolving, or that they are in hell. Some panic and try to run away from their illusions; there have been cases of people who jumped out of windows or ran in front of cars during such panic-stricken flights. There have been some suicides. Bad trips occur most often in uncontrolled circumstances—when the drug is taken by someone who is among strangers or among acquaintances he or she doesn't trust, or when it is taken by someone who is on the street or at a rock concert. Because the drug is illegal, the fear of getting caught can be greatly magnified by the drug's effects and may lead to a strong feeling of paranoia in some users. And if the user should be jailed while intoxicated by LSD, the result could be panic.

The fact that there is no way of being sure just how much LSD is contained in a tablet or a sugar cube purchased from a black market dealer adds to the hazards. While there are no known cases of people dying from overdoses of LSD, an overdose does increase the likelihood of adverse reactions. Another risk is that LSD obtained illegally is often adulterated with other drugs that can contribute to undesired ill-effects. People who swallow LSD unwittingly, as when someone secretly spikes a bowl of punch, are particularly likely to suffer from frightening effects, since they have no idea why such bizarre things are happening to them. Fortunately, there are drugs that can cut short a bad trip. There have been some reports that niacin was effective in mitigating the effects of LSD. Above all, people need someone they trust to talk them down, to stay with them, and to offer comfort and reassurance that the nightmare is only a chemical effect, that it will wear off, and that everything is all right.

Flashbacks   Some people, days or months after taking LSD, experience inexplicable recurrences of illusions that include all of the perceptual distortions and all of the vividness of the original experience. These flashbacks come on suddenly, without warning, and can happen at any time or in any place. They can be very frightening. The cause of flashbacks is not known, and there is no medication or treatment to prevent them. Most people who experience flashbacks find, however, that they occur with decreasing frequency as time passes, and they eventually stop.

Other Adverse Effects   To a borderline psychotic—a person whose grip on reality is precarious—an LSD experience could cause him or her to slip into long-term psychosis. In the late 1960s some researchers reported evidence found in laboratory studies that LSD could damage chromosomes, thus raising the possibility that such damage could result in birth defects among babies whose parents had taken LSD. Subsequent studies have indicated that the incidence of birth defects is no higher among offspring of LSD users than among other infants, but the findings remain controversial.

A number of investigators have also reported evidence that heavy, long-term use of LSD can cause brain damage. While these findings, too, are controversial, there is no question that chronic users often undergo major personality changes. One characteristic of the heavy user is what has been called the *amotivational syndrome,* a complete lack of interest in work and a lack of any goals. This may involve the LSD user's "cosmic" conviction that the universe is perfect just as it is, and that there is no need to make any effort to change it. It also may be that the user wasn't interested in working to begin with, and being a chronic LSD user gives him or her an excuse to stop working.

LSD Dependence

Chronic LSD users may be psychologically dependent in the sense that they like being intoxicated and don't want to give it up. LSD use doesn't usually lead to dependence. As William H. McGlothlin and David O. Arnold, psychologists at the University of California at Los Angeles, concluded after a study of LSD users: "Compulsive patterns of LSD use rarely develop; the nature of the drug effect is such that it becomes less attractive with continued use and in the long term, is almost always self-limiting."

The reasons given by McGlothin and Arnold for decreased use of hallucinogens over time "is to be found in the characteristics of the drug effect. The major effect of hallucinogens is to temporarily suspend the normal mode of perception and thinking. The utility of the experience lies in the uniqueness of the new modes of perception and thought which become available under these conditions. However, as one repeats the experience many times, what was initially unique becomes more commonplace and there is a process of diminishing returns. The effect of hallucinogens is indeed 'a trip,' and trips tend to lose their appeal when repeated too often."

LSD as Medicine

Before LSD became illegal in the 1960s, many psychiatrists gave the drug to patients as a therapeutic tool. There were conflicting reports on the results but few therapists find any use for the drug today. It is still used by some therapists in other countries. Experimental use of LSD to ease the pain, anxiety, and depression of terminal cancer patients had some success when combined with careful psychological preparation. One such patient reported after an LSD experience:

> . . . All noticed a change in me. I was radiant, they said. I seemed at peace, they said. I felt that way too. What has changed for me? I am living now, and being. I can take it as it comes. Some of my physical symptoms are gone. The excessive fatigue, some of the pains. I still get irritated occasionally and yell. I am still me, but more at peace. My family senses this and we are closer. All who know me well say that this has been a good experience.

Acid Art

The idea that LSD might be an aid to creativity, because of the novel sensory experiences and cosmic insights, has been a motive for some drug taking. The psychedelic poster art of the 1960s, with its vivid colors and complex patterns, may have been inspired, in part, by LSD trips. And there are musicians who believe that such drugs improve their playing, but it could be that the intoxicated musician only *thinks* the music sounds better, just as some nonmusicians think records sound better when they have taken LSD.

Since the quality of art is largely a matter of subjective judgment, it is difficult to prove that a painter or a musician performs better or worse after taking "illusogenic" drugs. Writers, however, have often found that the written records of their profound insights boiled down, in the cold, gray light of dawn, to nothing more artistic than the result of Oliver Wendell Holmes's experiment with ether, "A strong smell of turpentine prevails throughout."

Marijuana and Hashish

Many workers in Jamaica, in India, and in Africa use marijuana much as the Andes Indians use coca leaves, or as American office workers use coffee: to reduce fatigue, to make working easier—in other words, as an "upper." On the other hand, many people in other parts of the world use marijuana to help them relax, or even to help them sleep, as they might use alcohol or a tranquilizer or a barbiturate—in other words, as a "downer." In America, nowadays, the drug is often used to alter sensory perceptions, to provide insights, to expand consciousness—or, as what we have called an "illusogen" or "turn-arounder."

Marijuana is one of those drugs that defies precise classification; some investigators say it is in a class by itself. Perhaps more than any other drug, marijuana is apt to produce the effects expected by the user, although there is certainly no guarantee that the effects will be those expected or desired; some users are surprised, not always pleasantly. We have placed marijuana in this chapter because it has multiple effects but predominantly alters consciousness.

The "Weed"

Marijuana is the name popularly used in the United States for the Indian hemp plant, botanically *Cannabis sativa*. Once widely cultivated for its tough fibers, which were used to make rope, the tenacious plant now grows wild on thousands of acres in parts of this country, particularly in the Middle West, despite government efforts to stamp it out. It is also grown in many other parts of the world, where it is cultivated not for its fibers but for its psychoactive properties. It is known by a variety of names in other countries. *Marijuana,* Spanish for Mary Jane, is a name borrowed from Mexico, where Mary Jane was once a cheap kind of tobacco; how the name became attached to cannabis is not known.

In the United States, the name marijuana is applied both to the entire hemp plant and, particularly, to the dried leaves and flowering tops of female plants, which comprise the preparation also known colloquially as "grass" or "weed" or, to an older generation, "tea." It is also known as "pot," as in "a pot of tea." The resin from the hemp plant, when dried, is known in this country as *hashish* (or "hash"), a word said to have been derived from the Assassins (properly *hashishin*), a fanatical Moslem sect whose members, during the Crusades in the eleventh century, were believed to intoxicate themselves with cannabis resin before going out to murder their enemies.

The chief, if not the only, psychoactive ingredient in both marijuana and hashish is *tetrahydrocannabinol,* or THC, a complex chemical that can, with difficulty, be synthesized in the laboratory. Cannabis may contain other psychoactive chemicals, but, if so, they have not been identified as such. In the hemp plant, THC is concentrated most heavily in the resin, less in the flowering tops, still less in the leaves, and least in the seeds and stems, which accounts for the fact that hashish is much more potent than marijuana; the difference is analogous to the difference between strong whiskey and light wine. Contrary to a widespread belief, both male and female hemp plants contain THC. The psychoactive potency of cannabis preparations depends on the THC content. The hemp that grows wild in this country is usually low in THC, as compared to some of the varieties that grow in Mexico, the Caribbean, Africa, or India. However, it is not necessarily the soil or climate that makes the difference. Cannabis grown in the United States from seeds of more potent strains has proven to be equally high in THC content. Such celebrated strains as Acapulco Gold and Panama Red, which got their names from the localities in which they were originally grown and from the characteristic colors of their dried leaves (most marijuana is green or brownish green), gained their reputations because of their high THC content.

Cannabis in History

Cannabis has been used for both medical and nonmedical purposes in various parts of the world for thousands of years. In the United States, early in the twentieth century, cannabis preparations were prescribed by physicians for a number of ailments. Cannabis-based patent medicines, like the opiates, were legally available without prescriptions and were widely used, being valued for their euphoria-producing properties. Old apothecary jars labeled "Tincture of Cannabis" can still be found occasionally in antique shops. As a medicine, the drug was swallowed rather than smoked.

Relatively few people smoked marijuana in the United States before alcoholic beverages were temporarily outlawed following the First World War. Nonmedical use of marijuana, as an alternative to alcohol, began to increase in the 1920s. "Tea pads," where people could buy marijuana cigarettes (then called "reefers") much as people now buy alcoholic drinks in bars, sprang up in many places. Alarmed authorities claimed that the use of marijuana was responsible for any number of sensational crimes, and newspapers and magazines printed stories and editorials condemning the "killer weed." In the light of subsequent studies, which have shown no connection between marijuana use and crime (except that the possession, use, and sale of marijuana are now crimes), the stories were misleading. But they were generally believed, and many states passed laws against nonmedical use of cannabis. In 1937 such use became a federal crime. The law did not prohibit the prescription of cannabis by physicians, but it imposed a special tax on doctors who wrote such prescriptions and on pharmacists who filled them. Few paid the tax, and the use of cannabis as a medicine in this country became almost unknown, although doctors still prescribed cannabis preparations in other parts of the world.

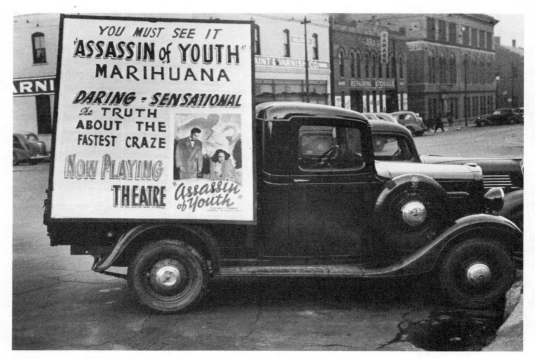

Movie poster, 1920s.

In recent years research has suggested that cannabis might be effective in treating some common diseases, including alcoholism, glaucoma (an eye ailment that can lead to blindness), and asthma. One study has even produced questionable evidence that cannabis, by affecting the body's immune responses, might inhibit the growth of certain kinds of cancer. The medical research continues.

Meanwhile, nonmedical use of marijuana spread explosively during the 1960s, despite its illegality. Estimates of the number of Americans who had at least experimented with marijuana ran as high as twenty million, or about a tenth of the population. Next to caffeine, nicotine, alcohol, and prescription medicines, marijuana has been the most-used psychoactive drug in this country in the 1970s.

Methods of Use

Among nonmedical users, marijuana and hashish are both eaten and smoked, and the way the drug is taken has a lot to do with the results. Smoked in pipes or cigarettes ("joints"), cannabis produces effects almost immediately. Experienced users learn to control their "highs" by controlling their intake; when they feel high enough, they stop smoking. When the drug is swallowed (whether baked in brownies, brewed in a beverage, sprinkled over salads, or simply gulped down raw—the way some people take hashish), absorption by the body takes longer, the effects are delayed, and there is no way to control the high. Thus, an accidental overdose is more likely when the drug is eaten than when it is smoked. THC also may be swallowed in tablet form, but the tablets sold on the street as THC are usually something else, often LSD. Marijuana smoking is by far the most common method of using cannabis in this country.

Marijuana's Effects

The most common effects of smoking marijuana in small doses are euphoria, suppression of inhibitions, distortion of the sense of time, and an apparent heightening of sensory perceptions. These effects are often accompanied by some of the altered awareness of sensory stimuli and thought processes, and the feeling of portentousness associated with LSD (see p. 173), although these feelings are usually less pronounced in the marijuana smoker. Users thus think of marijuana as consciousness expanding for the same reasons LSD users think of *their* drug that way; a *narrowing* of awareness seems to the intoxicated mind to be the opposite. Many users think of marijuana as a sociable drug, saying that it makes everyone feel closer when taken in a congenial group. The ritual of sharing a joint, passing the cigarette from person to person, along with the idea of being co-conspirators in a semiclandestine activity, may contribute to that feeling; so may the effect, on minds made suggestible by intoxication, of being told that marijuana is a sociable drug.

Marijuana, like alcohol, may contribute to sociability by suppressing inhibitions; and by suppressing inhibitions, impair social judgment. Like alcohol, marijuana produces nausea and vomiting in some users. It does not, however, cause hangovers, although users often feel fatigued after an evening of heavy smoking. Some people who experiment with marijuana notice no effects at all. Others become anxious and uncomfortable. Even many regular users acknowledge that they sometimes experience a mild, nagging paranoia. Some find that marijuana seems to intensify whatever mood they are in before they take the drug; if they are feeling anxious, they become *more* anxious.

All of these subjective evaluations are consistent with the fact that the subjective effects of marijuana are known to depend to a great extent on the "set" of the user's mind. Setting also plays an important part; a user who enjoys marijuana when alone or in a group of friends may have an unpleasant experience when he or she takes the drug in anxiety-provoking surroundings. Marijuana often affects short-term memory during intoxication; users finds themselves in the middle of a sentence and can't remember what they started to say. In large doses, the drug can produce perceptual distortions in some users like those produced by LSD; such effects are more likely when cannabis is used in the potent form of hashish. Overdoses of cannabis can cause hallucinations and panic reactions. However, there are no documented cases of long-term psychoses attributable to marijuana, and there is no known lethal dose of the drug.

Inexperienced users are likely to find that marijuana affects their physical coordination, making it difficult to perform complicated tasks. Research indicates that the ability to perform physical tasks after taking a moderate dose of marijuana may improve as the user becomes more experienced, but the results vary among individuals. Since there is no simple way to measure the amount of THC in the blood, it has been impossible to establish scientifically any statistical relationship between marijuana use and auto accidents. The perceptual and time distortions associated with marijuana use, however, suggest that driving under its influence is dangerous, as driving under the influence of *any* drug is dangerous.

Long-Term Effects   The chronic, heavy user of marijuana may, like the heavy user of LSD, develop the so-called amotivational syndrome, for the same reasons. In India, where heavy marijuana use is more common than in the United States, studies by Colonel Sir R. N. Chopra, director of the Drug Research Laboratory, Jammu and Kashmir, and his son, I. C. Chopra, a pharmacologist, led to the conclusion that "indulgence in cannabis drugs, unlike alcohol, rarely brings the habitué into a state of extreme intoxication where he loses entire control over himself. As a rule, the intoxication produced is of a mild nature, and those who indulge in it habitually can carry on their ordinary vocations for long periods and do not become a burden to society or even a social nuisance."

There is no evidence that marijuana smoking, like tobacco smoking, causes cancer or emphysema. Even daily users smoke much less marijuana than the amount of tobacco consumed by the average cigarette smoker. Because of the common practice of inhaling marijuana smoke as deeply as possible and holding it in the lungs, however, heavy marijuana smoking may cause irritation of the respiratory system. Whether or not heavy, long-term use of marijuana might cause organic damage is a matter of continuing controversy. Some researchers have suggested that heavy use can reduce the production of male sex hormones, reduce the individual's resistance to infections, and possibly cause organ damage. Other researchers disagree. There is no evidence that occasional marijuana use as practiced by most users in America causes physical or mental damage.

Habituation

Cannabis does not produce any physical dependence in users. It does not seem to produce tolerance. Some users, in fact, develop a reverse tolerance, finding that with experience they become intoxicated on less of the drug. The user's desires and expectations account for that effect. In laboratory tests, some regular marijuana smokers have reported that they were high after smoking marijuana from which the THC had been removed. They wanted to get high so they did; no drug was required as long as they *thought* they were smoking unprocessed marijuana.

Marijuana, like many other things, may produce psychological dependence in the sense that the user likes the effects of the drug and wants to keep using it. Even daily users, however, usually have no difficulty doing without marijuana if, for one reason or another, they can't get it.

Marijuana and Other Drugs

Some studies have shown that people who use tobacco and alcohol are more likely to use marijuana than those who do not use those other drugs. Studies have also indicated that people who use heroin have more often than not used tobacco, alcohol, and, to a lesser extent, marijuana. However, there is no evidence that the use of any of those

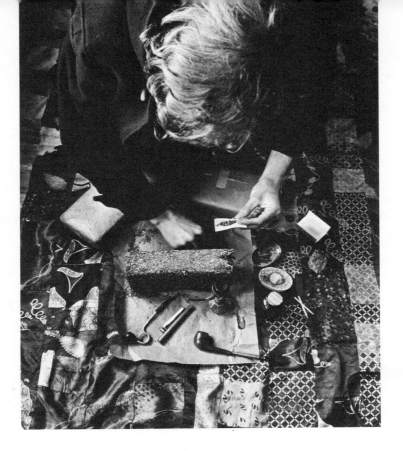

drugs *leads* to the use of any of the others. Following an extensive study, a government commission in Canada reported that "it appears that heavy use of sedatives (alcohol and barbiturates) rather than cannabis has most frequently preceded heroin use.

The Drug Controversy

"Okie From Muskogee," Merle Haggard's hit record of 1969, neatly captured the attitudes shared that year by a great many people throughout the country. In millions of minds, marijuana and LSD were associated with the burning of draft cards by young men opposed to the war in Vietnam, with campus demonstrations, with sexual promiscuity, with long hair, beads, and peace symbols, and with all kinds of things that were seen as threats to established ways and beliefs. Hardly anyone seemed to notice the irony in the song's association of "living right" and "Ol' Glory" with "the biggest thrill of all," *white lightning*—bootleg whiskey—an illegal drug.

It wasn't, of course, that people thought of bootleg whiskey as patriotic. The irony slipped right by those who applauded the sentiments expressed in the song, because alcohol was considered, if not good, at least familiar, even traditional, while marijuana was definitely bad, representing an unknown, frightening future, or so it seemed in that year of revolution. In a divided society in which new patterns of drug use coincided with spectacular social turmoil, drugs had become symbols of social philosophies. While greater issues were at the heart of the schism, the revolution of the 1960s was, on one level, a battle between "pot heads" and "juice heads." Since young people tended to use pot, while their parents continued to drink alcohol, drugs also became symbols of what was popularly called a generation gap.

By the mid-1970s, as we noted in the previous chapter, the revolution seemed to be fading into the past, and drug-use patterns were changing again as more and more young people began to drink alcohol. But millions of Americans were still using marijuana and other illegal drugs, and controversy over public policy regarding the use of such drugs continued. The controversy is considered briefly here because of the light it throws on individual and social psychology, and on the interrelatedness of social attitudes and individual health.

Drugs and "Nondrugs"

The National Commission on Marihuana and Drug Abuse reported in 1973 that, according to the results of a national public attitude survey conducted for the commission, "the public tends uniformly to regard heroin as a drug, as well as other substances associated with the drug problem, such as marijuana, cocaine, the amphetamines and the barbiturates. Some psychoactive substances, such as alcohol and tobacco, are generally not regarded as drugs at all. In neither public law nor public discussion is alcohol regarded as a drug. It may be called a beverage, a food, a social lubricant or a relaxant, but rarely is it called a drug."

> The imprecision of the term "drug" has had serious social consequences. Because alcohol is excluded, the public is conditioned to regard a martini as something fundamentally different from a marijuana cigarette, a barbiturate capsule or a bag of heroin. Similarly, because the referents of the word "drug" differ so widely in the therapeutic and social contexts, the public is conditioned to believe that "street" drugs act according to entirely different principles than "medical" drugs. The result is that the risks of the former are exaggerated and the risks of the latter are overlooked.

Robert S. de Ropp, a member of the commission, declared as long ago as 1957, "Just why the alcoholic is tolerated as a sick man while the opiate addict is persecuted as a criminal is hard to understand." The difference is explained, as the National Commission on Marihuana and Drug Abuse found, not by any essential difference between alcoholism and heroin dependence, but by differences in the ways people *think* about the drugs—or "nondrugs."

Marijuana and Prohibition

All laws which can be violated without doing any one an injury are laughed at. Nay, so far are they from doing anything to control the desires and passions of men that, on the contrary, they direct and incite men's thoughts the more toward those very objects. . . . He who tries to determine everything by law will foment crime rather than lessen it.

Just forty years before the National Commission on Marihuana and Drug Abuse wrote its report, a federal law was passed against the sale of alcoholic beverages, but no such law was passed against the sale of marijuana. Between 1920 and 1933, the manufacture and sale of illegal alcohol became a huge industry that created a highly organized network of crime. Many people drank more than ever, in speakeasies that were open twenty-four hours a day and completely unregulated, since they were outside the law. Contaminated and adulterated liquor killed, blinded, or otherwise crippled more than a few drinkers. An army of police officers and prohibition agents was helpless against the Niagara of bootleg booze. In 1933 Prohibition was repealed as a failure; people had simply refused to obey the law.

By the 1970s many authorities agreed that marijuana prohibition, in force since 1937, also had failed. There were millions of marijuana smokers of every age and in every social and economic class. In many jurisdictions, police had all but given up trying to enforce laws against simple possession and use of marijuana; it was impossible to arrest, prosecute, and imprison possibly a tenth of the population, especially when most marijuana users had committed no other crime. The National Commission on Marihuana and Drug Abuse recommended in 1972 that penalties for possession and use of marijuana be eliminated—a recommendation that was rejected by then-President Richard Nixon. A similar government commission in Canada proposed a more radical step, legalizing the cultivation and sale of marijuana under regulations similar to those governing the manufacture and distribution of alcohol. It, too, was rejected.

Opponents to such steps argued that decriminalization of marijuana would imply that the government condoned use of the drug, and would thereby encourage even greater use. It was argued that more research was needed to determine the effects of long-term use of marijuana. The huge social cost of alcoholism was cited as the strongest argument against making other drugs more easily available.

In recent years, many states, as well as the federal government, have reduced penalties for possession and use of marijuana, and an experiment in the states of California and Oregon has been watched with great interest. People found in possession of less than an ounce of marijuana have been given citations, similar to traffic tickets, rather than being arrested. They may be fined up to one-hundred dollars, but not jailed, and they do not incur criminal records. No great increase in the use of marijuana has been detected since the program began.

Drug Addiction: Crime or Disease?

Drug addiction, like prostitution and like liquor, is not a police problem; it never has been and never can be solved by policemen. It is first and last a medical problem, and if there is a solution it will be discovered not by policemen, but by scientific and competently trained medical experts. . . .

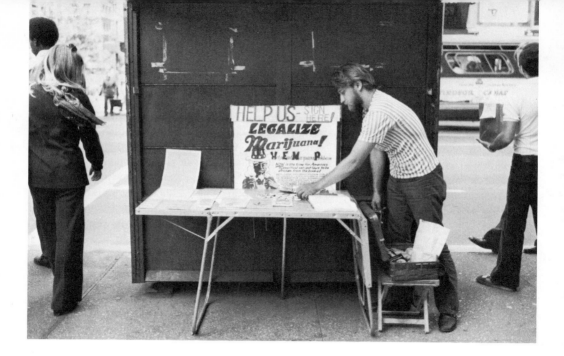

That declaration was made not by a physician but by a police officer, August Vollmer, former police chief in Berkeley, California, former professor of police administration at the Universities of California and Chicago, and past president of the International Association of Chiefs of Police. He made the statement in 1936. Since then, as before, the question of whether the drug dependent is a criminal or a sick person has been much debated. Law enforcement officials have tended to side against their former colleague, Chief Vollmer; physicians tend to agree with him.

Jerome H. Jaffe wrote in 1965: "Much of the ill health, crime, degeneracy, and low standard of living [among heroin dependents] are the result not of drug effects, but of the social structure that makes it a criminal act to obtain or to use opiates for their subjective effects. . . . It seems reasonable to wonder if providing addicts with a legitimate source of drugs might not be worthwhile, even if it did not make them our most productive citizens and did not completely eliminate the illicit market but resulted merely in a marked reduction in crime, disease, social degradation, and human misery."

The arguments against decriminalization of dependence-producing drugs are much the same as those against legalization of marijuana, but they are usually stated more strongly, since marijuana does not produce dependence. Would making heroin legally available to dependents encourage more heroin use? Would we become a nation of dope fiends?

Still, many people wonder, as Dr. de Ropp did in 1957, "Just why the alcoholic is tolerated as a sick man while the opiate addict is persecuted as a criminal. . . ."

We have devoted so many pages to psychoactive drugs because, in this society, they are among the most common health-affecting factors over which an individual has control.

The pressures to use psychoactive drugs of one kind or another are immense, the controversies confusing. As the National Commission on Marihuana and Drug Abuse wrote of the drug laws: "Implicit in present policy is the concern that many individuals cannot be trusted to make prudent or responsible decisions regarding drug-taking. . . . Most people are not accustomed to thinking about drug effects in terms of probabilities and uncertainties, of dose-response curves, of multiple effects (some desirable and some undesirable), of reactions which vary from individual to individual and from time to time in the same individual."

Familiarity with and careful consideration of drug effects in those terms, even when they are legal and socially approved drugs, can help the individual avoid the consequences of drug abuse. All psychoactive substances *are* drugs, and all drugs *can* be dangerous. It is the individual who decides whether or not to take a drug, how much of it to take, and under what conditions.

Summary

"Turn arounders" is an informal term for psychoactive drugs that produce effects unlike those associated with "uppers" and "downers." The "turn arounders" alter the functioning of the central nervous system and the physical state of the mind. They are sometimes called psychedelics or hallucinogens.

Examples include mescaline (from a cactus) and psilocybin (from Mexico's "magic mushrooms"). But the best known is the drug called LSD, or "acid." It's colorless, odorless, tasteless, and has tremendous power to produce great euphoria, heightened sensory perceptions and hallucinations or, more accurately, illusions. Mescaline, LSD, and related drugs are said to expand the mind, the consciousness, but many users have had bad experiences and some have killed themselves. The use of LSD in psychiatric therapy has been controversial, and is now illegal in the U.S.

Marijuana and hashish are considered nonaddictive drugs. Some states have decriminalized marijuana, and now simply issue citations to persons carrying an ounce or less. Possession of more than an ounce of marijuana or any amount of hashish is a felony. Both produce euphoria and heightened perceptions, and both can intensify joy—or depression.

References

p. 170 Carlos Castaneda, *The Teachings of Don Juan: A Yaqui Way of Knowledge* (Berkeley, 1968), pp. 97–98.

p. 171   Edward M. Brecher and *Consumer Reports* Editors, *Licit and Illicit Drugs: The Consumers Union Report on Narcotics, Stimulants, Depressants, Inhalants, and Marijuana—Including Caffeine, Nicotine, and Alcohol* (Boston, 1972), pp. 347–48.

p. 173   Sidney Cohen, "Psychotherapy with LSD: Pro and Con," *The Use of LSD in Psychotherapy and Alcoholism,* ed. Harold A. Abramson (Indianapolis, 1967), pp. 581–82.

p. 173   Ibid.

p. 173   Daniel X. Freedman, "On the Use and Abuse of LSD, " *Archives of General Psychiatry,* No. 18 (March 1968), p. 331.

p. 173   Brecher and *Consumer Reports* Editors, *Licit and Illicit Drugs,* p. 351.

p. 175   William H. McGlothlin and David O. Arnold, "LSD Revisited—A Ten-Year Follow-Up of Medical LSD Use," *Archives of General Psychiatry,* No. 24 (January 1971), pp. 35–49.

p. 175   Ibid.

p. 175   Sidney Cohen, "LSD and the Anguish of Dying," *Harper's,* No. 231 (September 1965), pp. 69–78.

p. 180   I. C. Chopra and R. N. Chopra, "The Use of Cannabis Drugs in India," *United Nations Bulletin on Narcotics,* No. 9 (1957), p. 13.

p. 181   *Interim Report of the Commission of Inquiry into the Non-Medical Use of Drugs* (Ottawa, 1970), p. 85.

p. 182   *Drug Use in America: Problem in Perspective, Second Report of the National Commission on Marihuana and Drug Abuse* (Washington, D.C., 1973), p. 10.

p. 182   Ibid., pp. 10–11.

p. 182   Robert S. de Ropp, *Drugs and the Mind* (New York, 1957), pp. 157–58.

p. 183   Baruch Spinoza (1632–1677), quoted by Joel Fort in *Utopiates: The Use and Users of LSD–25,* ed. Richard Blum et al. (Chicago, 1964), p. 205.

p. 183   August Vollmer, *The Police and Modern Society* (Berkeley, 1936), pp. 117–18.

p. 184   Jerome H. Jaffe, *The Pharmacological Basis of Therapeutics,* 3rd ed., ed. Louis S. Goodman and Alfred Gilman (New York, 1965), pp. 292–93.

p. 184   de Ropp, *Drugs and the Mind,* p. 157.

p. 185   *Drug Use in America, p. 23.*

PART V
The
Communicable
Diseases

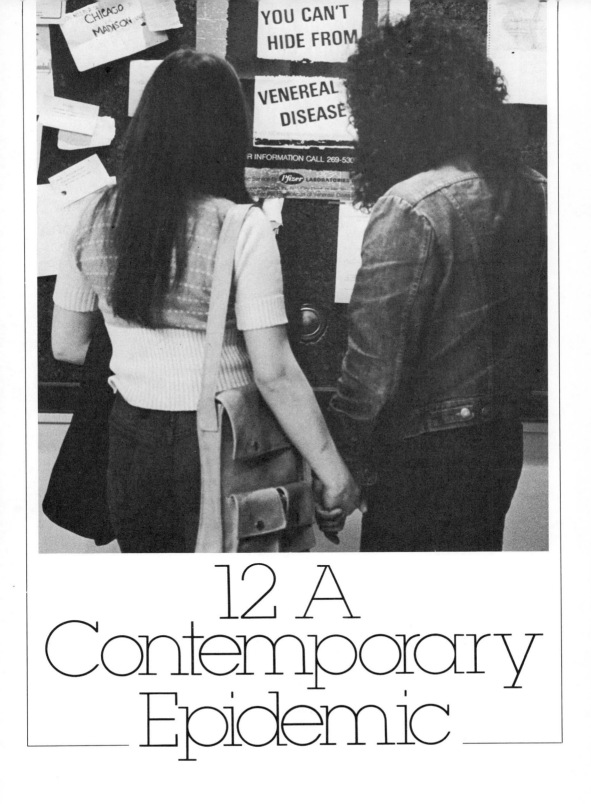

12 A Contemporary Epidemic

It's Monday morning in the dormitory. Leonard drapes a towel over one shoulder, shuffles sleepily to the lavatory, approaches a urinal. In the next second he is wide awake, startled by unexpected pain. Back in the privacy of his room, Leonard conducts a rudimentary examination. A drop of thick, yellowish pus oozes from his urethra, the urinary canal. Later, at a clinic, a smear containing some of the urethral pus is placed under a microscope. Beneath the lens, several pairs of globular shapes come into focus. A doctor is viewing some of the countless microorganisms, or microbes (from the Greek *mikros,* small, and *bios,* life), that share our environment—billions of which, indeed, make our bodies *their* environment.

The difficult task is to identify the particular kind of organism whose privacy has been violated by the user of the microscope. An incredible variety of living things, most of them invisible to the naked eye, many too small to be seen under an ordinary microscope, infest the air, the earth, our skin, and other parts of our bodies. Usually, we are unaware of their presence because we live in ecological harmony with most of them, most of the time. For example, certain kinds of organisms that live in human intestines help with digestion and so are actually beneficial. But some are dangerous.

What have we here? A *bacterium?* It's too large to be a *virus.* A *fungus?* A *protozoan?* There are hundreds, perhaps thousands, of different kinds of parasites that may take up residence in our bodies. The word *parasite* (from the Greek *para,* beside, and *sitos,* corn, bread, food) referred originally to a person who frequented another's table and offered nothing in return. Microbial parasites, or germs, come in many shapes and sizes. Each variety has its peculiarities. Some abuse our hospitality in the worst way. Leonard's pain and the pus, for example, are evidence that these beings now being examined under the microscope have violently attacked their host, invading and damaging his body cells. The entry of the microbes into his body was an *infection.* The damaging result is *disease,* literally dis-ease.

After certain tests, the doctor recognizes Leonard's attackers. Their kind has been identified with wearisome frequency by this doctor. Leonard has become another link in a biological chain, stretching back through the ages, of people who have been infected by *gonococcus,* the bacterium that causes gonorrhea.

The Mobile Microbes

The gonococcus has shared a most intimate relationship with humankind since ancient times. The disease it causes was given its name by the Greek physician Galen (130–200 A.D.), who called it gonorrhea (from the Greek *gonos,* seed, and *rheein,* to flow) out of an understandable confusion. To Galen, the pus that commonly flows from the urethra of the male victim looked like semen, the male seed.

Through the centuries the gonococcus has been responsible for untold human suffering, both physical and emotional, as well as some of history's oldest jokes. It has killed some, crippled many, embarrassed millions, destroyed marriages, and precipitated murders. It has ignited vast public health campaigns, employing thousands of people in unavailing efforts to stamp it out. The peculiar relationships between the gonococcus, as part of the environment, and the human body, the victim's emotions, and society make this microbe an apt focus for a study of communicable disease.

A disease is described as *communicable,* or *contagious* (from the Latin *con-,* together, and *tangere,* to touch), when the organism that causes it can be transmitted— or communicated—from one person to another. Someone coughs, expelling droplets of moisture, aswarm with viruses, into the air. You inhale. The viruses enter your respiratory tract. You are infected. If you develop the familiar symptoms, you say you have ''caught'' a cold. In fact, you have contracted a communicable disease.

Microbes may enter the body in other ways as well: through breaks in the skin, or in the food we eat. Each kind of microbe has its own environmental requirements and method of operation. Some can thrive almost anywhere—on a dirty sidewalk, on a shoe, or on an unfastidious waiter's finger. Others can survive only in a very special kind of environment and die quickly if they are removed from it. The gonococcus is one of these. It lives only in the bodies of humans making itself at home in the warm, moist mucus membranes that line the urethra, vagina, cervix, rectum, and, not infrequently, the throat. If left, somehow, on a toilet seat, washcloth, or doorknob, the gonococcus dies almost immediately and is harmless. But it can migrate from one person to another when their respective mucus membranes come into direct contact. So, in virtually every case, gonorrhea is transmitted during sexual intercourse. That is why it is called a sexually transmitted disease (abbreviated here to STD) or a venereal disease (VD), referring to Venus, the Roman goddess of love.

The Gonorrhea Epidemic

When unusually large numbers of people in a given population are infected with a communicable disease, an *epidemic* (from the Greek *epi,* among, and *demos,* the people) is said to exist. Influenza epidemics break out in parts of this country every two years or so. One person infects half a dozen others, who each infect half a hundred, and so on in a rapidly widening circle of illness until the outbreak runs its course or is brought under control by public health measures. Most epidemics are short-lived. Not so for the tenacious gonococcus. Beginning with the dawn of the 1960s, there was an explosive increase in the number of gonococcal infections throughout the United States. Authorities agree that the disease reached epidemic proportions before the end of that decade, and was still spreading at a furious pace in the mid-1970s.

In 1960, 246,697 new cases of gonorrhea were reported to public health officials across the country. In 1974, 999,937 new cases were reported. But that was only a fraction of the actual number. Doctors are required by law to report every new case of gonorrhea to the authorities, so that the patients' sexual contacts—and *their* contacts, and so on—can be located and treated, in hopes of preventing them from infecting still

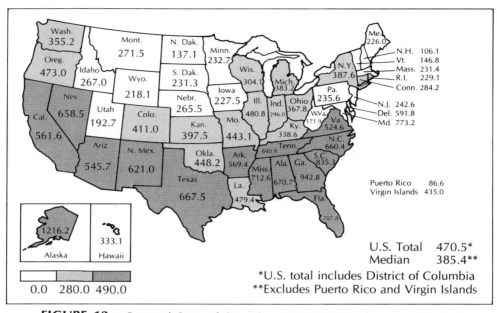

FIGURE 12-a *Reported Cases of Gonorrhea per 100,000 Population by State, Calendar Year 1976.*
Source: Morbidity and Mortality Report, Annual Summary (Atlanta: Center For Disease Control, 1977).

others. Such contact tracing is supposed to be carried on under strict rules protecting the privacy of everyone concerned. But many doctors, possibly concerned about the confidentiality of physician-patient relationships, fail to make the reports. In 1974 public health officials made "conservative" estimates that the true number of new cases had exceeded *two million annually* since 1970. Among communicable diseases, only common colds outnumbered the cases of gonorrhea in this country.

Until the 1960s gonorrhea had been regarded as a relatively minor problem so far as the general population was concerned. Its incidence had dropped sharply after the Second World War, when penicillin made its appearance on the medical scene. A shot of penicillin was a quick cure in almost every case. The disease, some thought, was on its way to extinction. What happened?

Sexual Freedom and STD

At a 1974 doctors' conference on gonococcal infections, one of the participating specialists reported: " . . . Young adults between the ages of 15 and 29 are at greatest risk of contracting gonorrhea. Their permissiveness and casual attitude about venereal disease contribute to the problem. . . ."

TABLE 12-1 Reported Cases of Gonorrhea in the United States, 1975–1976*

Age Group	Male 1975 Cases	Rate	Male 1976 Cases	Rate	Female 1975 Cases	Rate	Female 1976 Cases	Rate	Total 1975 Cases	Rate	Total 1976 Cases	Rate
0–14	2,980	10.9	2,978	11.1	9,442	35.9	8,889	34.6	12,422	23.2	11,867	22.6
15–19	115,504	1,121.5	110,760	1,061.5	151,109	1,462.4	150,740	1,445.8	266,613	1,292.2	261,500	1,253.6
20–24	236,561	2,659.8	234,910	2,574.1	155,196	1,631.4	154,656	1,596.4	391,757	2,128.3	389,566	2,070.6
25–29	135,132	1,674.7	138,854	1,635.7	57,424	676.1	59,008	661.7	192,556	1,162.6	197,862	1,136.7
30–39	77,214	635.0	81,263	653.4	25,819	198.3	25,266	190.2	103,033	409.2	106,529	414.2
40–49	19,022	171.6	20,005	181.8	4,998	42.4	4,863	41.6	24,020	105.1	24,868	109.6
50+	7,341	30.3	7,843	31.9	2,195	7.4	1,959	6.5	9,536	17.6	9,802	17.8
TOTAL	593,754	581.3	596,613	579.9	406,183	371.6	405,381	368.2	999,937	472.9	1,001,994	470.5

*Figures are per 100,000 population.
Source: *Morbidity and Mortality Report, Annual Summary* (Atlanta: Center for Disease Control, 1977).

How permissive are today's young people? Certainly, a great deal has been said and written about the new sexual freedom. Since its advent was proclaimed in the 1960s, the sexual revolution has been explored by newspapers and popular magazines to the point of satiety. And, clearly, young people (and a lot of older ones) are more publicly candid about their sexuality than people were twenty years ago. But is sexual promiscuity rampant? The question is arguable. One textbook analysis of assorted studies of sexual activity among college students concluded that "there is considerable reason to question seriously the highly advertised notion that premarital sexual intercourse without commitment is more prevalent than formerly, that it is occurring with greater frequency among those who do practice it, and that promiscuous sexual behavior without rules is the way of life among young people today."

Nevertheless, those same studies confirm, in case there was any doubt, that a great many college students are sexually active. And the various revolutions, sexual and otherwise, of the 1960s and the early 1970s didn't all take place on college campuses. Many of the social phenomena of that era manifested themselves in the streets of San Francisco's Haight-Ashbury and New York's East Village, which were gathering places for those seeking the new freedom. Thousands of dropouts and runaways in their teens and early twenties wandered the streets. They floated from commune to crash pad; they smoked, swallowed, or injected whatever drugs were available; they paid little attention to personal hygiene, and spread gonorrhea like wildfire from one casual bed partner to the next. Whether it was because of ignorance, drug-induced euphoria, or aversion to establishment medicine, many never sought treatment. In Boston, a physician who helped run a mobile medical unit that offered aid to the young street people told a colleague that those who contracted gonorrhea "tend to think it's nothing more than a cold in the penis and laugh it off."

The search for the new freedom involved, among other things, mobility. Hitchhikers formed clusters at freeway ramps. Vans and buses equipped for sleeping, cooking, and socializing roved the interstate highways, Denver this week, Los Angeles the next. And it was not only the dropouts who were on the move; vacationing students, young people from all strata of society, hit the trail. There was much mingling. Many spent a summer traveling around the country and then went back to their middle-class homes. Many of the street people themselves tired of the lifestyle and returned to the suburbs. How much all that may have contributed to the spread of gonorrhea throughout the country has not been established, but it certainly provided some ideal conditions for an epidemic.

Gonococcus versus Penicillin

The decade of the 1960s was remarkable in many ways. There were tremendous social upheavals, widespread changes in personal lifestyles, and fantastic technological strides. There were also changes at the microbial level.

Whether through old-fashioned evolutionary survival of the fittest or through mutation, a tougher breed of gonococci appeared. The new ones were resistant to the

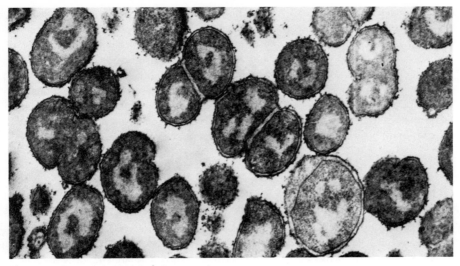

Electron micrograph of Neisseria gonorrhoeae.

effects of penicillin. The relatively mild doses that formerly cured nearly every case of gonorrhea no longer did the job. Some particularly hardy gonococci turned up halfway around the world, in Vietnam. By 1970, according to one report, 20 to 25 percent of the American soldiers in Vietnam had venereal disease, in most cases gonorrhea. Black market penicillin was easily available there, and many of the soldiers treated themselves—ineffectively. Inadequate doses of penicillin immunized the microbes instead of killing them. As a result, some of the veterans came home carrying penicillin-resistant strains of gonococci.

While tetracyclines and other antibiotics were used as substitute treatments—and the gonococci began to develop resistance to them, too—penicillin remained the most effective treatment. But larger and larger doses were required. Whereas 160,000 units of penicillin were more than adequate to cure almost any case of gonorrhea in the 1940s, the recommended dosage had risen by 1974 to 4.8 million units—a dosage so large that doctors took to dividing the dosage into halves and giving the patient a shot in each buttock.

"As gonococcal antibiotic resistance continues," one specialist wrote in mid-1974, "conventional therapy will no longer be effective."

Birth Control and STD

Still another development that may have made life easier for the gonococcus was the availability of birth control pills, which became the favored method of contraception in the 1960s. Before the popular acceptance of the pills, the most commonly used contraceptives were the condom and the diaphragm, the latter widely used in combination with sperm-killing jellies or foams. While far from foolproof, the physical barrier provided by the condom does offer considerable protection against the transfer of microbes. And the spermatocidal jellies and foams also tend to kill at least some gonococci and other germs likely to be transmitted during intercourse.

However, hormones in birth control pills cause changes in vaginal secretions that, it appears, actually help gonococci survive. So people who rely on pills, while less likely to be confronted by unplanned pregnancies, may be more susceptible to venereal diseases than those who favor the older methods of contraception.

The Hidden Microbes

Almost everything seems to favor the proliferation of the gonococci, including their own secretive ways. Leonard, the account of whose urethral drip opened this chapter, had a case that was easily diagnosed. Many other cases are not. In a large majority of females who are infected, and in a substantial percentage of males, the gonococcus causes no symptoms, in no way betrays its presence—at least in the early stages of the infection. Furthermore, "The laboratory diagnosis of gonorrhea is a difficult procedure, and the best available methods detect only about 50 to 75 percent of infections," a microbiologist reported at a 1974 medical conference.

There is no way to tell, then, just how many people may have gonorrhea without knowing or even suspecting it. Estimates run to many hundreds of thousands. And those people are capable of infecting others.

STD and Emotions

"Tell me, please, will my parents find out I was here?" The anxious young patient was questioning a doctor at a venereal disease clinic in New York City. It was not an unfamiliar question.

> Often couples come for a checkup together; not so much, it seems, for treatment as to find out who infected whom. . . .
> "You better tell him that I don't have it! He won't believe me!" a girl with a black eye implores.
> And I tell him. (Sometimes I lie.)

Will my parents, my wife, my boyfriend find out? Who gave it to whom? Anxiety, jealousy, guilt—the emotional problems stirred up by the gonococcus and its ilk are endless. Everyone who has venereal disease got it from someone else, and everyone knows how. Sexual revolution or no, the possibility that A might learn that B has become sexually active, or that C might discover that D has had sexual intercourse with someone besides C may seem more terrifying to the gonorrhea victim than the disease itself. B may avoid seeking treatment at all, risking serious complications. D may decide not to tell C about the symptoms that have appeared. And C, who also hasn't told D about a relationship with E, may become one of those asymptomatic carriers who unknowingly spreads the infection. And so it all meshes—microbes, people, emotions, society—and an epidemic grows.

The Effects of Gonorrhea

As the 1970s passed their midpoint, the gonorrhea epidemic showed no signs of abating. Just what is this stubborn disease? What does it do to people? In many cases, there are few ill effects, especially if the disease is diagnosed and treated early. In many others, however, gonorrhea is much more serious than just "a cold in the penis."

In Males

In a majority of cases, the gonococcus announces its presence about two days to two weeks after its arrival. The usual symptoms are a sometimes severe burning sensation during urination and a discharge of pus (the drip) from the urethra. If untreated, the disease may spread through the reproductive system, including the prostate gland, causing painful inflammation. This inflammation may lead ultimately to sterility. In a significant number of cases, gonorrhea becomes *systemic,* that is, it enters the bloodstream or lymph channels and spreads to other parts of the body. The most common result of that development is *gonococcal arthritis,* which can cause serious damage to joints. Less commonly, the liver, the heart, or the membrane covering the central nervous system may become infected.

In Females

Although gonorrhea usually produces no early symptoms in females, some are alerted by a urethral discharge and a burning during urination. Those who do not receive treatment may develop any of the systemic complications mentioned in the preceding paragraph, as well as those involving the female reproductive organs. In many cases, untreated females develop acute infections of the uterus, Fallopian tubes, and ovaries. Low abdominal pain and fever result. Sometimes the lining of the abdominal cavity becomes inflamed. Occasionally the symptoms may become so severe that they simulate acute appendicitis. Abscesses frequently scar the Fallopian tubes and ovaries. Surgery may be required to repair the damage, though often it can't be repaired. Gonorrhea has been described as "the leading preventable cause of sterility in women."

In pregnant women the gonococcus may be involved in such complications as premature birth. And, although gonorrhea does not infect babies while they are in the womb, they may become infected by direct contact while passing through the cervix and vagina during birth. Formerly, many infants were blinded by such infections. Now state law requires that every newborn baby receive silver nitrate in its eyes, and cases of infants blinded by gonorrhea are rare. However, babies may still receive gonococcal infections of the genitals, rectum, or mouth during birth.

In adults, gonococcal infections of the rectum and throat have become increasingly common. Rectal gonorrhea occurs with particular frequency among male homosexuals. *Gonococcal pharyngitis* (infection of the mucous membrane in the throat) results most often from oral-penile, and less often from oral-vaginal, contact. Gonorrhea is rarely, if ever, transmitted by mouth-to-mouth kissing.

More Sexually Transmitted Microbes

The gonococcus is just one of the disease-causing microbes whose environmental preferences make indiscriminate sexual activity a kind of Russian roulette. Other sexually transmitted infections are caused by an assortment of bacteria, viruses, protozoa, fungi, and other microorganisms.

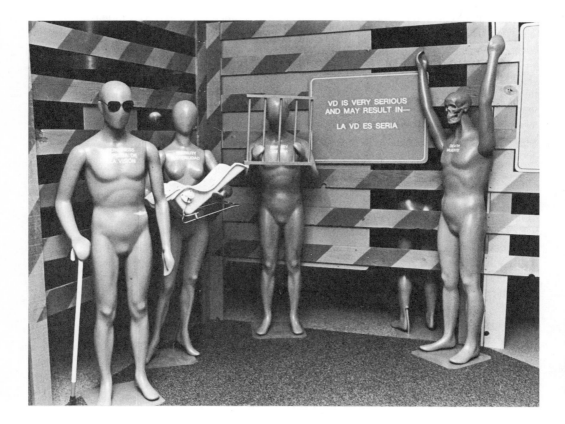

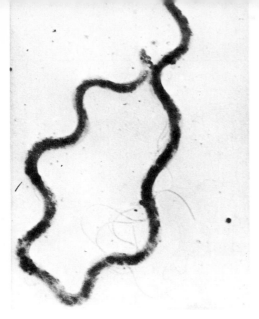

The spirochete that causes syphilis.

Syphilis

A *spirochete,* or corkscrew-shaped bacterium, called *Treponema pallidum* is responsible for syphilis. Although less common than gonorrhea, syphilis is the most dangerous of the venereal diseases. And it, too, began to appear with increasing frequency in the 1970s. In 1974, 25,561 new cases were reported to public health authorities in the United States. How many more cases went unreported is, of course, unknown.

The first sign of syphilis may be a painless *chancre,* or sore, at the point of infection. In males it is most often on the penis. In females it may be inside the body, and it therefore may go unnoticed. Or there may be no chancre at all. If there is one, it disappears without treatment after some days or weeks. Weeks or months later, secondary symptoms may (or may not) appear—sores on the body, a fever, sometimes a rash. Those, too, go away, and the disease becomes latent. It may cause no further trouble, but in many victims it does cause trouble, years later. It can damage the bones, the liver, and other organs; it can cause heart failure, paralysis, brain damage, blindness. Unlike gonorrhea, syphilis can infect a baby in the womb. In some cases, syphilis can be transmitted mouth-to-mouth, as well as by other sexual contact.

Treatment of Syphilis

Syphilis can be treated effectively with penicillin and other antibiotics, although in the early 1970s the spirochete began showing signs that it, like the gonococcus, was becoming resistant to penicillin.

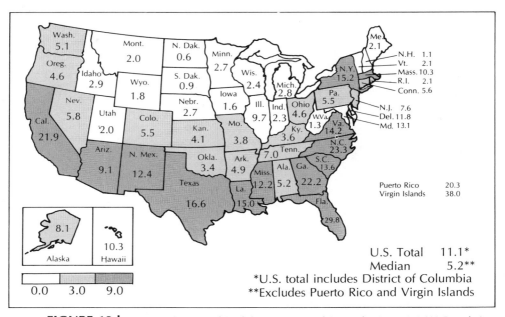

FIGURE 12-b *Reported Cases of Syphilis (Primary and Secondary) per 100,000 Population by State, Calendar Year 1976.*
Source: Morbidity and Mortality Report, Annual Summary (Atlanta: Center For Disease Control, 1977).

Other Sexually Transmitted Diseases

Chancroid and *granuloma inguinale,* both caused by bacteria, and *lymphogranuloma venereum,* caused by an organism classified somewhere between a bacterium and a virus, are venereal diseases that are common in tropical and subtropical climes. They are encountered infrequently in most parts of the United States.

Usually not dangerous, but frequently quite painful or irritating, are a number of other venereal infections that are common throughout this country. *Trichomoniasis* is caused by a protozoan, a one-celled animal with a whiplike tail. *Moniliasis,* also known by other names including *thrush,* is a fungus (yeast) infection. A type of *herpes* virus, related to the kind that causes cold sores around the mouth, is responsible for some infections of the genitals and surrounding areas. Another kind of virus causes *genital warts. Nonspecific urethritis,* a mild infection of the urethra, is transmitted by some as yet unidentified microbe or microbes.

Such infections—all sexually communicable—produce a variety of symptoms that may include discharges of pus, burning or itching, sores on, in, or around the genitals and sometimes on the thighs and buttocks, fever, swollen lymph nodes, and other manifestations. Sometimes the symptoms mimic those of gonorrhea or syphilis. Attempts at self-diagnosis are unwise. *Any* unusual symptoms call for medical attention.

Finally, leaving the world of the microbes for the moment, there are still other organisms that commonly migrate from one person to another during sexual contact. One is a mite, a tiny insect, that burrows into the skin and causes *scabies,* an infuriating itch that may spread all over the body. And then there is the *pubic louse,* or "crab," that often travels from the pubic region to armpits, chest hair, beards, mustaches, and even eyebrows. Proper medication and scrupulous cleanliness will dispose of these pests. Both, incidentally, can sometimes be picked up through nonsexual contacts. A person *can* get crabs from a toilet seat.

Preventing Sexually Transmitted Disease

Two or more people who confine their sexual activities exclusively to each other are presumably safe from venereal disease, *if* the relationship remains exclusive, and *if* no one involved was infected—asymptomatically or otherwise—before it began.

For those who are sexually active, there is no certain way of avoiding venereal infections. There are no vaccines that will prevent gonorrhea or syphilis and no prospects that any will be developed in the near future.

As mentioned earlier, the condom and spermatocidal jellies and foams provide some protection. Thorough washing of the male genitals after coitus may be helpful. There is some question about the advisability of postcoital douching for females, since it may only reduce the acidity of vaginal fluids and provide an even more favorable environment for infectious microbes.

A shot of penicillin or one of the other antibiotics before or after sexual intercourse might help prevent infection, but it might also have undesired results. In addition to contributing to the gonococcus's increasing resistance to antibiotics, indiscriminate use of antibiotics can lead to serious allergic reactions in some people.

Unlike measles and some other diseases, gonorrhea and syphilis do not produce future immunity in those who have been infected. The same person can be infected over and over again. It isn't unusual for an individual to get cured and then reinfected by the same person who passed on the first infection. Unless everyone who has been exposed is contacted and treated, whether or not there are any symptoms, the disease is likely to go on and on. As that doctor in the New York clinic wrote:

> The patients come in a constant flow. Some have syphilis, some gonorrhea, some have both. But it seems only accidental: if it weren't for a chain of coincidences, they wouldn't be here; they would not have been contaminated. . . .
>
> As a general rule they blame someone for "giving it" to them. He blames her, she blames him. . . .
>
> It seems that no one can be blamed personally, individually. Often three or four persons are involved, and it becomes a circle. . . .
>
> This vicious circle can be broken only by an absolute stop, a radical abstention (besides penicillin), a six-week moratorium for everyone involved. How clear seem to me the scientific and beneficial implications of Lent! And yet a doctor is reluctant to speak about abstention. It sounds moralistic.

TABLE 12-2 Reported Cases of Primary and Secondary Syphilis in the United States, 1975–1976*

Age Group	Male				Female				Total			
	1975		1976		1975		1976		1975		1976	
	Cases	Rate	Cases	Rate	Cases	Rate	Cases	Rate	Cases	Rate	Cases	Rate
0–14	82	0.3	71	0.3	164	0.6	139	0.5	246	0.5	210	0.4
15–19	1,886	18.3	1,890	18.1	1,833	17.7	1,714	16.4	3,719	18.0	3,604	17.3
20–24	5,063	56.9	4,648	50.9	2,263	23.8	1,947	20.1	7,326	39.8	6,595	35.1
25–29	4,341	53.8	4,233	49.9	1,272	15.0	1,204	13.5	5,613	33.9	5,437	31.2
30–39	4,556	37.5	4,230	34.0	1,103	8.5	924	7.0	5,659	22.5	5,154	20.0
40–49	1,822	16.4	1,547	14.1	394	3.4	373	3.2	2,216	9.7	1,920	8.5
50+	679	2.8	682	2.8	103	0.3	129	0.4	782	1.4	811	1.5
TOTAL	18,429	18.0	17,301	16.8	7,132	6.5	6,430	5.8	25,561	12.1	23,731	11.1

*Figures are per 100,000 population.
Source: Morbidity and Mortality Report, Annual Summary (Atlanta: Center for Disease Control, 1977).

Other Types of Venereal Disease

In addition to the reported cases of syphilis and gonorrhea during 1976 in the United States (see Tables 12-1, 12-2), there were also 300,000 reported cases of herpes simplex virus–2; 2.5 million cases of nongonococcal urethritis; and 3 million cases of trichomoniasis. Herpes simplex virus–2 is the first venereal disease to be identified as a probable cause of cancer in women. A woman with herpes–2 is eight times more likely to develop cancer of the cervix than the woman who has not had the infection. Six percent of the women who contract HSV–2 of the cervix develop cervical cancer, and for a pregnant woman with HSV–2, there is one chance in four that her newborn child will be seriously damaged or will die.

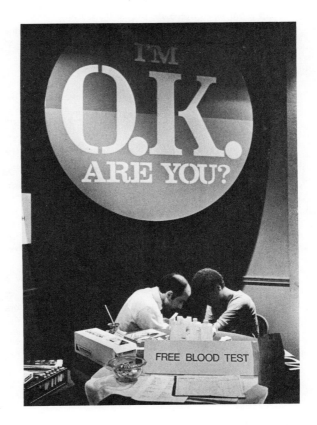

Summary

We share our environment with many different kinds of microorganisms, or microbes. Some of them cause disease. When a disease-causing microbe can be transmitted from one person to another, the disease is described as communicable or contagious.

Organisms that cause communicable diseases thrive in different kinds of environments and can enter the human body in different ways. Some survive best in the mucus membrane lining the urethra, vagina, cervix, rectum, and mouth. These include the gonococcus, a bacterium that causes gonorrhea. It is a venereal disease—meaning it is transmitted during sexual intercourse.

An epidemic of gonorrhea began spreading throughout the United States in the 1960s and continued in the 1970s. A variety of social and other factors may be involved. The spread of the disease is difficult to control, partially because the gonococcus is becoming increasingly resistant to penicillin and other antibiotics.

Gonorrhea can have serious complications. So can some other venereal diseases, especially syphilis. For sexually active people, there is no certain way of avoiding infection, although there are precautions that provide some protection. Contacting and treating everyone who has been exposed to venereal disease is the only way to stop its spreading.

References

p. 192 Thomas F. Keys, "Gonococcal Infections," *The Western Journal of Medicine,* Vol. 120, No. 6 (June 1974), pp. 459–61.

p. 192 Stewart M. Brooks, *The V.D. Story* (Cranbury, N.J., 1971), p. 14.

p. 192 Keys, "Gonococcal Infections," pp. 459–61.

p. 194 Benjamin A. Kogan, *Health: Man in a Changing Environment,* 2nd. ed. (New York, 1974), p. 447.

p. 194 John W. Grover, *VD: The ABCs* (Englewood Cliffs, N.J., 1971), p. 26.

p. 195 Keys, "Gonococcal Infections," pp. 459–61.

p. 195 Keys, "Gonococcal Antibiotic Resistance in Los Angeles," *The Western Journal of Medicine,* Vol. 120, No. 6 (June 1974), pp. 452–55.

p. 196 Robert N. Yoshimori, "Gonococcal Infection," *The Western Journal of Medicine,* Vol. 120, No. 6 (June 1974), pp. 456–58.

p. 196 Basile Yanovsky, *The Dark Fields of Venus* (New York, 1973), p. 23.

p. 196 Ibid., p. 15.

p. 197 Grover, *VD,* p. 52.

p. 202 Yanovsky, *The Dark Fields of Venus,* p. 219.

p. 202 Ibid., p. 73.

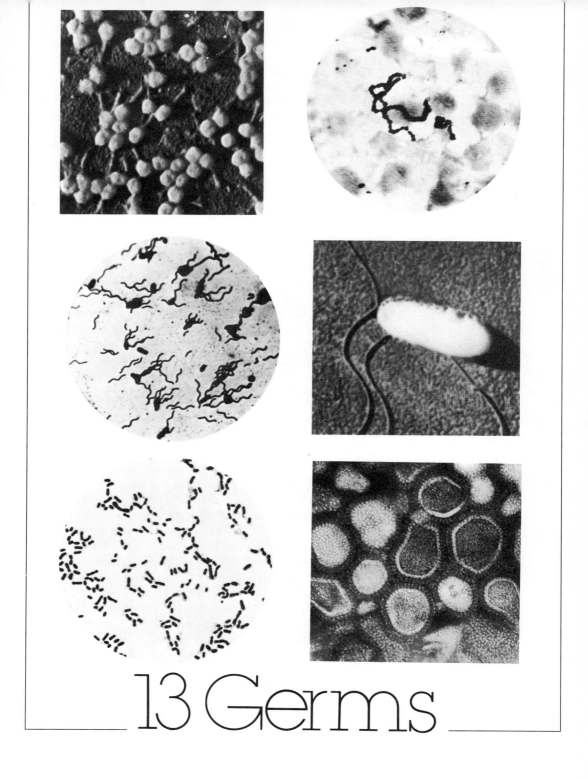

13 Germs

Eighteenth-century physicians used to speak metaphorically of the *germ* of a disease. The word, from the Latin *germen,* a sprout, implied the existence of some unknown seed from which illness sprouted, as it does from poison ivy. The old-time doctors also thought of disease as being caused by some kind of *virus,* the Latin word for poison. Later, when it was established that certain microscopic organisms caused many diseases, the microorganisms or microbes (Greek *mikros,* small, and *bios,* life) were called germs.

There are many different kinds of microbes. For some of them, the word germ seems particularly appropriate because they are, in fact, tiny vegetables. These include the *fungi* (Latin for mushrooms), such as those that cause athlete's foot. Also usually classified as vegetables are the *bacteria* (from the Greek *bakterion,* a little stick). Some bacteria are cylindrical, like sticks, while others are spherical, and still others are shaped like corkscrews. *Protozoa* (from the Greek *protos,* first, and *zoion,* animal) are another kind of microbe—among them are those that cause malaria. They are one-celled animals, presumably much like the first animals on earth. The word *virus* has been attached to the smallest and oddest of the germs. The virus seems to be neither vegetable nor animal; it is a kind of borderline microbe between animate and inanimate matter.

Countless germs of all kinds, invisible to the naked eye, share our environment. They infest the air, the earth, even the nuclei of some raindrops. Indeed, billions of them make our bodies *their* environment. Usually, we are unaware of their presence.

Infection and Resistance

Germs can get into our bodies through openings created by wounds, such as cut fingers or scratches caused by fingernails; they can be passed from person to person. Sneezes spray germ-laden droplets into the air we breathe. Contaminated fingers sometimes transfer germs to food. A hand used to stifle a cough lifts a telephone receiver; the next caller picks up germs along with the receiver. Casual sexual intercourse may pass *gonococci* (see Chapter 12) from one partner to another. Diseases spread in such ways have already been described as *communicable* or *contagious* (see p. 191). Fortunately, only certain kinds of germs cause disease, and only under certain conditions.

Different kinds of germs thrive in different environments. Some are harmless when swallowed but can cause trouble if they are in an open wound. Some can penetrate the tough mucus membranes lining our inner passages; others can't. *Infection* occurs when microbes take up residence in the body under environmental conditions that favor the development of disease. Whether or not the infection results in disease depends on the *virulence,* or disease-causing potential, of the particular germs, and on the *resistance* of the individual body.

The term *resistance* refers to the efficiency of the body's natural disease-fighting mechanisms. The degree of resistance varies among individuals and in the same person at different times. High resistance is usually associated with general good health.

Resistance may be lowered by excessive stress as a result of poor nutrition, fatigue, or other physical or psychological factors. Resistance tends to be relatively low in infants, old people, and people who have chronic diseases.

Evidence of the body's disease-fighting systems in action can be seen when bacteria get into a cut or an abrasion. The area around the injury becomes red, swollen, and painful. This is *inflammation.* It is not caused directly by the germs, but by the body's reaction to injury. Among other things, tissue swells and new tissue forms, creating a physical barrier against the microbial invaders. At the same time, in a separate reaction, white blood cells attack the germs. This is the *immune response.* The pus that forms is the debris of battle, containing microscopic corpses of white blood cells and vanquished bacteria.

A Viral Invasion

Germs attack the body in different ways. Some bacteria break down the walls of cells. Other bacteria, such as those that cause tetanus and diphtheria, release *toxins*— poisonous chemicals. The viruses, much smaller than bacteria, are also more difficult to detect. Consider, for example, the common cold.

A virus, transported perhaps on a wayward fingertip, arrives in the nostril of an unsuspecting human. Its arrival goes unnoticed, the virus being an entity so small that it is invisible under the most powerful optical microscope—an electron microscope, enlarging the image to hundreds of thousands of times its actual size, gives us but a hazy view of the virus. What we have here in this enormously magnified image is a very strange thing. Learned people earnestly debate the question: Can or cannot a virus properly be regarded as a living being? All it seems to consist of is a minute speck of crystalline nucleic acid encased in a dab of protein—it is a tiny blob. Isolated, the virus shows no signs of life. It doesn't move or eat or reproduce. When the virus is placed amid living tissue, however, things begin to happen. The virus finds or creates an opening in the wall of a cell, and then insinuates itself into the cell's interior. From the viewpoint of the virus, the cell is quite a large structure housing a number of smaller structures.

To make any sense of the astonishing event that next takes place, we need to know a little bit about the nucleic acids of which viruses are largely composed.

The Genetic Code

Deoxyribonucleic acid (DNA) is what genes are made of; it is the structural material of the chromosomes in the nucleus of every cell. It carries in its molecular structure the genetic code—the chemical script that tells each member of each new generation how to grow a body. DNA determines, among thousands of other details, the colors of eyes and the shapes of noses and whether a person will be tall and skinny or short and plump. We don't know yet exactly how all that works. We do know, though, that every living thing, plant or animal, has DNA in the nucleus of its cells and that the DNA of every living thing is made up of the same four building blocks, molecules called nucleotides. It is the number of nucleotides and the order in which they are arranged along the strands of DNA that determine whether an organism will be a human or, for instance, an artichoke.

Ribonucleic acid (RNA) performs a number of functions in the cells, including the transmission of instructions from the genes to the ribosomes, which are cellular workshops where the many different products that keep the organism operating and in good repair are fabricated. Inside its protein sheath, each virus is composed entirely of either DNA or RNA, never both. The particular virus we are concerned with, the one we left infiltrating a cell in someone's nostril, is of the DNA variety.

Now comes the astonishing part.

Viral Replication

Once inside the cell, the virus sheds its protein coating, bares its DNA, and starts giving orders, so to speak, passing its own genetic instructions (a complex chemical process) to the cell's RNA for transmission to the ribosomes. If it were an RNA virus, it would operate somewhat differently, but the final result would be the same.

A ribosome has just finished manufacturing, say, a bit of protein to be used as part of the material for constructing a new cell. Another order arrives. The ribosome obediently assembles . . . a *virus*. That's right. The virus which slipped in through the wall has put its host cell to work manufacturing more viruses. One by one they emerge from the ribosomes, each an exact replica of the original, complete with protein coating. It is as though some secret agent had inserted a new program into the computer in charge of an automated assembly line, causing a Chevrolet factory to start turning out robot soldiers.

For a while, there is confusion. The cell's own DNA is still issuing instructions, too, and the ribosomes are filling orders from first one source, then the other, working overtime. The cell is filling up with a variety of products, including a large number of viruses. Finally, there is no more room. The cell walls burst open, and the newly

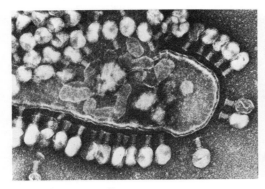

Virus attacking a cell.

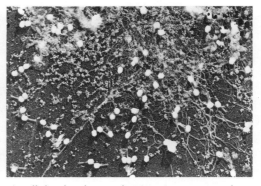

A cell that has burst releasing viruses created in the old cell.

manufactured viruses come out, each potentially capable of infiltrating and taking over another cell, making that cell build more viruses, and so on. Soon, at another level of reality, the owner of the invaded nostril is seized with a sudden impulse to sneeze.

The Body's Response

A sneeze. The beginning of a cold. The viruses are spreading out, attacking more cells. Some *lymphocytes*—white blood cells—drift by. Then one lymphocyte stops. If lymphocytes had noses, we might imagine this one sniffing inquisitively, as though it had detected a familiar scent. It has, in fact, sensed the presence of the one particular *antigen* for which it has been waiting all its life.

An antigen (antibody generator) is a certain molecular configuration on the surface of a body such as a bacterium or a virus. There are hundreds of different kinds of viruses, and each kind has its own unique antigen, a sort of molecular signature. Lymphocytes of a certain type are equipped with molecular configurations called *receptors*. The receptor of each lymphocyte is a perfect match, atom for atom, for one and only one antigen.

> Lymphocytes, like wasps, are genetically programmed for exploration, but each of them seems to be permitted a different, solitary idea. They roam through the tissues, sensing and monitoring. Since there are so many of them, they can make collective guesses at almost anything antigenic on the surface of the earth, but they must do their work one notion at a time. They carry specific information in their surface receptors, presented in the form of a question: is there, anywhere out there, my particular molecular configuration? . . .
>
> Lymphocytes are apparently informed about everything foreign around them, and some of them come equipped for fitting with polymers that do not exist until organic chemists synthesize them in their laboratories. The cells can do more than predict reality; they are evidently programmed with wild guesses as well. . . .
>
> When the connection is made, and a particular lymphocyte with a particular receptor is brought into the presence of the particular antigen, one of the greatest small spectacles in nature occurs. The cell enlarges, begins making DNA at a great rate, and turns into what is termed, appropriately, a blast. It then begins dividing, replicating itself into a new colony of identical cells, all labeled with the same receptor, primed with the same question.

We have, by now, quite a mob scene. First there were all those newly assembled viruses, each wearing the distinctive antigen inherited from the original virus that was deposited in a nostril several pages back. Then came the lymphocyte, which swelled up and divided itself into two new cells, called *plasma cells*. These cells then divided themselves into four, then eight, and so on until a swarm of lymphocyte offspring is crowded around the viruses. Now another odd thing happens.

The plasma cells begin releasing *antibodies,* little bits of protein that, one by one, attach themselves to the viruses. Each of the antibodies carries on its surface a receptor that is a perfect match for the viral antigen. Receptor meets antigen, molecules mesh, and antibody and virus become solidly locked together, a single entity bound by molecular ties. The virus is neutralized for good.

Meanwhile, the body has brought other weapons into play. There are other lymphocytes, a different kind, that do not produce antibodies; instead, they engulf the viruses, swallow them up, and digest them. Infected, dying cells release chemicals that block the advance of the viruses. Other chemicals, histamines and the like, cause blood vessels to dilate, and more blood rushes to the scene, bringing emergency supplies of oxygen and nutrients to the embattled cells. Some blood fluid leaks into surrounding tissue, and the nose, which is the scene of conflict, swells and reddens. Mucus flows, capturing viruses in a gluey stream, and irritated cells produce a reaction that expels viruses along with mucus—a sneeze.

Sniffling, red-nosed, stuffed-up, bleary-eyed, a miserable human goes to bed. By morning the cold is better. Within a few days it is gone. The body has healed itself.

Complications

The scenario just unfolded is typical of the way the body defends itself against all kinds of infections. The outcome, however, is not always the same. The common cold is not a disease. It is not caused by a particular kind of virus. It is a *syndrome,* a pattern of signs and symptoms associated with an infection of the upper respiratory tract by any of hundreds of different kinds of viruses (colds are only occasionally caused by bacteria), including those that can cause serious disease.

Poliovirus The virus in our drama might have been, for example, one of the *polio-viruses.* If a person infected with one of these potentially dangerous viruses has very high resistance, the infection might product no symptoms at all. If the body's resistance is a bit lower, the result might be a cold like the one just described. If resistance is very low, the virus might overwhelm the defenders and spread through the body, causing paralyzing *poliomyelitis.*

Respiratory Infection Complications that can result from respiratory infections, if resistance is low or if the invading microbes are especially virulent, include *pneumonia, encephalitis, meningitis,* and *carditis.* These are not the names of diseases, but words that refer to infections affecting particular parts of the body. The suffix *-itis* denotes inflammation.

Inflammation Encephalitis (from the Greek *en,* in, and *kephale,* the head) is an infection of the brain, or "brain fever." Meningitis is an infection of the meninges (Greek *meninx,* membrane), the membrane covering the brain and spine. Carditis (Greek *kardia,* the heart) is an inflammation of the heart. Pneumonia (Greek *pneumon,* the lung) is another name for pneumonitis.

Such inflammations may result from infections by many different kinds of viruses or bacteria. The *measles* virus, for example, causes encephalitis in about one out of a thousand cases. Most victims recover, but a few suffer permanent brain damage. *Mumps* is one of many common infections that can lead to either encephalitis or meningitis. Viral meningitis usually runs its course and goes away, leaving no lasting effects, but *meningococcal meningitis,* or spinal meningitis, caused by a particular kind of bacteria, is often fatal. *Streptococcus* bacteria, which are responsible for strep throat and scarlet fever, among other things, can cause a variety of complications, including rheumatic heart disease. Numerous kinds of viruses, as well as some bacteria, can be responsible for pneumonia, the most common complication resulting from respiratory infections.

These complications, however, are exceptions. Most respiratory infections, even by potentially dangerous germs, go no further than the common cold stage. The cold is a kind of border skirmish, which the body usually wins. And usually, for reasons described in the next section, the first encounter with a particular kind of germ is the last time it poses a threat.

Natural Immunity

Measles, mumps, and the like are known as childhood diseases because, although people of all ages can get them, most of us have them as children, if at all, and never get them again. But one can be infected by the measles virus over and over again. Why doesn't the same person get measles every year?

The answer lies in the antibody-producing plasma cells created by lymphocytes during the initial infection. On first contact with the measles virus, the disease may develop before the lymphocytes have time to produce enough plasma cells to stop the infection. Once the infection has run its course, however, a large number of plasma cells, carrying measles-specific antigen receptors, remain in the body. In effect, they "remember" the measles virus. The next time that particular antigen is detected, a whole fleet of plasma cells begins producing antibodies immediately, and the viruses are neutralized before they can do any harm. The body has become permanently immune to that particular kind of virus. In like fashion, the body can create its own natural immunity to many other kinds of germs.

For reasons that are not completely understood, the body is unable to create immunity against certain microbes. The same person can have gonorrhea, for example, over and over again. The body does, however, become immune to most viruses and many bacteria after an initial infection—and in many cases it isn't necessary to have the disease or even a cold in order to become immune.

The Immortal Cow

Late in 1975, the World Health Organization announced that *smallpox,* a disease that in earlier years killed people by the millions, had been all but eradicated throughout the world. The disease was still a problem in a small section of Ethiopia, and a few cases turned up in Bangladesh. Otherwise, not a single case of smallpox was reported anywhere in the world.

Centuries ago, before anything was known about viruses, the Turks had discovered that a person could be protected against smallpox by injecting into one of his or her veins a bit of matter taken from one of the sores on the body of a smallpox victim.

Usually, the recipient became slightly ill, recovered, and thereafter was immune to the disease. It was a risky business, however. Some recipients became very sick and died. In 1796 a surgeon's assistant named Edward Jenner was told by a milkmaid, who knew from experience, that people who had been infected with cowpox never got smallpox. Cowpox, a disease of cattle, usually causes nothing worse than a mild infection in humans. In the interests of science, Jenner conducted some rather dangerous experiments on a small boy and found that inoculation with matter from one of the sores on a cow infected with the pox did, in fact, confer immunity against smallpox. And this method, as it turned out, was much safer than the Turkish way.

Vaccine

Doctors didn't know exactly why it worked, but for some time inoculation with a preparation containing matter from cowpox sores was the standard method of preventing smallpox. The preparation was called *vaccine,* from *vacca,* the Latin word for cow. Later, scientists discovered why the vaccine worked. Injection of a few cowpox viruses caused the body to respond in exactly the same way it would respond to any infection. The cowpox antigen triggered the production of lymphocytes of cowpox-specific plasma cells and antibodies. After the initial contact, the body was immune to cowpox. By a lucky accident, it was also immune to smallpox. The virus that causes the latter disease is so closely related to the cowpox virus, their antigens so nearly identical, that antibodies effective against one are also effective against the other. An unusual case, since most antibodies are so specific in their responses that they will pass up every virus except one. The vaccine that in recent years has come so close to conquering smallpox throughout the world has been made with a hybrid virus related to both cowpox and smallpox.

Since Jenner's time, vaccines that prevent a number of diseases, both viral and bacterial, have been developed. Although all are called vaccines, in honor of those long-gone cows, they have nothing to do with cowpox. They contain the viruses or bacteria, or in some cases bacterial toxins, of the particular diseases they prevent. In some the germs are dead, and in others they are weakened. In any case, vaccination introduces into the body enough germs to trigger the production of antibodies, but not enough to cause a serious infection. After vaccination, the body is as immune as it would be if it had actually had the disease. In some cases, immunity is permanent. In others, booster shots are needed periodically.

The Immunization Crisis

"I think the fact that we still have about 30,000 cases of measles and about 30 deaths from its complications every year, with outbreaks occurring in many parts of the country, is more than we should be willing to tolerate."

That exasperated comment was made in 1974 by John J. Witte, director of the immunization division of the National Center for Disease Control. With some adjusting of the figures, it could apply to any recent year. In a 1973 survey of preschool children, a particularly vulnerable group, the Center for Disease Control found that only 72.6 percent had been immunized against diphtheria, pertussis (whooping cough), and tetanus; only 61.2 percent against regular measles (rubeola); only 60.4 percent against poliomyelitis; only 55.6 percent against German measles (rubella); and a mere 34.7 percent had been immunized against mumps. And it seemed that the percentages were becoming smaller year by year.

Unnecessary Risks

Ironically, the success of earlier vaccination programs apparently has lulled young parents into thinking that such diseases are no longer a threat, that there is no need to have their children—and themselves—vaccinated. They don't remember the annual outbreaks of polio that used to cripple thousands of children and adults annually. A president of the United States, Franklin Roosevelt, governed from a wheelchair because he was crippled by polio. They also don't remember when there were thousands of cases each year of diphtheria, a deadly disease, and hundreds of thousands of cases

TABLE 13-1 Vaccination Schedule

Disease	Number of Doses	Age for First Series	Booster
Diphtheria	4 doses	2 months	At 4 to 6 years—before
Tetanus		4 months	entering school. As recom-
Whooping Cough		6 months	mended by physician.
		18 months	
Polio (Oral vaccine)	4 doses	2 months	At 4 to 6 years—before
		4 months	entering school. As recom-
		6 months	mended by physician.
		18 months	
Rubella (German measles)	1 vaccination	After 1 year	None
Measles	1 vaccination	After 1 year	None
Mumps	1 vaccination	After 1 year	None

This vaccination schedule is based on the recommendations of the American Academy of Pediatrics and the American Medical Association. A first test for TB (tuberculosis) may be recommended at one year. The family physician may suggest a slightly different schedule of vaccination based upon the child's individual needs. As knowledge of diseases' causes and prevention expands, vaccination recommendations may change from time to time.

Source: Metropolitan Life Insurance Company.

annually of measles, mumps, and whooping cough, all of which had the potential for fatal complications. The fact is that people still get all of those diseases, and, with so many people unvaccinated, serious outbreaks could still occur. People who leave their children and themselves unvaccinated are risking illness or even death from diseases that need not occur at all.

For women of childbearing age, immunization against German measles is particularly important. Although this disease causes only mild illness in children and adults, it can cripple an unborn baby if the mother becomes infected during pregnancy. Since immunization against German measles may not be permanent, even women who were vaccinated against the disease when they were children may need to be vaccinated again; doctors can arrange for a laboratory test to determine whether or not a woman is immune. Women who are already pregnant should *not* be vaccinated against German measles during pregnancy; even the mild infection caused by vaccination can endanger the fetus.

Flu Vaccine

"A touch of the flu" is one of the most common conclusions reached by people who diagnose their own illnesses. More often than not, what these people have is not *influenza* at all, but a respiratory infection caused by some other virus—a common cold, perhaps, with symptoms more severe than usual.

The word *influenza* is Italian for influence; centuries ago, Europeans attributed epidemics to some supernatural *influenza*. Actually, influenza is a respiratory infection caused by particular strains of viruses. It affects the entire respiratory tract, and may lead to complications, such as pneumonia. Influenza and its complications cause a considerable number of deaths each year in this country, mostly among the old and the chronically ill, who have low resistance. Every few years, some new strain of flu virus turns up, is spread around the world by travelers, and becomes known by the name of the place where it first broke out; thus we have "Spanish flu" or "Hong Kong flu" or "London flu."

Antiflu vaccines have been available for a number of years, but so far they have had limited value. One reason is a peculiar tendency of the flu viruses to undergo frequent mutations—changes in their molecular structure that alter their antigens, so that antibodies developed in response to one strain are ineffective against new, mutant strains. Just as frequently, the vaccines have to be changed to include the latest strain of viruses, which takes time. And the immunity conferred by the vaccines is of limited duration. Also, influenza vaccines, which are made with weakened viruses, are not effective in all cases, and many people have had unpleasant side effects from antiflu vaccinations.

Each fall, as the flu season nears, public health officials recommend that those most susceptible—the old and the chronically ill—get flu shots, but no effort is made to inoculate the general population. Whether or not people other than those in the most vulnerable categories should have flu vaccinations is something to be decided by the individual and his or her doctor.

Hepatitis

The National Institutes of Health announced in 1975 that a vaccine to prevent *hepatitis B,* otherwise known as *serum hepatitis,* had been proven safe and effective when tested in laboratory animals, and that tests in humans were about to begin. The announcement indicated that it might soon be possible to immunize people against a disease that has caused much suffering and thousands of deaths.

Serum Hepatitis

Serum hepatitis (from the Greek *hepatos,* liver) is an inflammation of the liver caused by a virus that is carried in the blood of those infected. It is usually transmitted from one person to another in blood transfusions or by the use of unsterilized hypodermic needles. Drug users who share needles are particularly susceptible. Victims are likely to suffer fatigue, loss of appetite, nausea, and abdominal discomfort, and they may lose their taste for cigarettes and coffee. As the disease progresses, patients frequently develop jaundice, a yellowing of the skin. Symptoms may last for weeks or months, sometimes becoming quite severe. Among the old and the ill, who are likely to require blood and blood products more often than others, serum hepatitis is sometimes fatal.

Infectious Hepatitis

The virus that causes *hepatitis A,* or *infectious hepatitis,* has not yet been isolated, so there is still no vaccine to prevent this disease. Infectious hepatitis often occurs in epidemics, particularly where large numbers of people live close together, as in military barracks or college dormitories. The elusive virus appears to be present in the feces of people who are infected, and the disease may be spread when food is contaminated by inadequately washed hands.

Infectious hepatitis occurs most frequently in adolescents and young adults. The lingering symptoms are similar to those of serum hepatitis, but are usually less severe, and fatalities from infectious hepatitis are rare. A person who has the disease once is thereafter immune.

Mononucleosis

Another disease that most often affects adolescents and young adults is *infectious mononucleosis,* sometimes called the "college disease" or the "kissing disease." It is believed to be caused by a virus, as yet unidentified, that may be carried in the throat and spread by close personal contact. The symptoms, usually mild though sometimes severe, include headaches, malaise, fatigue, fever, and sore throat. Jaundice develops in a small percentage of cases, and some victims have a measleslike rash. Enlargement of the spleen occurs in many patients, and in extremely rare cases the spleen ruptures, causing severe abdominal pain and requiring immediate hospitalization and surgery. Except in those rare cases of splenic rupture, infectious mononucleosis is hardly ever fatal. There is, at present, no known way to prevent the disease.

It is believed that many children have both infectious hepatitis and infectious mononucleosis in "subclinical" forms; that is, they have no symptoms, but develop a natural immunity against these diseases.

The Common Cold

As we have seen, colds can be caused by any of hundreds of different viruses, so there is little likelihood that we will ever have vaccines that would prevent all colds.

People who have colds usually develop immunity to the particular kinds of germs that have infected them, and those who have been vaccinated against polio, measles, mumps, and so forth are protected against any colds that might be caused by those viruses. As for the rest, it seems inevitable that we will all have to put up with a certain number of colds.

Treatment

There are no drugs that will cure a cold once a person has become infected. Antibiotics, for reasons described in the following pages, are ineffective against ordinary colds. And

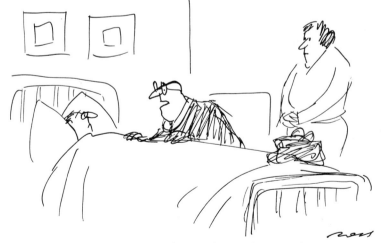

Drawing by Ross; © 1975 The New Yorker Magazine, Inc.

"You've got whatever it is that's going around."

cold tablets and other preparations that are so widely advertised on television do not kill germs. Some of them may help to relieve some cold symptoms, but even that is questionable in most cases. Cold sufferers who claim that they felt better after taking a patent medicine probably would have felt better anyway, although they may have received a psychological lift simply because they thought they were doing something about their colds.

Aspirin may help reduce the achiness and fever that sometimes accompany colds, but it may also reduce the body's germ-fighting efficiency. Some research has indicated that people who take aspirin for their colds "shed" more viruses than other people, and therefore may be more likely to spread their colds to others. In an experiment reported in 1975, researchers at the University of Illinois infected a group of volunteers with some relatively innocuous viruses. Between 60 and 70 percent of the volunteers "caught" colds.

> The doctors then gave aspirin to only some of their ailing subjects. It produced "some amelioration of symptoms," though nothing spectacular.
> But daily nasal samplings showed that the aspirin users produced up to a third more viruses than nonusers.

Aspirin should be taken for a cold only on the advice of a physician.

There have been conflicting reports about the effectiveness of large quantities of Vitamin C in preventing or reducing the severity of colds. Some researchers say that Vitamin C seems to have some anticold effect; others disagree. There is concern about the possibility that taking unusually large quantities of any vitamin might have untoward effects not yet suspected.

The only universally recognized treatment for a cold is to get a lot of rest, so that the body can use its energy to fight the infection. It is also important to drink a lot of fluids to replace those lost in sneezing, coughing, and sweating. The soundest advice is still that given by the sixteenth century English physician who wrote, "The beste and moste sure help in this case is not to meddle with anye kynde of medicines, but to let nature worke her operacio."

Antibiotics: Bacteria's Enemy

Trying to dredge a bit of humor out of the misery of a cold, an ill-informed wag remarks, "I wish this cold would turn into pneumonia. They can cure that."

The belief that a shot or two of penicillin is a sure cure for pneumonia or almost anything else is widespread—and largely erroneous. While penicillin and other antibiotics are invaluable weapons against the bacterial infections that used to be major killers, the antibiotics are not effective against viruses.

The reason is simple. Bacteria attack cells from the outside, and there they can be reached by antibiotics; viruses work inside the cells, and the antibiotics cannot reach them. If pneumonia, for example, is the result of a bacterial infection, it can usually be cured with the help of antibiotics. If it is the result of a viral infection, antibiotics won't help. Fortunately, most viral infections are self-limiting; the body heals itself.

Overuse of Antibiotics

Because antibiotics are ineffective against viruses, including the viruses that cause most colds, it is pointless to ask one's doctor for a shot of penicillin for every case of sniffles. And there are strong arguments against the indiscriminate use of antibiotics. One is based on the fact that some people become allergic to certain antibiotics. Unnecessary use of an antibiotic may sensitize the patient, causing an adverse and possibly dangerous reaction the next time that particular antibiotic is used—and perhaps making it impossible to use the drug when it is really needed. Another argument against unnecessary use of antibiotics is based on the fact that some bacteria, as a result of repeated exposure, become resistant to the effects of drugs, just as people become immune to germs to which they have been exposed. In some hospitals, bacteria that have become resistant as a result of continual exposure to antibiotics pose a serious problem when patients and staff members become infected. The use of antibiotics in cases of severe respiratory infection is appropriate when it appears that bacteria may be involved. This is a matter of judgment on the part of the doctor.

Interferon: Virus's Possible Enemy

There are a few chemicals that are effective against certain kinds of viral infections, but in most cases chemicals that might destroy viruses can't be used because they would also destroy the cells. One promising area of research, which could result in a weapon effective against many kinds of viruses, involves *interferon,* a protein produced naturally by infected cells. Interferon is so named because it interferes with the spread of viruses from infected to healthy cells. Researchers have reported encouraging results in the experimental use of interferon against several kinds of viral infections. So far, studies have been limited by the very high cost of preparing it from human cells, but efforts are under way to produce the protein synthetically, which may eventually make interferon widely available—possibly even as an effective treatment for the common cold.

Food-Borne Illness

And the swine, though he divide the hoof, and be clovenfooted, yet he cheweth not the cud; he is unclean to you.

Of their flesh shall ye not eat, and their carcase shall yet not touch; they are unclean to you.

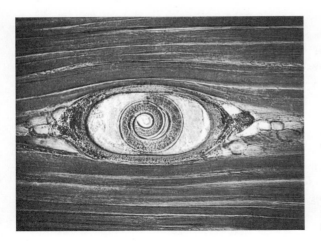

Trichinae cyst in muscle tissue.

The Old Testament injunction against eating pork, still observed by Orthodox Jews and by Moslems, may have been one of the world's first public health laws. The elders of the time had no doubt observed that some people who ate the flesh of swine became very ill; some went blind, and some died. Presumably, the victims had eaten their pork raw or undercooked. The flesh of animals, particularly hogs, is sometimes infected with the larvae of tiny intestinal worms called *trichinae*. If the meat is not cooked long enough to kill the larvae, people who eat it may get *trichinosis*. The disease is relatively rare in this country, but a few cases are reported every year. The danger is eliminated by thorough cooking of all meats.

Much more common are illnesses caused by certain kinds of bacteria often found in foods. It is estimated that there are as many as ten million cases a year in the United States of food-borne infection. Nobody knows for sure just how many cases there are because the stomach cramps, vomiting, diarrhea, and, sometimes, fever that result from such infections are usually dismissed as "something I ate" and are not reported to public health authorities.

Salmonellosis

Many of the infections are caused by bacteria of the *Salmonella* family, which are especially likely to turn up in raw or undercooked eggs. Outbreaks frequently occur during or just after outings at which egg salad sandwiches or other foods containing eggs or egg products, such as mayonnaise, are left unrefrigerated for a few hours; the germs multiply very fast under those conditions. Most Salmonella infections are not serious, but rarely, a patient may die.

Most food-borne infections can be avoided if all foods are thoroughly cleaned before cooking, if they are cooked at temperatures of at least 140 degrees Fahrenheit, and if they are either eaten right after being cooked or kept well-refrigerated (below 45 degrees Fahrenheit). Germs tend to multiply at temperatures between 45 and 140 degrees, and foods should not be kept at temperatures in that range any longer than necessary. These precautions do not apply, of course, to fresh fruits and vegetables, which are usually safe if they are clean.

Botulism

Botulism, a deadly disease caused by the toxin of certain bacteria that sometimes grow in improperly canned foods, is quite rare. In recent years, however, with the renewed popularity of home canning there has been an increase in concern about this disease. People who can homegrown foods should be sure to read up on the safe procedures. Literature is available from the U.S. Government Printing Office, among other sources.

Summary

Communicable diseases are carried by germs, which may be animal, vegetable, or something in between. They are variously called microbes, bacteria, and viruses and are so tiny that they are invisible. Most germs don't harm us, and some even help us, but some of them can cause serious or fatal disease.

Germs may pass into the body through a cut or a scratch; they may be swallowed in food or drink; they may be transmitted by sex or a sneeze. Infection can occur unless the body's resistance is high enough to reject the disease, and unless its genetically programmed white blood cells can neutralize a virus and subdue a disease. Sometimes the body can make itself immune and sometimes immunity is achieved by use of a vaccine.

References

p. 209   Lewis Thomas, *The Lives of a Cell* (New York, 1974), pp. 93–94.

p. 211   *San Francisco Chronicle* (November 24, 1975), p. 38.

p. 213   Ibid. (September 30, 1974), p. 24.

p. 215   Ibid. (March 20, 1975), p. 3.

p. 217   Ibid. (March 25, 1975), p. 4.

p. 217   Thomas Phaire, *The Boke of Chyldren,* quoted by John M. Adams, *Viruses and Colds: The Modern Plague* (New York, 1967), p. 135.

p. 218   *Medical World News* (February 22, 1974), p. 12.

p. 218   Leviticus 11:7–8.

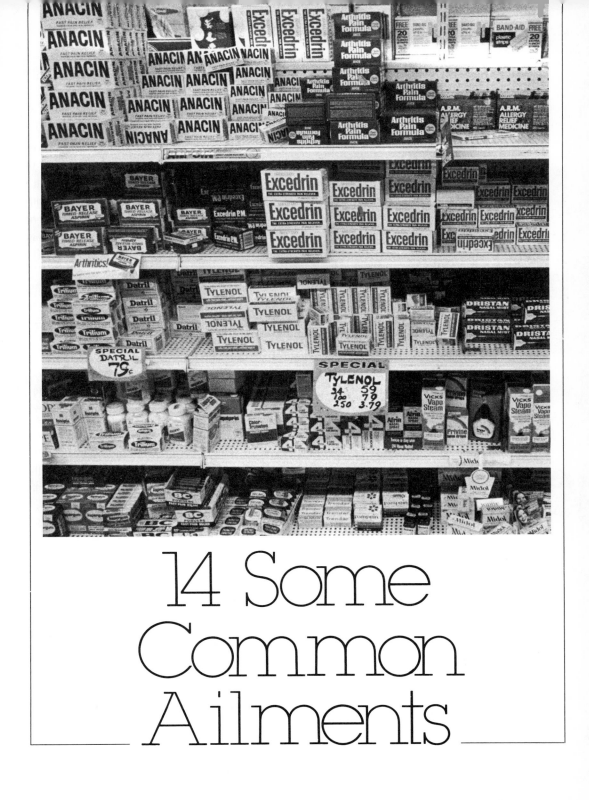

14 Some Common Ailments

To judge by television commercials, Americans do more worrying about their bowel movements than about economic instability, crime in the streets, and the threat of nuclear disaster. Life is just one personal crisis after another. If it isn't constipation, it's diarrhea, hemorrhoids, headaches, acid indigestion, or pimples. The television sponsors, of course, know their audience. All of us are, from time to time, plagued by one or more of these common afflictions. Among them, they cause more minor discomfort than any major disease. Consequently, there is a ready market for anything that promises relief.

This chapter describes the causes of some of these ailments, and explains that while some of the advertised remedies might be helpful, others are useless, and some can even be harmful.

Acne

Around the roots of body hairs are little glands that secrete a white, fatty substance called *sebum* (Latin for tallow). Bacteria residing in the hair follicles produce an enzyme that breaks down some of the sebum, turning it into free fatty acids. The acids apparently damage the linings of the follicles. Dead cells mixed with sebum and bacteria plug up pores, causing *comedones,* otherwise known as "whiteheads." Exposed to air, "whiteheads" may become "blackheads." Inflammation turns them into *papules,* or *pustules*—pimples, in the vernacular. The outbreak of pimples is common acne, or, to give it the traditional Latin rendering, *acne vulgaris.*

Acne most often affects the face and back, because the sebacious (sebum-secreting) glands are more active in those areas. People of all ages get acne, but adolescents are most vulnerable because the increased activity of sex hormones in their changing bodies stimulates the production of sebum.

Treatment

Most cases of acne are relatively mild and disappear in time, leaving no traces. Occasionally, however, severe acne leaves a face permanently scarred and pockmarked. Anyone with severe acne should see a doctor; treatment with antibiotics, with Vitamin A acid, or with certain drugs may prevent permanent skin blemishes. Such treatment may have to be continued over a considerable period of time, since acne is resistant to all kinds of therapy.

For the usual, mild cases of acne, dermatologists (physicians who are skin specialists) usually recommend washing affected areas several times a day with ordinary soap and warm water. The washing won't cure the acne, but it removes oils and other materials that might add to the clogging of pores. Oily hair should be kept off the face,

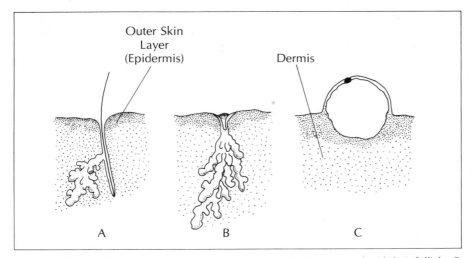

FIGURE 14-a *Formation of a pimple. A. Sebaceous gland associated with hair follicle; B. Blackhead blocking duct to sebaceous gland of the skin, as over the nose; C. Sebaceous cyst. The continued secretion of sebaceous material enlarges the duct of the gland to form a cyst, and the gland itself is drawn upward, compressed, and largely contained by the cyst. The black mark indicates the opening of the duct closed by a blackhead.*

and greasy hair dressings should be avoided, as should face creams and lotions. Cosmetics may cover pimples, but they may also help create more of them by clogging pores.

Diet

Foods containing iodides and bromides appear to contribute to flare-ups of acne in some cases. Those foods include iodized salt, saltwater fish, shellfish, spinach, cabbage, lettuce, and artichokes. Some drugs and vitamin preparations also contain iodides and bromides; labels should be read carefully. Beyond this, researchers have found no connection between diet and acne. Yet many people still think their acne gets worse when they eat such things as chocolate, sweets, and fried foods. If that seems to be the case, a simple test is to give up the suspected food for a while and see if it makes any difference.

Medication

Among the dozens of different preparations advertised as acne treatments and sold without prescription, some may help in certain cases. Others either contain no ingredients recognized as effective against acne, or contain too little of the effective ingredients to do any good. Some of the creamy treatments may do more harm than good—by clogging pores. The antibiotics contained in some of the preparations are not known to be effective against acne when applied to the skin, and could cause allergic reactions in some people. The wisest course is to consult a doctor before using any of the over-the-counter preparations.

Finally, however great the temptation, squeezing and picking pimples should be resisted in order to avoid spreading infection and causing scars.

Headaches

Final exams, traffic jams, lovers' quarrels, all kinds of stressful situations—including unconscious anxieties—can produce physical responses. One response is contraction of the neck and scalp muscles and dilation of the blood vessels around the skull: a "tension headache." Most headaches fall into this category. The best treatment is to relax, if possible, and take aspirin, which often helps. Unfortunately, there is little else to be done in the way of medication. For people who are allergic to aspirin, or who find that it irritates their stomachs, *acetaminophen* is about equally effective. Acetaminophen can be purchased under its generic name or under various trade names. Most

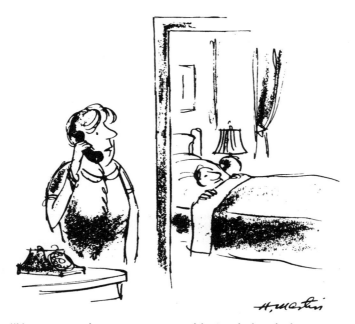

"He seems to have a common cold, simple headache, and minor aches and pains."

authorities agree that analgesic (pain-relieving) compounds, most of which contain aspirin combined with other ingredients, are no more effective than aspirin alone, although they may be much more expensive.

Migraines

The vicious *migraine* headaches that strike some people periodically are seldom helped by aspirin, but may be relieved by certain prescription drugs. The causes of migraine headaches are still under investigation. Psychological problems, allergies, or other factors may be involved.

Some headaches are caused by uncorrected vision problems or other disorders requiring professional attention. Unusually frequent or persistent headaches call for a visit to the doctor.

Indigestion

Indigestion is a quite unscientific word that can mask many different problems, some of them serious. Usually the word is taken to mean the occasional stomach upsets that may result from too much food and drink or from emotional strain. An excessive amount of hydrochloric acid, one of the digestive juices, pours into the stomach, causing irritation. Some of the acid may get up into the esophagus, causing the symptom usually described as heartburn. In such cases, distress may be relieved by taking an antacid—a chemical that neutralizes the hydrochloric acid. A teaspoonful of bicarbonate of soda—baking soda—in a glass of water is often an effective antacid. Some of the most highly advertised commercial antacids contain bicarbonate of soda, sometimes in combination with aspirin—a combination that the Food and Drug Administration has called "irrational," since aspirin is an acid too.

Often, the symptoms that sufferers self-diagnose as indigestion are really caused by bacteria in contaminated food (see Chapter 13). Sometimes, the symptoms are caused by ulcers, by other diseases of the digestive tract, or even by heart disease; symptoms dismissed as heartburn frequently accompany heart ailments, especially in middle-aged men. In such cases, self-prescribed medication could be dangerous. Medical attention should be sought if the symptoms of indigestion are unusually severe, if they persist for more than a day or so, or if they occur frequently.

Constipation

Regularity is a word heard most often in laxative advertisements. Nobody exactly says so, but the impression people receive is that anyone who doesn't have a bowel movement every day is in serious trouble.

The fallacy of this impression was revealed in an experiment supervised by Dr. Walter C. Alvarez. A group of healthy young medical students swallowed sets of gelatin capsules containing many small glass beads. The results were interesting. Two of the students passed about 85 percent of the beads in 24 hours; most took four days to eliminate three-fourths of the beads; some passed only half of the beads in nine days.

Dr. Alvarez further observed that those who passed the majority of the beads in twenty-four hours had pooly formed stools containing undigested material. Those with a slower rate usually had well-formed stools showing evidence of good digestion. Some of the participants with the slower rates had believed they were constipated.

There is no scientific basis for the notion that everyone should defecate daily. Normal frequency of evacuation varies among individuals. Some healthy people have bowel movements only once every two or three days. They are not constipated. Temporary constipation may occur occasionally for any of a number of reasons, including emotional upsets, travel, or changes in work schedules. Usually, bowel movements return to normal within a few days, without medication.

Laxatives

Chronic constipation can result from certain diseases, but this is rather unusual. More often, chronic constipation is a result of repeatedly ignoring the urge to defecate because it isn't convenient to go to the toilet for one reason or another; if the signals are ignored often enough, the body may stop sending them. In such cases, a doctor may prescribe a laxative—and future obedience to calls of nature. Paradoxically, one of the most common causes of chronic constipation is overuse of laxatives. People obsessed with the idea of regularity may purge themselves so often that the muscles of the bowel become weakened, making bowel movements increasingly difficult. Giving up laxatives frequently returns these people to normal within a short time.

Sometimes, laxatives can be dangerous. There have been cases, for example, in which people mistook the pain of appendicitis for constipation, dosed themselves with laxatives, and suffered ruptures of the appendix because of the delay in treatment. In a 1975 report to the Food and Drug Administration, a panel of researchers concluded that only half of the ingredients in numerous brands of nonprescription laxatives they studied were definitely both safe and effective. "Prolonged laxative use," the panel said, "can in some instances seriously impair normal bowel function. Use of laxatives for acute abdominal pain, vomiting and other digestive tract symptoms can lead to serious life-threatening situations."

Diarrhea

Like constipation, diarrhea is often brought on by emotional upsets. Many people, in fact, suffer from "irritable colons," which respond to emotional ups and downs by

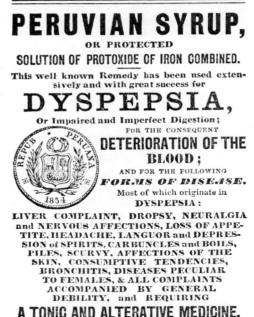

Nineteenth-century advertisement

alternating constipation and diarrhea. Diarrhea may also be caused by certain kinds of infections, contaminated food, some medications—even, in some people, by Vitamin C. A common cause of diarrhea is the lack of an enzyme needed to digest milk products.

No treatment is required for occasional, uncomplicated bouts of diarrhea. However, the patient should drink lots of liquids to replace lost fluids. One of the nonprescription antidiarrheal preparations available at drug stores might be helpful. If the attack lasts more than a day or two, or if it is accompanied by severe abdominal pains, fever, or bloody stools, the patient should see a doctor.

Hemorrhoids

Hemorrhoids (piles) are varicose (dilated) veins in the anus or lower rectum frequently associated with chronic constipation. They may be caused by too much straining to force bowel movements. In pregnant women, pressure by the fetus on rectal veins may cause hemorrhoids. People whose occupations require them to sit constantly are often victims. Hemorrhoids can be very painful.

The hemorrhoids associated with constipation usually disappear when bowel movements return to normal. While some of the ointments sold in drug stores may help relieve discomfort, none of them cure hemorrhoids, regardless of what the advertisements may say. In severe cases, local injections, which shrink the hemorrhoids, or surgery may be required.

Rectal bleeding is sometimes caused by ruptured hemorrhoids. The bleeding usually stops without treatment. Any rectal bleeding, however, is reason to see a doctor; it could be a sign of something more serious than hemorrhoids.

Summary

There are a number of commonplace ailments that, taken together, probably cause more widespread misery than any major disease. Sufferers anxiously seek relief, often from widely advertised remedies which may or may not be safe or effective.

Among these ailments are acne, headaches, "indigestion," constipation, diarrhea, and hemorrhoids.

References

p. 225 *Consumer Reports* Editors, *The Medicine Show: Some Plain Truths about Popular Products for Common Ailments* (Mount Vernon, N.Y., 1974), p. 83.

p. 226 Ibid., pp. 94–95.

p. 226 *San Francisco Chronicle* (March 21, 1975), p. 1.

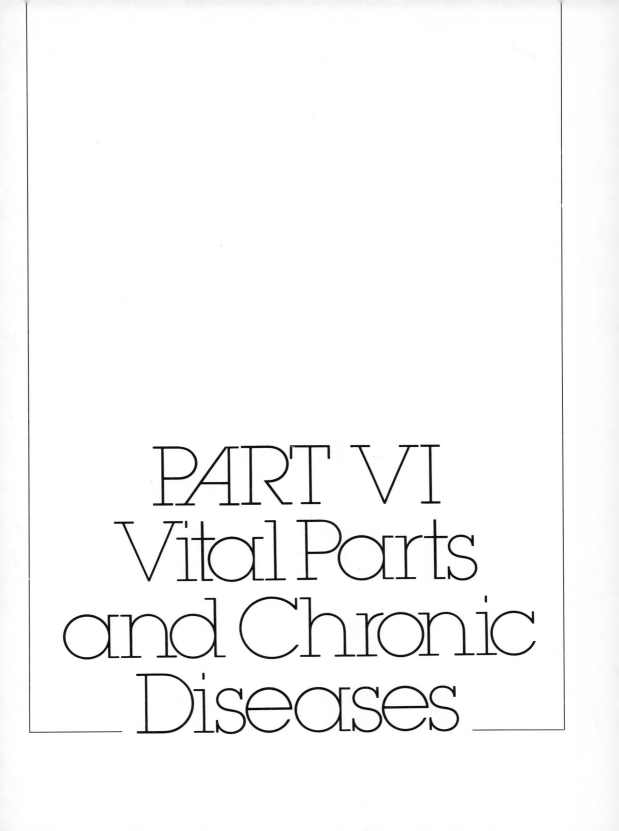

PART VI
Vital Parts and Chronic Diseases

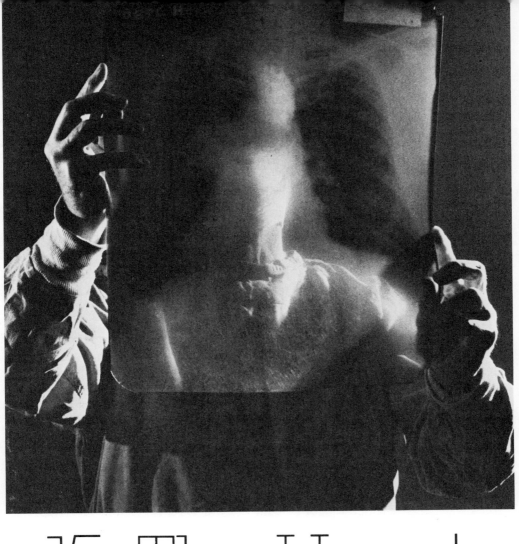

15 The Heart, Blood Vessels, and Kidneys

Between the disappearance of a salad awash in bleu cheese and the arrival of a nicely marbled top sirloin, Harvey sucks hungrily at a cigarette, one of forty or more he would burn on an average day. Not today, though. He doesn't know it, but this will be his last smoke for some time.

Harvey's mind isn't on the cigarette or even on the food. He has his pen out, scribbling on the tablecloth, eagerly explaining to his luncheon companions the business deal he hopes to consummate before dessert. At forty-five, Harvey is intent on pushing his way to the top, and if he doesn't have much time for exercise, if his paunch bulges over his belt a bit, he seldom gives it more than a passing thought. The waiter is placing his steak in front of him when Harvey freezes in midsentence, grimacing. As his companions stare incredulously, the pen slips from his fingers, and he clutches his chest. His breath is coming in short gasps. Sudden, searing pain stabs through his chest and down his left arm. He slumps forward, unconscious.

What Is a Chronic Disease?

You may have viewed a scene something like that in the movies or on television. They are all too common in real life—so common you've already guessed that Harvey has suffered a heart attack. Why Harvey? That will be explored in detail in the following pages. For the moment, it is enough to say that Harvey is a victim of a disease that develops slowly, and that may have long-lasting effects. Such a disease is described as chronic, from the Greek word *chronos,* time. Chronic diseases kill far more people in the United States each year than all other causes combined, including infectious illnesses, accidents, crimes, and natural disasters. This wasn't always true. The primary reason for the change sounds paradoxical: Most people now die of chronic diseases because people live longer than they used to.

Increased Prevalence of Chronic Disease

A few generations ago, most people in this country died young by today's standards. Influenza, pneumonia, and tuberculosis, diseases caused by an outside agent, were among the major killers. Advances in medicine have dramatically reduced the mortality rates from those and many other illnesses. Since 1900 the average life expectancy of Americans has increased from about fifty years to about seventy years. With longer life came greater risks of becoming a victim, eventually, of a slow-developing chronic disease. Such diseases most often reveal themselves in the middle years or later, even though they may have their beginnings early in life. Their causes are still being investigated, and they have become the prime targets of medical research.

The Heart's Function

Why Harvey? While he had occasionally noticed mild chest pains and shortness of breath, the hard-driving businessman, whose heart attack opened this chapter, had never before felt seriously ill. Yet his sudden attack was the result of a condition that had been developing since early childhood—and it quite possibly could have been avoided. To understand what happened to Harvey, it will help to take a brief look first at the way the heart and blood vessels—the *cardiovascular system*—normally function.

The Cardiovascular System

The heart, that remarkable, fist-sized machine quietly doing its work inside your chest, is essentially a double pump. Specialized cells inside the heart send out bursts of electrical impulses that control the rhythmic beat. They cause regular contractions of the heart muscle, which sends blood pulsing out through the arteries. Between contractions, the muscle relaxes, allowing blood to flow back into the heart through the veins. The right side of the heart pumps blood into the lungs, from which the blood, enriched with oxygen, flows back to the larger left side of the heart. From there it goes coursing out to every extremity, from the brain cells to the toes. It rushes through the arteries to the arterioles (the arteries' smallest endings) and then feeds into tiny capillaries. From capillaries the blood enters venules (the veins' beginnings) and then the veins, and so back to the right side of the heart to begin the circuit anew.

As well as fresh oxygen from the lungs, the blood's red cells carry nutrients, hormones, and other necessities to every bit of body tissue. And they carry away from the tissues waste materials, some in the form of carbon dioxide to be exhaled by the lungs, and others to be eliminated by the liver and kidneys.

Atherosclerosis: The Slow Squeeze

If something goes wrong with one part of the intricate circulatory system, other parts may be seriously—even fatally—affected. In Harvey's case, as in most heart attacks, what went wrong resulted from a condition called *atherosclerosis.* The term (from the Greek *athero,* soft, and *skleros,* hard) refers to the condition that arises when parts of the inner linings of the arteries first become soft and weak, then become covered with hard, inflexible deposits. The condition, really a long-term process, is commonly known as hardening of the arteries.

The causes of atherosclerosis are not clearly understood, but the process is associated with the presence of certain fatty materials in the blood. One of those materials, cholesterol, is under particularly intensive investigation by scientists as a likely factor in the genesis of atherosclerosis. The fatty substances appear to irritate the linings of the

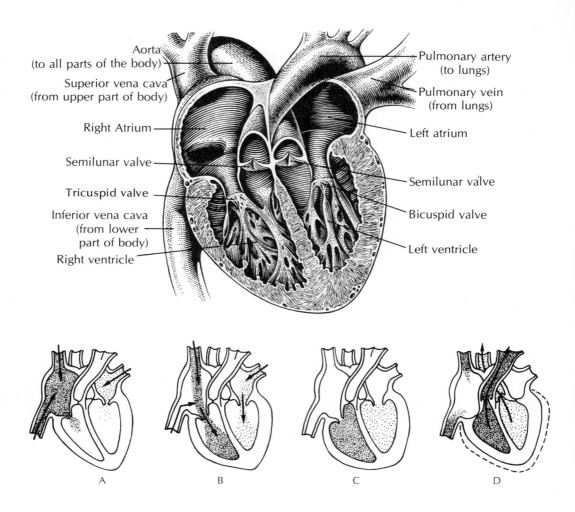

FIGURE 15-a *The human heart and its pumping cycle. The upper figure shows the detail of the heart's four chambers and its valves. A, B, C, and D are successive stages in the pumping cycle. A. The atria fill with blood as their walls relax. B. The relaxation of the ventricles causes blood to flow into them from the atria. C. Contraction of the atria completes the filling of the ventricles. D. Contraction of the ventricles drives blood from the ventricles into the aorta and pulmonary artery. The blood is prevented from returning to the atria by the bicuspid and tricuspid valves. During the relaxation stage, it is prevented from returning to the ventricles from the arteries by the semilunar valves.*

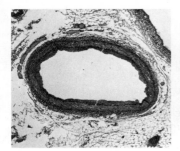

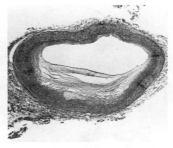

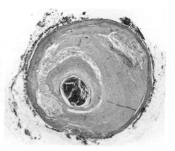

Cross-section of a normal artery.

Cross-section of artery with atherosclerotic deposits in inner lining.

Narrowed channel of artery blocked by blood clot.

arteries, causing lesions, or sores. When the lesions heal, scar tissue forms. Calcium deposits build up on the scars, causing the arteries to lose their flexibility and gradually narrowing the passages through which blood flows.

Imagine yourself watering some flowers with a garden hose. Gradually, you squeeze the hose. When you first begin to squeeze, the flow slackens, but the petunias are still getting some water. If you keep squeezing until the hose is tightly kinked, the water is completely cut off. Something like that happens to an artery affected by atherosclerosis. And when an artery is completely closed, it is not petunias, but a part of the human body that is deprived of life-giving fluid. If it happens to be a *coronary artery,* one of those through which the heart pumps blood to its own muscle, the results can be devastating—as Harvey discovered. The heart's muscle would fail to contract, thus ceasing the flow of blood to the body.

You may think of hardening of the arteries as being synonymous with old age. But the fatty streaks that mark the beginning of atherosclerosis are sometimes found in the arteries of small babies. And autopsies on the bodies of American soldiers killed in the Korean war revealed that more than 77 percent had atherosclerosis, some of them in advanced stages. Their average age was twenty-three. It is not because young people are unaffected, but because the process is usually so slow that relatively few people feel the results of atherosclerosis before middle age.

Angina Pectoris: An Early Warning

Like the flow through the gradually squeezed water hose, the flow through Harvey's diseased coronary artery wasn't cut off all at once. Long before his heart attack, he had received faint warning signals that there might be serious trouble ahead. Those occasional pains in his chest and the shortness of breath that he had noticed from time to time were gentle flare-ups of *angina pectoris* (Latin for a choking in the chest), which may range in severity from mild discomfort to agonizing pains in the chest and left arm, sometimes spreading into the neck.

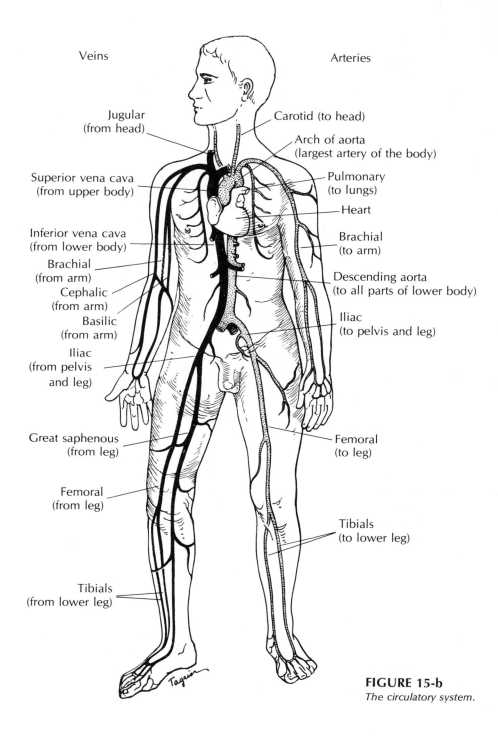

Veins

Arteries

Jugular
(from head)

Carotid (to head)

Arch of aorta
(largest artery of the body)

Superior vena cava
(from upper body)

Pulmonary
(to lungs)

Heart

Inferior vena cava
(from lower body)

Brachial
(to arm)

Brachial
(from arm)

Cephalic
(from arm)

Descending aorta
(to all parts of lower body)

Basilic
(from arm)

Iliac
(to pelvis and leg)

Iliac
(from pelvis
and leg)

Great saphenous
(from leg)

Femoral
(to leg)

Femoral
(from leg)

Tibials
(to lower leg)

Tibials
(from lower leg)

FIGURE 15-b
The circulatory system.

Angina attacks frequently follow bouts of exercise, anxiety, heavy eating, or anything else that increases the heart's workload, but they may come on for no readily apparent reason. Angina indicates that the heart is already suffering from an insufficient supply of blood because of narrowed arteries. Not all heart attacks are preceded by angina symptoms. And not all chest pain is angina, of course, but severe or repeated symptoms should call for a visit to a doctor. One major study has indicated that one out of four men who suffer from angina pectoris will have a heart attack within five years.

What Is a Heart Attack?

Finally, one of Harvey's coronary arteries, narrowed over the years by atherosclerosis, was suddenly blocked, or occluded, by the formation of a blood clot (*thrombos* in Greek). That occurrence is what doctors call a *coronary occlusion,* or a *coronary thrombosis;* it is the way most heart attacks happen.

When the blockage cut off the blood supply to a part of his heart, Harvey suffered a *myocardial infarction* (from *myocardium,* or heart muscle, an *infarct,* an area of dead tissue). This means that part of the heart muscle, deprived of oxygen and nutrients, literally began to die. That was when Harvey collapsed facedown into his lunch.

Heart attacks like Harvey's may have different results. The heart may stop beating, in which case the victim will die unless prompt emergency treatment restarts the beat. If the patient survives, the body's own healing system will reroute blood around the blocked artery through other vessels, setting up what is called collateral circulation. Damage to the specialized cells that regulate the heartbeat may cause *arhythmia,* a sometimes wildly irregular beat that is often fatal. Arhythmia also occurs in many cases when there has been no occlusion, but a narrowed artery is simply unable to deliver enough oxygen.

TABLE 15-1 Deaths in the United States Due to Major Cardiovascular Diseases, 1974

Cause	Rate per 100,000
Diseases of the Heart:	
Active rheumatic fever and chronic rheumatic heart disease	6.3
Hypertensive heart disease	5.7
Ischemic heart disease	314.5
Chronic disease of the endocardium	2.3
All other forms of heart disease	20.4
Hypertension	3.3
Cerebrovascular Disease	98.1
Arteriosclerosis	15.3
Other Diseases of Arteries, Arterioles, and Capillaries	12.4
Total	478.3

Source: Statistical Abstract of the United States, 97th ed., 1976, p. 65.

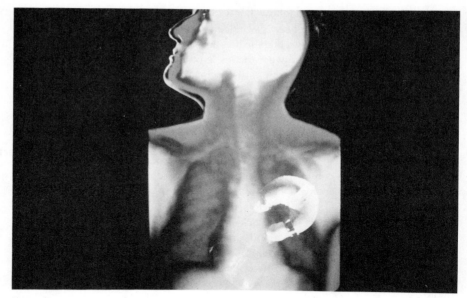

X-ray showing artificial aorta.

There are other kinds of heart trouble that affect significant numbers of people. They include birth (congenital) defects and rheumatic heart disease and damage to the heart valves brought on by childhood streptococcus infections. But the greatest health menace by far is heart attacks resulting from atherosclerosis. They kill more people in the United States each year than any other single cause. They temporarily or permanently disable a great many more.

Stroke

Atherosclerosis does more than cause heart attacks. If Harvey's blood clot had blocked a narrowed *cerebral* (brain) artery instead of a coronary artery, the result might have been a stroke. A blood clot in a brain artery is called a *cerebral thrombosis,* and the resulting closure of the artery is called *cerebrovascular occlusion.* The blood supply to a part of the brain is cut off, and the nerve cells in that part of the brain are damaged. Most strokes—though not all of them, as we shall see—are brought on by the clogging of arteries as a result of atherosclerosis.

A stroke may also result from a *cerebral hemorrhage,* which occurs when a weak spot in the wall of one of the small brain arteries balloons out and bursts. Such weak spots are called *aneurysms.* They result either from a congenital lack of muscular coating on an artery or from the punishing effects of *hypertension* (high blood pressure), a very widespread and mysterious disorder that will be discussed later in this chapter.

Many strokes kill; many more cripple. The nerve cells in the brain control thinking, sensation, and most body movements. When some of the cells are destroyed, the functions they control are lost. This can result in paralysis, inability to speak, loss of memory, inability to think clearly.

The effects of a stroke may be transient or permanent, mild or severe, depending on the extent and location in the brain of the cell damage and on how quickly the body can repair itself by rerouting blood through other channels or by transferring functions of the damaged cells to other cells.

Hypertension

If you think of the heart as a water tower that is one story high under normal circumstances, and then imagine it being jacked up to two stories, you may get some idea of what happens to the blood pressure under hypertension. Earlier, we compared the flow of blood through the arteries to the coursing of water through a garden hose. Now we may think in terms of the high-pressure stream jetting through a fire hose.

Hypertension develops when the arterioles, those tiny ends of arteries leading into the capillaries, become abnormally narrow, making it hard for blood to get through and building up pressure in the arteries as the heart pumps harder to make the blood circulate. In a relatively few number of cases, high blood pressure results from kidney disease or tumors. But in the majority of cases—more than 90 percent—the cause of hypertension simply isn't known.

Whatever the cause, about one out of four Americans has some elevation of blood pressure. About half of those affected, according to some surveys, are not aware of their hypertension. Like atherosclerosis, it can be present for many years without revealing itself by any symptoms. It is often present in teen-agers.

We have already seen how hypertension causes strokes. But that isn't all it does. Its punishing pressure on artery walls predisposes the victim to atherosclerosis, further increasing the dangers of both heart attacks and strokes. Furthermore, the extra work that hypertension forces the heart to do can damage the heart muscle, causing *hypertensive heart disease.* And the constant pressure can also damage arteries in the kidneys, causing those vital organs to fail.

Improving the Odds Against Heart Disease

The mythical Harvey, the middle-aged, sedentary, overweight, cholesterol-eating, two-pack-a-day smoker whom we left crumpled over the luncheon table a few pages back, was invented as a typical example of what the American Heart Association calls the "coronary profile" of a likely candidate for a heart attack. He was also, as we have seen, a prime candidate for a stroke, so closely interrelated are the causes of those leading killers and cripplers.

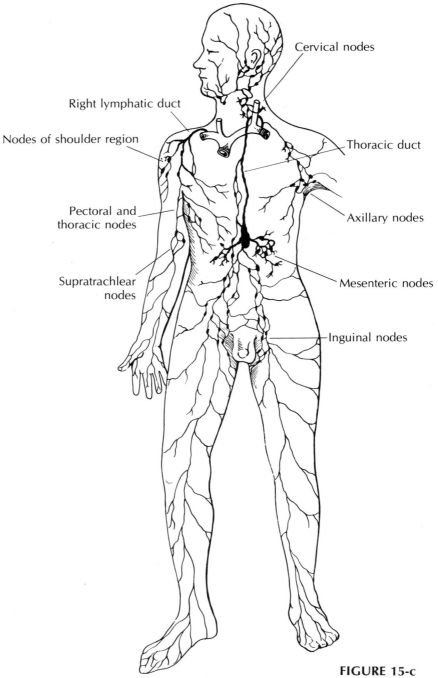

Cervical nodes

Right lymphatic duct

Nodes of shoulder region

Thoracic duct

Pectoral and
thoracic nodes

Axillary nodes

Supratrachlear
nodes

Mesenteric nodes

Inguinal nodes

FIGURE 15-c
The lymphatic system.

What is meant by a coronary or a stroke profile? Various studies, particularly a famous one involving the long-term observation of residents of Framingham, Massachusetts, by the U.S. Public Health Service, have shown that certain factors are closely associated with the risk of suffering a heart attack or a stroke. The more of those factors found in an individual, the more likely he or she is to become a victim. Here are some of the major risk factors.

Cigarette Smoking   People who smoke cigarettes have more heart attacks and strokes than those who do not, and the more a person smokes, the greater the danger. The incidence of heart attacks and strokes increases in direct proportion to the number of cigarettes smoked. People with hypertension, in particular, should not smoke because smoking constricts arteries, further increasing the blood pressure.

Diet   People who are overweight and people whose diets are rich in saturated fats and cholesterol may have more heart attacks and strokes than those who limit their weight and their fat intake. What constitutes a healthy diet is described in this book in the chapters on nutrition and physical fitness (pp. 298–331).

Exercise   People who get little or no exercise have more heart attacks than those who exercise regularly.

Stress   People who are subject to a lot of stress are likelier to become victims than those whose lives are more relaxed. Stress is difficult to avoid, but examination of one's personal values and life-style may reveal ways of reducing the strains.

Those are the factors that the individual can do something about. There are others that can be controlled with the help of a physician.

Hypertension   We already know what high blood pressure can do, but prompt treatment is effective in reducing its damaging effects. Studies in veterans hospitals have shown that patients who have been treated for hypertension have fewer strokes than those who have not been treated. Treatment is primarily with drugs that reduce blood pressure. The emphasis is on *prompt* treatment, which means early detection of hypertension—a simple matter of having a doctor measure your blood pressure.

Cholesterol   A high level of cholesterol in the blood may be a factor in the development of atherosclerosis. A doctor can measure a person's cholesterol level and prescribe drugs or a diet—if necessary—to reduce it.

Diabetes   People with diabetes, a common disorder affecting sugar metabolism, or people with a familial tendency toward diabetes, run an increased risk of suffering a heart attack or a stroke. Detection and treatment of diabetes by a doctor can reduce those added risks.

Other Factors   There are also some factors that are beyond anyone's control—sex, for example. Men have more early heart attacks than women. The incidence of heart attacks among women has been rising rapidly in recent years, however, possibly because more women have taken up cigarette smoking and because more women are competing for high-level jobs. Among black people in the United States, hypertension is twice as common as it is among whites. Black people have more strokes, and more severe strokes, and often have them at relatively early ages. We don't know why. Heredity, too, seems to play a role that is not understood. It is known that people whose families have a history of heart attacks or strokes run greater risks of suffering them than those with no such family history.

Emergency Care and Treatment

Every heart attack, every stroke, is an emergency. That means speed is all-important. Every minute of delay in getting professional help for the victim increases the danger. About half of all deaths from heart attacks in the United States occur within an hour after the appearance of the first symptoms. And a majority of those deaths occur outside of hospitals. Chances of survival are being improved by the growing use of specially equipped "cardiac ambulances" staffed by medical or paramedical personnel specifically trained to deal with such emergencies. Aboard the ambulances are drugs and machines that can be used to restore breathing, restart the beating of a heart that has

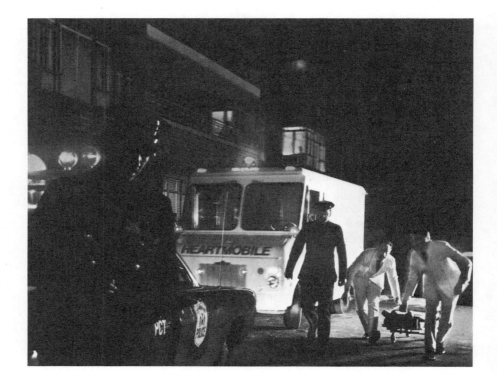

stopped, and monitor and regulate the heartbeat, all while the patient is on the way to a hospital.

More and more hospitals, particularly the larger ones, now have special coronary care units in which the patient's heartbeat is monitored twenty-four hours a day by equipment that automatically triggers an alarm, summoning immediate help, if there is any significant change in the heart rhythm. An increasing variety of drugs, surgical techniques, and technological advances are used in the treatment of heart and stroke patients. Because it dilates the arteries, nitroglycerine has long been used to ease the pain of angina pectoris. Medicines such as digitalis and quinidine help stabilize the heart's rhythm. Digitalis can also increase the effectiveness of the heart's pumping. Anticoagulant drugs reduce the chances of additional blood clots forming and bringing on repeated heart attacks or strokes.

Heart-lung machines, which temporarily take over the functions of those organs, make it possible for surgeons to perform open-heart surgery. They can repair heart valves deformed by birth defects or rheumatic heart disease or they can replace them with artificial valves. In many cases, damaged segments of arteries can now be surgically replaced by artery transplants or by installing flexible synthetic tubing. An important advance is the development of a surgical technique for bypassing a clogged coronary artery to relieve the pain of angina. The possibility that such operations may reduce the danger of heart attacks is being investigated.

Opaque dye injected into an artery and X-rayed can reveal spots where the artery has been dangerously narrowed by atherosclerosis. This technique is particularly useful in the possible prevention of a major stroke in a patient whose vulnerability has been established by transient stroke symptoms. The X-ray *arteriogram* can disclose the location of atherosclerotic plaques in the carotid arteries of the neck. Such plaques sometimes break up and release debris, which floats upstream to block a brain artery. Once discovered, they can be cleaned out of the carotid artery with a device resembling a tiny RotoRooter.

Also helpful are electronic pacemakers implanted under the skin that can take over the regulation of the heartbeat when the heart's own regulatory cells have been damaged.

Rehabilitation

For many a survivor of a heart attack or a stroke, life will never be the same again. A damaged heart must be pampered, and a damaged brain may leave a limb permanently lifeless, a tongue unable to form words, a mind confused forever. But a survivor is one who is still alive, and even a different life can be fulfilling. Some people who recover can return to their jobs and to most of the activities that were interrupted by their crises. Some can't. Determining the highest level of activity the patient can return to, helping him or her learn to accept new realities, and giving him or her as much support as possible—sympathetically but without demeaning pity—are the goals of rehabilitation. It should be a group effort involving doctors, nurses, possibly counselors, therapists of various kinds, and—most of all—the patient and his or her family.

The patients, particularly if they are physically or mentally impaired stroke victims, may need professional help in dealing with possible emotional problems. They may need to be convinced of their own worth and given motivation to recover as completely as possible. Their doubts about their ability or inability to work, to socialize, to perform sexually must be dealt with. They may need the help of physical and, sometimes, speech therapists. Prosthetic devices may be required to help them walk, or to grasp things.

For the survivors of heart attacks, a test of cardiac reserve capacity can help determine just how much physical and mental stress their damaged hearts can stand. If their former jobs seem too strenuous, they, like many stroke victims, may need retraining and help in finding a suitable new job.

With prompt emergency care, modern hospital treatment, and proper rehabilitation, someone like our friend Harvey may still look forward to a long and satisfying life.

The Kidneys

Bones can break, muscles can atrophy, glands can loaf, even the brain can go to sleep without immediate danger to survival. But should the kidneys fail, neither bone, muscle, gland nor brain could carry on.

The heart, the body's pump, keeps the blood circulating. The kidneys, the organs that act as the body's washing machines, keep the blood clean. Earlier, it was mentioned that kidney disease sometimes causes high blood pressure and that high blood pressure, in turn, can result in kidney failure. Atherosclerosis, too, can damage the kidneys by choking off their blood supply. So closely interrelated are the cardiovascular system and the kidneys that they merit discussion in the same chapter.

The human body has two kidneys, one on either side of the spine, behind the other abdominal organs at the bottom of the rib cage. They are marvelously complex. Each contains about seventy miles of filters and tubes in about one million miniscule units called *nephrons*. Through this intricate filtering system, all of the blood in the body passes every twenty minutes. Wastes are separated out and about 99 percent of the fluid, thoroughly cleansed, is returned to the bloodstream. The other 1 percent is dispatched to the bladder to be flushed out of the body as urine. Either kidney can

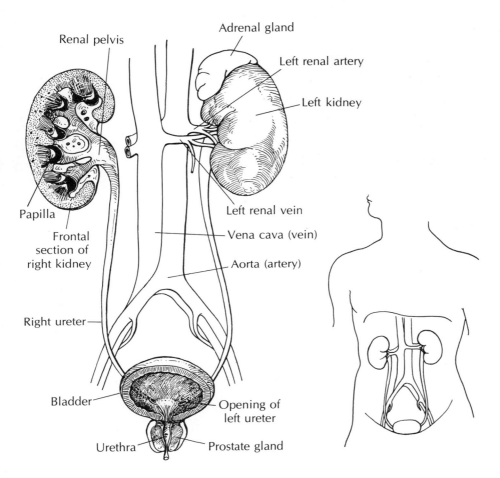

FIGURE 15-d *The human urinary system: Frontal view. Insert shows position in body.*

function independently of the other. If one is lost, the other can keep its owner alive and well. If both stop working, the results may be fatal. About 100,000 people in this country die of kidney diseases each year.

Common Kidney Diseases

Pyelonephritis   This is an infectious inflammation of kidney tissue; affects more people of all ages than any other kidney ailment. Attacks may range from mild to severe, and the condition can become chronic. Early detection and treatment usually leads to complete recovery.

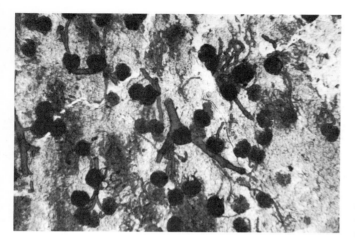

Section of human kidney tissue injected with dye to show glomeruli.

Nephrosis A disease found most often in children, but sometimes in adults. The kidneys allow protein molecules to escape from the blood into the urine, and the loss of protein results in water accumulating in the body, bringing on generalized swelling. The cause of the disorder is unknown, but drugs can often suppress the disease.

Acute Glomerulonephritis It is a noninfectious inflammation affecting the *glomeruli*, tiny tufts of capillaries within the nephrons. Usually occurring after streptococcal infections, it is most common in children and young adults. Destruction of nephrons by the inflammation hampers kidney function. Most patients recover within a few weeks.

Chronic Glomerulonephritis This can develop from acute glomerulonephritis or from unknown causes. It can bring about progressive damage over many years before betraying its presence, and it leads to uremia. There is no known cure.

Polycystic Kidneys These result from congenital defects in the nephrons. Cysts in the kidney tissue may affect the kidney function, produce symptoms of uremia, and require hospitalization.

Uremia This is not a disease but a condition that may result when the kidneys fail from any cause. Wastes accumulate in the blood, often causing serious illness or death.

Treatment of Kidney Disease

The various kidney diseases may announce their presence through a variety of symptoms—a burning sensation during urination, too-frequent urination, blood or coffee-colored urine, swelling of the face, feet, or abdomen, low back pain, headaches, or fatigue.

Many kidney ailments can be combated with drugs. Antibiotics are useful against pyelonephritis. Diuretics, which help the kidneys do their work, can relieve swelling. Cortisone suppresses the effects of nephrosis, although how it works isn't understood.

Dialysis   Not many years ago, complete failure of both kidneys meant almost certain death within a matter of weeks. That is no longer true. Two developments have saved the lives of thousands of people whose kidneys stopped functioning. One is the successful transplantation of healthy kidneys from either live or dead donors (since only one kidney is really necessary, healthy donors can give one up without endangering their own lives). The other development is the artificial kidney (dialysis) machine, which can be attached two or three times a week to the blood vessels of a patient to perform the blood-washing function of the kidneys.

Transplants of kidneys or other organs, unless from a very close relative, once had a relatively small chance of success because of the body's natural defense system. The antibodies would attack and try to destroy the foreign substance "invading" the body. The technique of "tissue typing," which matches the tissue of the kidney donor as closely as possible to that of the recipient, along with immuno-suppressive drugs that restrain the antibodies, have made kidney transplantation a common and increasingly successful operation.

Artificial kidney machines are still so expensive, and personnel trained to operate them so scarce, that their benefits are denied to many who need them. Much research is being directed toward developing simpler and cheaper artificial kidneys.

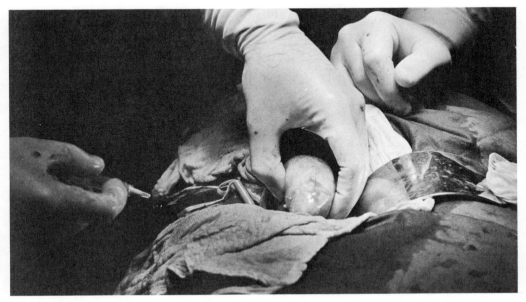

Kidney transplant.

Summary

Chronic diseases—those that usually develop over a long period of time and have long-term effects—have become the major killers and cripplers in the United States. Chief among them are diseases affecting the heart and blood vessels, brought on in most cases by atherosclerosis.

Atherosclerosis is a process in which substances deposited on the linings of arteries gradually narrow the blood passages, often blocking them entirely. Blockage of a coronary artery can cause a heart attack. Blockage of an artery feeding blood to the brain can cause a stroke.

Hypertension (high blood pressure) also causes many strokes, contributes to heart attacks, and, sometimes, leads to kidney failure.

The risks of suffering a heart attack or a stroke can be reduced by proper diet, exercise, and avoidance of cigarette smoking, among other factors. Developments in emergency care, surgery, and technology are improving the survival chances of those who do fall victim.

The kidneys are the "blood-washing" organs. A number of little-understood diseases may affect their functioning. Many victims of those diseases are being helped by drugs, kidney transplants, and artificial kidney machines.

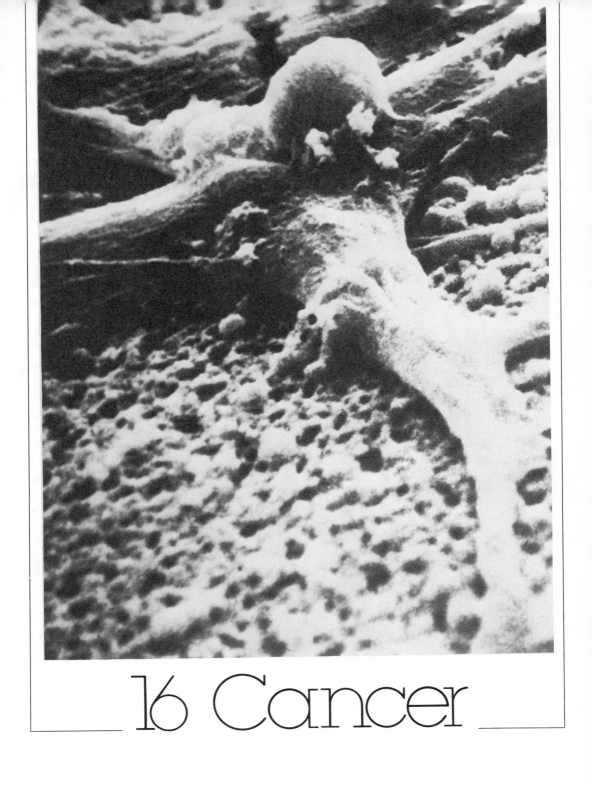

16 Cancer

A number of years ago a syndicated newspaper horoscope writer announced that people born under the astrological sign of the crab would be identified in the column from that time forward as "moon children." The innovation, the writer explained, was intended to spare those people the discomfort of being associated with the word *cancer*. Such delicacy demonstrates the extent to which that mysterious group of diseases, which share the Latin name of the inoffensive crab, holds sway over the imagination. In many minds, cancer equals death.

The notion is not groundless, to be sure. Cancer is second only to heart disease in the number of deaths it causes in the United States each year. But tens of thousands of cancer victims recover, and the chances of recovery are increasing steadily as more effective means of treatment are developed. "We are saving one out of three persons who get cancer," the American Cancer Society reports. "But we could be saving one out of two, with the means we have on hand today, with early diagnosis and prompt treatment."

What Is Cancer?

Cancer is cells gone wild. Normally, the cells that make up the body behave in strict obedience to the instructions carried in their genes. They divide and redivide in accordance with some law passed down through the evolutionary chain, each cell formed for a purpose, each one carrying out that purpose—rebuilding some worn-out tissue, fighting an infection—in exquisite harmony, like soldiers in a perfectly disciplined army. Then, in one cell, a mutation takes place (it would be carrying the army analogy too far to call it a mutiny, although the words have the same Latin root). Somehow the cell breaks the genetic restraints. It grows out of control, invading the tissue around it. As it grows, it divides into other cells like itself (often somewhat crab-shaped, hence the name), that continue the uncontrolled growth, destroying normal cells as it spreads.

Some cancers are tumors (swellings, or lumps); but not all tumors are cancer. A *benign* tumor is one in which cells grow out of control, but do not destory the surrounding tissue. Benign tumors do not spread to other parts of the body, and are rarely a threat to life. A *malignant* tumor is cancerous. If its growth continues unchecked, it will not only destroy the tissue in its immediate vicinity but may invade blood vessels or lymph channels, which will carry the destructive cells to other parts, a process called *metastasis* (from the Greek *methistanai,* to place in another way).

While some kinds of cancer may spread to different parts of the body by metastasis, others are "generalized" from the beginning. These include *leukemia,* which affects the white blood cells.

There are many kinds of cancer. Some run their deadly course in a matter of weeks; others may be present for years before any symptoms appear. Some respond well to existing methods of treatment, others less well.

250

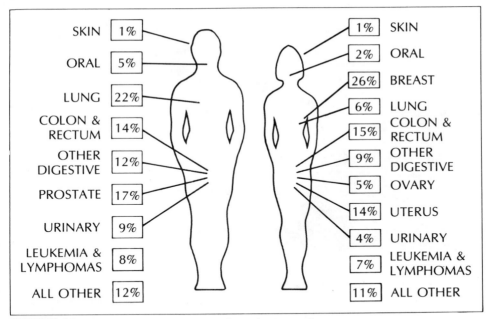

SKIN	1%			1%	SKIN
ORAL	5%			2%	ORAL
				26%	BREAST
LUNG	22%			6%	LUNG
COLON & RECTUM	14%			15%	COLON & RECTUM
OTHER DIGESTIVE	12%			9%	OTHER DIGESTIVE
PROSTATE	17%			5%	OVARY
				14%	UTERUS
URINARY	9%			4%	URINARY
LEUKEMIA & LYMPHOMAS	8%			7%	LEUKEMIA & LYMPHOMAS
ALL OTHER	12%			11%	ALL OTHER

FIGURE 16-a *1977 Estimates: Cancer Incidence by Site and Sex.*
Source: American Cancer Society, *Cancer Facts and Figures,* 1977.

The Causes: Cancer from "Outer Space"

Exactly what takes place at the molecular level inside a cell, just how the genetic signals get switched to set a cell off on a destructive rampage, is not yet clear. In many cases, however, cancerous growth is triggered by agents from outside the body, including certain chemicals and radiation. To use a fanciful comparison, it is as though invaders from another galaxy took over our minds, causing us to run amok. In fact, the most common cancers—those of the skin—are actually caused in most cases by "invaders" from space, the ultraviolet rays from the sun. This radiation can in some way alter the chemical structure of a cell, turning it malignant. Fortunately, skin cancer is usually curable (and the right kind of screening lotion, which a doctor can recommend, will protect the sunbather from most of the ultraviolet rays).

That other kinds of radiation can cause cancer has been demonstrated by the unusually high rate of leukemia among survivors of the atomic bombings of Hiroshima and Nagasaki and of lung cancer among some uranium miners—and these are only a couple of examples. There is solid evidence, too, that some chemicals cause cancer, as shown by the high incidence of certain types of cancer among workers in particular industries and proven by extensive research with animals. Some asbestos workers, for example, are prone to getting a type of cancer, *mesothelioma,* from breathing tiny

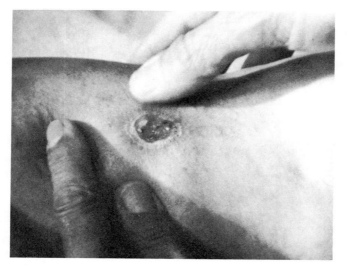

Skin cancer lesion.

asbestos fibers. And people who work with certain dyes are threatened with cancer of the bladder. These are only a few of the known cases of cancer-causing chemicals. More are being discovered all the time.

Smoking and Cancer

It is suspected, though not yet proven, that some of the chemicals in the polluted air breathed by most of us are *carcinogens* (cancer causers). And there is no longer any doubt that one kind of pollution—cigarette smoking—is largely responsible for the fact that more men die of lung cancer than from any other kind of malignancy. Like the heart attack rate, the lung cancer rate in men increases in direct proportion to the number of cigarettes smoked. An increase in lung cancer, as well as in heart attacks, among women in recent years may be a result of more women having adopted the cigarette habit. (There are fewer cases of lung cancer among pipe and cigar smokers. But they, as do cigarette smokers, risk cancer of the mouth, throat, and bladder.)

Viruses and Cancer

Do viruses cause cancer? In animals, they do. A great deal of research has established that beyond question. There is even evidence that some kinds of virus-caused cancer may be contagious among cats and chickens, although there is no indication that the viruses involved can be passed on to humans. There is certainly no evidence that you can catch cancer from being around another person who has it. It has not been proven that any human cancers are caused by viruses, but studies strongly suggest that possibility. The search for a link between viruses and human cancer is rooted in the hope of someday developing anticancer vaccines.

Is cancer hereditary? Only a few kinds are, and they are rare ones. But members of some families have a familial tendency to suffer from certain types of cancer, including leukemia, and those cancers of the breast, colon, stomach, prostate, and lung. Why such cancers appear to run in some families is not understood.

Early Detection: The Key to Cure

Some people die of ignorance, some of indifference. Fear probably kills a considerable number. A few may even die of modesty. These are not, of course, the proximate causes of death. But they are among the reasons that cancer so often goes undetected until it is too late for effective treatment.

One person simply hasn't learned the warning signals of cancer. Another is too busy or just can't be bothered to have a physical examination. Still another has a suspicious swelling or a sore that doesn't heal, but he or she avoids going to a doctor for fear of discovering that it is, indeed, cancer. And some women actually find it too embarrassing to be examined by their doctor for possibly significant lumps in their breasts. These people may be among the thousands who die needlessly each year

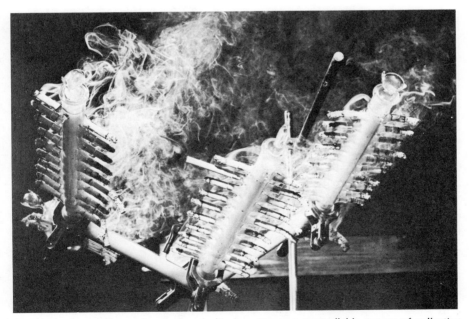

Smoking robot puffs on simultaneously lit cigarettes as a controllable means of collecting smoke residue. When painted on the backs of mice, the tars collected produce cancer.

TABLE 16-1 Reference Chart: Leading Cancer Sites, 1978*

Site	Estimated New Cases 1978	Estimated Deaths 1978	Warning Signals	Safeguards	Comment
Breast	91,000	34,000	Lump or thickening in the breast, or unusual discharge from nipple.	Regular checkup. Monthly breast self-exam.	The leading cause of cancer death in women.
Colon and Rectum	102,000	52,000	Change in bowel habits; bleeding.	Regular checkup including proctoscopy, especially for those over 40.	Considered a highly curable disease when digital and proctoscopic examinations are included in routine checkups.
Lung	102,000	92,000	Persistent cough, or lingering respiratory ailment.	80% of lung cancer would be prevented if no one smoked cigarettes.	The leading cause of cancer death among men and rising mortality among women.
Oral (Including Pharynx)	24,000	8,000	Sore that does not heal. Difficulty in swallowing.	Regular checkup.	Many more lives should be saved because the mouth is easily accessible to visual examination by physicians and dentists.
Skin	10,000 †	6,000	Sore that does not heal, or change in wart or mole.	Regular checkup, avoidance of overexposure to sun.	Skin cancer is readily detected by observation, and diagnosed by simple biopsy.
Uterus	48,000‡	11,000	Unusual bleeding or discharge.	Regular checkup, including pelvic examination with Pap test.	Uterine cancer mortality has declined 65% during the last 40 years with wider application of the Pap test. Postmenopausal women with abnormal bleeding should be checked.

TABLE 16-1 Reference Chart: Leading Cancer Sites, 1978*

Site	Estimated New Cases 1978	Estimated Deaths 1978	Warning Signals	Safeguards	Comment
Kidney and Bladder	45,000	17,000	Urinary difficulty. Bleeding—in which case consult doctor at once.	Regular checkup with urinalysis.	Protective measures for workers in high-risk industries are helping to eliminate one of the important causes of these cancers.
Larynx	9,000	3,000	Hoarseness—difficulty in swallowing.	Regular checkup, including laryngoscopy.	Readily curable if caught early.
Prostate	57,000	21,000	Urinary difficulty.	Regular checkup, including palpation.	Occurs mainly in men over 60. The disease can be detected by palpation at regular checkup.
Stomach	23,000	15,000	Indigestion.	Regular checkup.	A 40% decline in mortality in 25 years, for reasons yet unknown.
Leukemia	22,000	15,000	Leukemia is a cancer of blood-forming tissues and is characterized by the abnormal production of immature white blood cells. Acute lymphocytic leukemia strikes mainly children and is treated by drugs which have extended life from a few months to as much as ten years. Chronic leukemia strikes usually after age 25 and progresses less rapidly.		
Lymphomas	33,000	21,000	These cancers arise in the lymph system and include Hodgkin's disease and lymphosarcoma. Some patients with lymphatic cancers can lead normal lives for many years. Five-year survival rate for Hodgkin's disease increased from 25% to 54% in 20 years.		

Incidence estimates are based on rates from N.C.I. Third National Cancer Survey, 1969–1971.
*All figures rounded to nearest 1,000.   †Estimate new cases of non-melanoma skin cancer about 300,000.
‡If carcinoma in situ is included, cases total over 88,000.

Source: American Cancer Society, *Cancer Facts and Figures,* 1978. Reprinted by permission of the American Cancer Society, Inc.

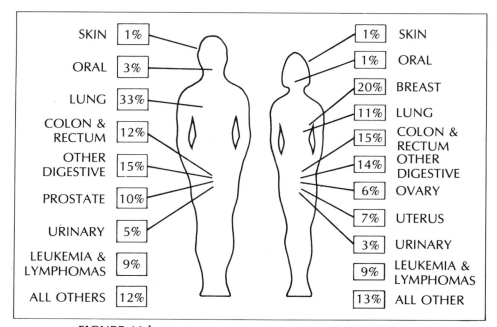

FIGURE 16-b *1977 Estimates: Cancer Deaths by Site and Sex.*
Source: American Cancer Society, *Cancer Facts and Figures,* 1977.

because they fail to take advantage of the most important weapons against cancer—
early detection and *prompt treatment.*

Cancer, you will remember, grows and spreads. The longer the delay in detecting and treating it, the smaller the chances for effective treatment. Studies have shown that 85 to 90 percent of the women whose breast cancers were detected while still localized were still alive five years later. Among women whose breast cancers had spread to other areas before being diagnosed, the five-year survival rate was only 40 to 45 percent. Similar figures resulted from studies involving other types of cancer.

How Is Cancer Detected?

Common warning signals that call for a visit to a doctor are changes in bowel or bladder habits, sores that do not heal, unusual bleeding or other discharges (particularly bleeding from the rectum), thickening or lumps in the breasts or elsewhere, frequent indigestion, difficulty in swallowing, obvious changes in warts or moles, and persistent coughing or hoarseness.

The best chance for a cure, however, comes when the cancer is discovered before any symptoms have appeared. And such discoveries are most likely to be made during regular annual physical examinations. Every physician is trained to detect signs of cancer, and a check for such signs is a routine part of every thorough examination. In addition to the more traditional methods of detecting breast cancer, the doctor may find

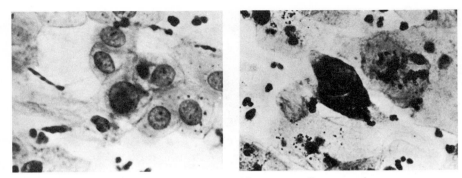

Pap smear: Normal cells.   Cancerous cells.

it advisable to order a mammography performed, a recently developed technique of diagnosis used when there are no lumps or other outward symptoms. The doctor may use a *proctosigmoidoscope,* a lighted tube, to examine the rectum and lower bowel. About 75 percent of all cancers of the rectum and colon can be detected in that manner; they are the most common internal cancers, and they are highly curable if they are diagnosed early and treated right away.

For women, a part of the regular examination is a Pap test (named for Dr. George Papanicolaou, who invented it), a simple, painless test for cancer of the uterus. A sample of vaginal fluid is examined under a microscope for cancer cells that might have been discharged from the uterus. The doctor can also teach a woman the proper technique for examining her own breasts. Every woman is advised to conduct a self-examination of her breasts once a month. Most lumps are not cancerous, but they do merit investigation.

What happens if the doctor suspects the presence of cancer? Normally, a tiny sample of tissue is taken from the area under suspicion and examined microscopically by a pathologist, a procedure called a *biopsy.* If the growth is malignant, treatment begins. If it is benign, the doctor has a very relieved patient.

Treating Cancer

Cancers are treated by surgery, drugs (chemotherapy), radiation, or a combination of these methods, depending on the type and location of the disease.

Surgery and Radiation

In some cases, sections of tissue containing malignant cells are simply removed. In others, cancer cells may be destroyed by certain of the growing arsenal of cancer-fighting drugs or by radiation therapy. The use of radiation is limited by the fact that it

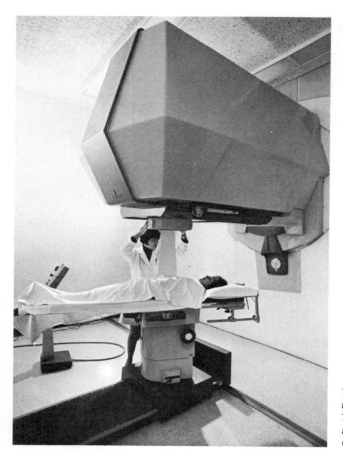

The world's most powerful Betatron, for treatment of cancer by radiation. This is installed at the Boston, Massachusetts, University Medical Center.

may also destroy normal cells, but its use has been highly successful against some kinds of cancer.

Immunotherapy

Some of the most promising research currently being carried on involves *immunotherapy*. This treatment attempts to stimulate the body's natural defense system to destroy cancer cells in the same way the germ-fighting white cells destroy invading bacteria. There is evidence that the natural immune response can kill cancer cells in some cases, which spurs hopes that eventually people will be able to get vaccinations to prevent cancer.

Summary

After heart disease, cancer is the second greatest cause of death in the United States, although an increasing number of cases can be treated successfully. Cancer is an uncontrolled growth of body cells in which the growth becomes malignant, destroys normal cells, and often spreads to different parts of the body through metastasis.

Certain kinds of chemicals and radiation are known to be among the causes of cancer. Some viruses cause cancer in animals and, possibly, in humans.

The earlier cancer is detected and treated, the better the chances that it can be cured. Regular physical examinations and prompt attention to suspicious symptoms lead to early detection. Cancer is treated by surgery, drugs, radiation or combinations of those methods.

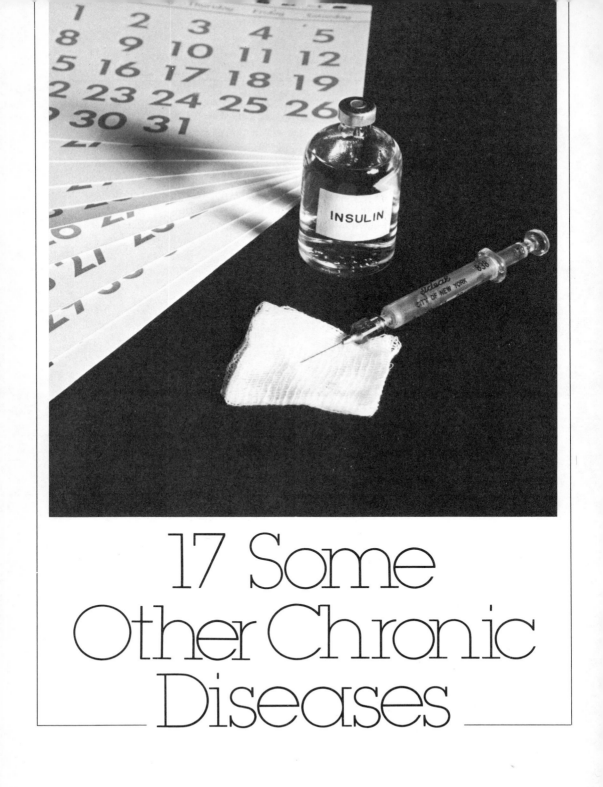

17 Some Other Chronic Diseases

> *And the Lord God formed man of the dust of the ground, and breathed into his nostrils the breath of life; and man became a living soul.*

Any time you're feeling isolated, as if you are an island cut off from the rest of the universe, there is a simple experiment that will remind you very quickly just how inseparable a human being is from his or her environment: Stop breathing. The Old Testament text equates breath with life. That hasn't changed. Without oxygen (which accounts for about 20 percent of the air we breathe, the rest being nitrogen, other gases, and myriad pollutants), the body begins to die within minutes. The job of getting oxygen into the bloodstream and of removing waste carbon dioxide, which results from the combination of oxygen with organic material in the body, falls to the lungs and their associated breathing apparatus. Together they make up the *respiratory system*.

The Respiratory System

The *diaphragm,* the large muscle between the chest and the abdomen, and the muscles of the chest wall work together like a bellows to force used air out of the body and draw fresh air into the lungs. The fresh air is warmed, moistened, and partially filtered as it flows through the upper respiratory system—the mouth, the nose, and the *trachea* (windpipe). From the trachea the air enters the *bronchial tubes,* which branch out into smaller and smaller passages forming the *bronchial tree.*

From the bronchial tubes, the air goes through even smaller *bronchioles* to the *alveoli,* the millions of tiny, delicate air sacs in which the lungs do their work. Through their thin walls, the alveoli feed oxygen into the blood that is flowing to the heart to be pumped out to the rest of the body. They then remove carbon dioxide from the blood being pumped back through the lungs after it delivers its oxygen supply to other regions. The used air is exhaled through the same tubes that bring the fresh air into the body.

The bronchial tubes are lined with specialized cells. Some of them secrete mucus, which lubricates and protects the tube linings and catches—like flypaper—much of the dust and other irritants in the inhaled air. Other cells have hairlike projections called *cilia,* which sway rhythmically, gently brushing dust-laden mucus toward the mouth. Usually, you dispose of this swept-up mucus by clearing your throat. If there is too much of it, you may cough. All kinds of things—colds and various irritants—can cause coughing. But if frequent coughing continues over a long period of time, the trouble may be more serious.

Chronic Bronchitis and "Smoker's Cough"

Bronchitis is an inflammation of the linings of the bronchial tubes. *Acute bronchitis,* caused by a virus infection, usually amounts to no more than a few days of fever, coughing, and general discomfort. Repeated infections or, more commonly, long-term irritation can result in *chronic bronchitis*. This is a condition in which excessive mucus is secreted constantly, narrowing the bronchial passages, interfering with the flow of air, and causing persistent coughing.

Because chronic bronchitis usually develops slowly, many victims don't even notice how much they cough. And if they do notice, since most of them are smokers, they are likely to dismiss it as "smoker's cough." Meanwhile, the irritated, mucus-clogged bronchial tubes make ideal breeding places for germs, and the victim becomes more susceptible to infections, such as pneumonia. Eventually, the condition can result in damage to the lungs or even to the heart.

Emphysema: A Deadly Kind of Inflation

Emphysema (inflation in Greek) is so closely associated with chronic bronchitis that the two are widely regarded as stages of the same disease. With the breathing passages clogged, air gets trapped in the lungs. Delicate air sacs balloon, burst, and are permanently damaged. After a time, the entire lung becomes enlarged, making it harder for the diaphragm and other breathing muscles to operate. Meanwhile, the destruction of walls between the alveoli, along with their capillaries, interferes with the transfer of oxygen and carbon dioxide between the lungs and the bloodstream. The heart may be

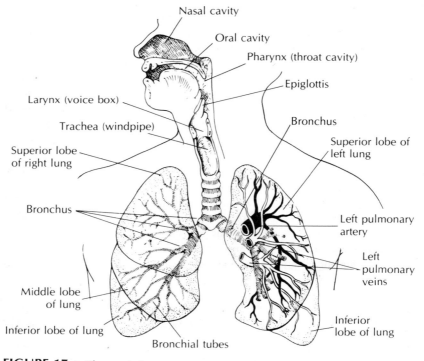

FIGURE 17-a *The respiratory system.*

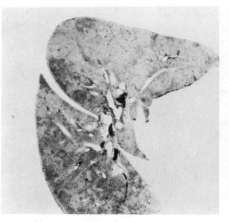

Normal lung tissue in which air sacs are too fine to be visible.

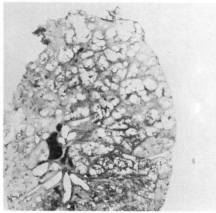

Lung tissue of heavy smoker, showing abundance of greatly enlarged air sacs.

affected because it must labor to pump blood through the lungs. Emphysema disables thousands of people and is often the cause of fatal heart failure.

Because the lungs have vastly greater capacity than is normally needed, the destructive process of emphysema can go on for years before the symptom—increasingly severe difficulty in breathing—becomes apparent. Men of fifty or older are most often affected, but the disease is likely to have had its beginnings much earlier.

The Causes

Some cases of chronic bronchitis, as we have noted, begin with infections. Air pollution apparently plays a role; the incidence of chronic bronchitis and emphysema is higher among those who live in smoggy cities. But by far the most common denominator among sufferers from chronic bronchitis and emphysema is cigarette smoking. Most victims are long-time smokers. And, as is the case with other chronic diseases associated with smoking, a growing number of women now get chronic bronchitis and emphysema, presumably because more women are smoking.

Antibiotics can be used to fight the infections associated with chronic bronchitis. Drugs that dilate the bronchial passages can ease breathing. Breathing exercises often help people with emphysema, though there is no known cure. The treatments vary. But one instruction is always the same: Give up smoking.

The Nervous System

The heart pumps. The kidneys filter. The lungs breathe. The brain . . .

The writer thinks: *The brain.* Fingers move below the field of vision, finding from memory hard, cool, round keys. *Clackety-clack.* T-h-e b-r-a-i-n. A faucet dripping, a

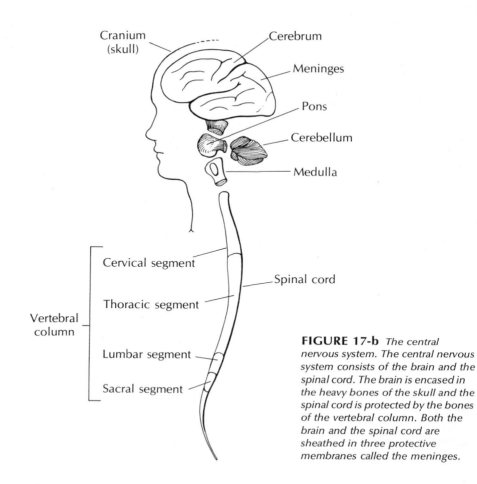

FIGURE 17-b *The central nervous system. The central nervous system consists of the brain and the spinal cord. The brain is encased in the heavy bones of the skull and the spinal cord is protected by the bones of the vertebral column. Both the brain and the spinal cord are sheathed in three protective membranes called the meninges.*

remembered sound identified (the writer thinks, as fingers blindly strike the keys, applying just the right amount of pressure, remembering spellings as if fingers had minds of their own). Fragrance of yellow roses on the table. . . . It's a little drafty here.

Abstract thoughts, tactile sensations, sounds, colors, odors, memories are all perceived, sorted out, classified; while muscles go on typing sentences, the brain thinks about itself. . . .

The foregoing was not just an unfortunate exercise in creative writing. It was a quick, unscientific exploration of a few of the things one human nervous system was dealing with more or less simultaneously. The same nervous system was performing countless other tasks at the same time, most of them beyond the threshold of awareness. Not only the thinking, such as it was, but all of the sensory perceptions and muscular activity that went into the preceding paragraphs were controlled, through little-understood processes, by electrochemical impulses traveling to, from, and within the brain, an organ weighing roughly three pounds (in an adult male) and containing billions of cells.

The basic cells of the brain and the rest of the nervous system are *neurons*. They contain fibers that carry electrically transmitted messages—like many microscopic telegraph wires. The fibers are sheathed in a protective, or insulating, material called *myelin*. The fibers of one cell are not connected directly to those of the next; They are separated by tiny gaps called *synapses*. When an electrical impulse traveling through a nerve reaches a synapse, a chemical is released to carry the impulse across the gap.

There is a dish of peanuts on the table in front of you. Light reflected from the peanuts stimulates your optic nerves. Along fibers and across synapses, the image is flashed to your brain. Through some mysterious, computerlike process, neurons in the brain compare incoming data with stored information and make the identification: Peanuts! Down the spinal cord and along the nerves of the arm, the brain sends instructions that set muscles in motion. Peanuts are transported to your mouth, where other instructions from the brain have meanwhile set digestive juices flowing. Taste buds send still more messages to the brain, where enjoyment is registered. But you barely notice it because you're busy watching television.

All that activity involves both the *central* and the *peripheral nervous systems*. The brain and spinal cord comprise the central nervous system. The rest of the nerves, a few connected directly to the brain and the rest to the spinal cord, make up the peripheral system. A few actions, such as the knee jerk reflex, are controlled by the spinal cord

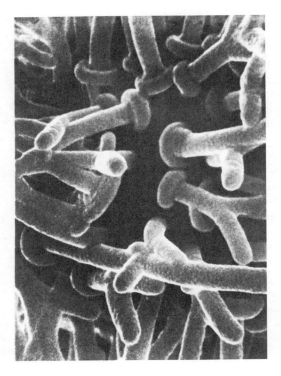

Nerve fibers and synaptic knobs. The knobs are believed to transmit nerve impulses from cell to cell.

without instructions from the brain. But the brain controls almost everything else that goes on in the body.

Autonomic Nerves

In a special category are those activities regulated by the *autonomic* (self-governing) nerves of the peripheral system, which are concerned with the heartbeat, breathing, digestion, and glandular functions—among others—and which were once thought to be beyond any conscious control. Lately, researchers have established that people can be taught to control some of those functions at will, lowering their body temperatures or slowing their heartbeats merely by concentrating on it. Many yogis have known for a long time how to do those things, but conscious control of autonomic functions is only now being seriously investigated by Western scientists.

Sympathetic and Parasympathetic Nerves   The autonomic nervous system is divided into *sympathetic* and *parasympathetic* nerves. The sympathetic nerves include masses called *ganglia,* which flank the spine. When you are calm, the parasympathetic nerves are in charge. Emotions, such as fear, stir the sympathetic nerves into action. They stimulate glands, speed up the heart, and instantly prepare you to run or fight or whatever else might be called for.

Some Common Disorders of the Nervous System

Like the wiring in some devilishly complex supermachine, the "wiring" of the nervous system sometimes becomes deranged in ways that can play havoc with the workings of the body.

Epilepsy   This disease, which included Julius Caesar among its famous victims, afflicts an estimated one out of every hundred people in the United States. For usually unknown reasons, groups of neurons in the brain discharge sudden bursts of uncontrolled electrical impulses—like showers of sparks from short circuits. The results may range from a momentary blackout or muscular twitching to a violent seizure in which the victim falls unconscious, froths at the mouth, and bites his or her tongue. Flickering or flashing lights have been found to bring on seizures in some cases—particularly the stroboscopic lights that became a popular accompaniment to rock concerts in the 1960s. A drug named phenytoin has proven highly successful in preventing epileptic seizures, apparently by blocking the transmission of those uncontrolled bursts of electricity. Most epileptics can now live normal lives.

Parkinson's Disease   This is associated with degeneration of the cells involved in the production of a chemical called *dopamine,* one of those essential transmitting substances that carries impulses across the synapses between neurons. Victims develop palsy (trembling). They may become partially paralyzed or lose the ability to speak.

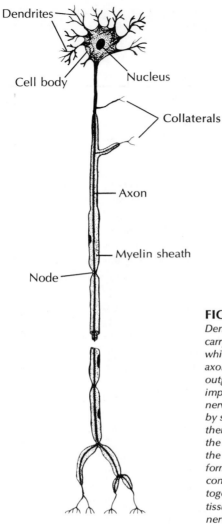

Dendrites

Cell body

Nucleus

Collaterals

Axon

Myelin sheath

Node

Terminal branches

FIGURE 17-c *A nerve cell. Dendrites are incoming fibers that carry impulses to the cell body, in which the nucleus can be seen. The axon, which may branch, is the outgoing fiber along which the nerve impulse is transmitted. In some nerve cells, the axon is surrounded by sheaths. In the illustration above, there is a sheath partly composed of the fatty substance myelin. In places the sheaths may be constricted, forming distinct nodes. A nerve consists of many nerve fibers packed together into bundles by connective tissues. Blood vessels penetrate the nerve, supplying it with food and oxygen.*

More than a million Americans are affected by this disease. Their symptoms can now be relieved in most cases by a drug called L-dopa, which stimulates the production of dopamine in the brain.

Multiple Sclerosis   MS is a disease of the central nervous system in which, unaccountably, the cells of the brain and spinal cord begin to lose their myelin sheaths. Scar tissue replaces the myelin, and the nerve tissue hardens. Gradually, the victim loses control over movements and may become paralyzed. Neither cause nor cure is known.

The Glands

You are walking through the woods. From behind a rock appears a very large, hungry-looking bear. Suddenly you find yourself in the upper branches of a tree, heart pounding. Never have you moved so fast, nor been so agile. What made it possible for you to scale the tree in such a hurry was a boost from your *adrenal gland.* This is only one example of the remarkable functions the body's glands perform.

The *exocrine* glands secrete fluids that are conveyed to internal cavities or to the outside of the body through tubes, or *ducts.* Their products include the milk secreted by the breasts as well as sweat, tears, mucus, saliva, and digestive juices.

The *endocrine* glands have no ducts. They manufacture complex chemicals called *hormones* (from the Greek *hormon,* to set in motion) that are released into the bloodstream to regulate a multitude of body functions, ranging from body growth to ovulation. Directly controlled by the central nervous system, the endocrine glands often respond to emotions, and in turn influence one's personality, as well as one's physical well-being. The adrenal gland, for example, responded to an emotion when you spotted that bear. Stimulated by the nervous system, it released *epinephrine* (also called *adrenalin*), which speeded up your heartbeat and increased your blood sugar, giving you the quick energy needed for your flight.

The *thyroid,* located in the throat, is another of the endocrine glands. It governs the rate of *metabolism* (from the Greek *metabole,* meaning change)—all of the chemical changes that take place in the cells, including the conversion of fuel into energy. A *hyperthyroidic* person is one whose thyroid is, for one reason or another, overactive. Such a person is likely to be nervous, jumpy, unable to sit still. He or she can't help it.

When Glands Malfunction

The *pituitary* gland, a pea-sized endocrine gland at the base of the brain, controls some of the other glands (including the *gonads,* or sex glands), and produces several hormones, including the growth hormone. Sometimes, because of hereditary or other factors, the pituitary gland makes too much or too little of the growth hormone, turning a child into a giant or a dwarf.

A more common glandular disorder is *diabetes,* a condition that seems to run in families. It occurs when the *pancreas* fails to provide enough *insulin,* which is needed to regulate the body's sugar metabolism. Sugar, normally used by the cells to produce heat and other energy, builds up in the blood and spills out in the urine. Meanwhile, the cells get their energy by burning protein, which instead should be used to build tissue and fats. When the fats are used to excess they produce a substance that can poison cells. Diabetics are further endangered by the fact that their condition contributes to the development of atherosclerosis, the most frequent cause of heart attacks and strokes.

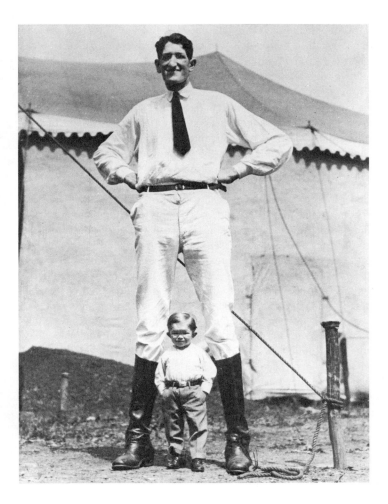

Results of pituitary dysfunction: gigantism and dwarfism.

Fortunately, regular injections of animal insulin can replace what the pancreas fails to supply. And, in many cases, drugs taken orally can stimulate the pancreas to produce more insulin. With the drugs or insulin injections and a careful diet, most diabetics are not disabled by their disease.

Genetic Diseases

Huntington's Chorea

In the early 1950s, when he was getting close to forty years old, Woody Guthrie began having trouble finding the right strings on his guitar with his fingers. The folk singer and composer wasn't well known then. And in the years that followed, as the growing popularity of his songs began to make his name famous, he wasn't able to take any bows. By the time he died in 1967 at the age of fifty-five, Woody Guthrie had been hospitalized for fifteen years, unable to control his muscles due to a steadily deteriorating condition.

His disease was *Huntington's chorea,* which, like some of the disorders described earlier in this chapter, attacks the central nervous system. But while the origins of some such diseases are unknown, we know where Huntington's chorea comes from: It is genetically transmitted—that is, it is carried in the genes from one generation to the next. Woody Guthrie's mother died of the same disease.

Genetic Transmission In some families there are abnormal genes, their chemical structures somehow gone wrong, that are passed from parents to children along with the normal genes. A number of diseases are transmitted this way. But not every child of parents with disease-bearing genes gets the disease. The chances vary, depending on the malady. In the case of Huntington's chorea, the chances that the child will be afflicted are one out of two.

The term *genetic* should not be confused with *congenital. Congenital* means existing from the time of birth, and a congenital condition, such as a heart defect, may have nothing to do with genetic transmission. On the other hand, a person may be born with a genetic disease but have no congenital symptoms. Like Woody Guthrie, most people whose parents had Huntington's chorea don't discover they have inherited the disease until they are in middle age. Like Woody Guthrie's son Arlo, they may be aware of their fifty-fifty chances, but they have to wait and see.

There is still no known cure for Huntington's chorea, which affects an estimated 100,000 Americans, but researchers have found evidence that it may be linked to a chemical imbalance in the brain, and they are trying to develop drugs to correct the imbalance.

Sickle Cell Anemia

Although sickle cell anemia is almost exclusively an affliction of black people in the United States, the reason is a matter not of race but of geography. Around the Mediterranean and parts of the Middle East, the disease is not uncommon among caucasians. The peculiarity in the red blood cells that marks the *sickle cell trait*—the genetic factor that predisposes one to the disease—is believed to have evolved as a defense against malaria epidemics that ravaged those regions and much of Africa many generations ago. The trait did provide resistance to malaria. But, passed along in the genes to successive generations, it created what has become one of the major health problems among Americans of African descent. About one of every ten black people in this country carry the sickle cell trait in their genes. Their red blood cells are abnormal, but, in most cases, not so abnormal as to cause any ill effects. However, if two people with the trait have a child, the chances are one out of four that the child will have sickle

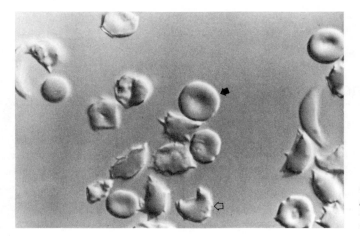

Red blood cells. Arrow at top points to a normal cell; arrow at bottom points to a sickle-shaped cell.

cell anemia—a painful, disabling, and life-shortening disease that affects more than 50,000 black Americans throughout their lifetimes.

Normal red blood cells—the ones that deliver oxygen throughout the body—are doughnut-shaped. They float easily through the small blood vessels. In victims of sickle cell anemia, the red blood cells become crescent-shaped—like a sickle. They tend to clump together, clogging capillaries and cutting off the supply of oxygen to some of the body's tissues. The results can be severe pain, swelling, and sometimes even failure of vital organs.

The average life of a normal red blood cell is more than one hundred days. Sickled cells usually last less than a month. The body cannot produce new red cells fast enough to replace them. With a shortage of oxygen-bearing red cells—anemia—people suffer from weakness, exhaustion, loss of appetite, susceptibility to infections. Children may be underdeveloped physically (although intelligence is not affected). Most victims of sickle cell anemia die young.

Gene Modification: A Hopeful Search

While intensive research is being directed toward finding specific treatments for Huntington's chorea, sickle cell anemia, and other genetic diseases, scientists are also working on the problem at a more fundamental level. They are trying to find ways of actually altering the structures of gene-carrying chromosomes. Much has been written about the possibility of someday creating "tailor-made" people in test tubes, of engineering chromosomes to produce someone's idea of a perfect physical specimen. That may be fantasy. But there is reason to hope that it may become possible, eventually, to remove defective genes from chromosomes, or to repair them, which could lead to the elimination of genetic diseases from the hereditary chain.

Joints, Muscles, and Bones

It is responsible for an annual loss of more than fourteen million work days in business and industry, plus uncounted days in other, nonremunerative pursuits . . . plus an estimated 1.5 billion hours of something loosely called "reduced efficiency." . . . It generates a yearly medical bill of one billion dollars—plus one billion, seven hundred million dollars in lost wages. It lies behind an estimated 12 percent of our welfare expenditures. . . . All in all, its total cost to our economy is believed to be in excess of nine billion dollars each year. . . . Not to mention the cost in human suffering. . . .

The popular picture used to be one of Grandma, hobbling on her cane toward her rocking chair, muttering about changes in the weather that she could foretell because her "rheumatiz" was acting up. Like many popular conceptions, it was very loosely based on reality. What Grandma called rheumatism would have been one of the dozens of rheumatic ailments, most of which are now generally grouped under the heading of arthritis, a word referring not to a specific disease but to a condition common to a variety of disorders. The word comes from the Greek *arthron,* which means joint, and *-itis,* a suffix indicating an inflammation. Thus, arthritis means an inflammation of a joint.

Arthritis in the United States

Arthritis is the nation's number-one disabling disease. An estimated fifty million people in the United States are afflicted with some form of arthritis; twenty million of these suffer severely enough to require medical care. And out of these twenty million, 3.5 million people are either wholly or partially disabled by arthritis.

There are over one hundred different types of arthritis, some with names such as tennis elbow, gout, and lupus, but the most dangerous and crippling forms of arthritis are rheumatoid arthritis and osteoarthritis. Rheumatoid arthritis attacks over five million people, usually aged between 20 and 45, while osteoarthritis, claiming twelve million victims, usually strikes older people—it is called the "wear and tear" disease. In addition, 250,000 people suffer from juvenile rheumatoid arthritis, and there are 600,000 new victims of arthritis in the United States every year.

Source: Interview, Arthritis Foundation, New York, N.Y.

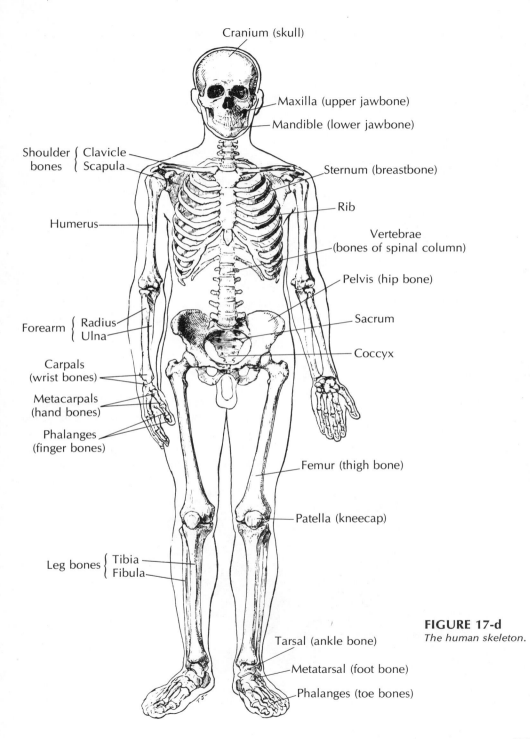

Cranium (skull)

Maxilla (upper jawbone)

Mandible (lower jawbone)

Shoulder { Clavicle
bones   { Scapula

Sternum (breastbone)

Rib

Humerus

Vertebrae
(bones of spinal column)

Pelvis (hip bone)

Forearm { Radius
        { Ulna

Sacrum

Coccyx

Carpals
(wrist bones)

Metacarpals
(hand bones)

Phalanges
(finger bones)

Femur (thigh bone)

Patella (kneecap)

Leg bones { Tibia
          { Fibula

FIGURE 17-d
The human skeleton.

Tarsal (ankle bone)

Metatarsal (foot bone)

Phalanges (toe bones)

At least 15 million Americans suffer, to one degree or another, from some form of arthritis. And, although the onset is more likely to come in the middle years, a great many of the sufferers are in their twenties and thirties.

Osteoarthritis

The most common form of arthritis, *osteoarthritis* is inaccurately named because it isn't an inflammation at all. It is a degenerative joint disease that eventually affects almost everyone if they live long enough. Most escape with only aches and stiffness, but many are disabled by the disease. Although it is usually blamed on gradual wear and tear on joints, it sometimes results from an infection, sprain, or fracture. One or more joints may be affected, but, unlike some of the more properly named varieties of arthritis, osteoarthritis doesn't move from joint to joint.

As osteoarthritis develops, first the fibrous, elastic cartilage that cushions the ends of the bones begins to erode. As the cartilage wears away, the bones themselves are affected, hardening and sometimes growing "spurs." The connecting ligaments and the muscles around the joint may also deteriorate. In many cases, nothing more complicated than aspirin is needed for treatment. If pain is acute, a doctor may prescribe other drugs. In extreme cases, surgery may be required. Surgeons can now replace entire hip joints with metal and plastic.

Rheumatoid Arthritis

The Arthritis Foundation estimates that about five million Americans suffer from rheumatoid arthritis, which most often attacks people before they reach the age of forty, and which affects about three times as many women as men. It usually starts with mild pain and swelling in one or two small joints, caused by inflammation of the *synovial membrane* lining the joints. Later, it may spread to other joints, and the pain may

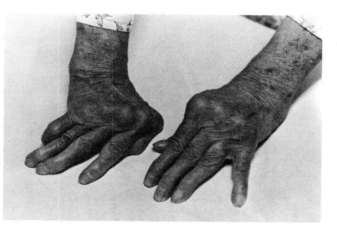

The results of severe arthritis.

become very severe. Spasms in the muscles around affected joints, a reaction to the pain, can pull the joints out of line and cause deformities—although that can usually be avoided if the disease is detected and treated early.

Rheumatoid arthritis comes and goes, its remissions interspersed with flare-ups, which apparently can be triggered by conditions ranging from stress to fatigue to changes in the weather (there *was* something in Grandma's predictions). What causes the inflammation is not clear. One theory is that some undiscovered virus is responsible. Another is that the disease results from an *autoimmune* reaction—the body turning its disease-fighting system on itself. Still another theory is that some kind of metabolic disorder is at fault. Research continues.

Pain-relieving and anti-inflammation drugs are used in treating rheumatoid arthritis. Physical therapy often helps. Surgery is used sometimes to remove the synovial membrane from a joint—it grows back eventually, but in the meantime the patient may be relatively free of pain for years.

Gout

The gout sufferer used to be a favorite of cartoonists, who pictured a man with one bandage-swathed foot propped on cushions, always somehow the object of ridicule. After all, it was the victim's own fault—or so the popular notion went. It was thought that gout was caused by too much rich food and strong drink. Actually, that excruciating inflammation of joints—usually starting with the joint of a big toe—is caused by a metabolic disorder, which results in an excess of uric acid in the blood. The acid forms crystals that are deposited in the joints. Certain foods can bring on attacks of gout, and alcohol can aggravate the condition, but they are not the causes. Fatigue, stress, or a stubbed toe can precipitate an attack.

Allergies

Cats, strawberries, wool rugs, chocolate, dandelions, aspirin, cashew nuts, hollyhocks, seafood, textbooks—the list of things that can start at least some people scratching or sneezing could go on endlessly. Eating certain foods or wearing particular kinds of fabrics makes some people break out in itchy hives. More commonly, a bit of plant pollen sets off a fit of sneezing. In either case, the reaction occurs because the individual has been sensitized to the offending substance sometime in the past.

During an earlier encounter, the body's defenses created specific antibodies—or *allergens*—to fight the foreign substance as though it were a germ. Now each contact with the allergen rallies the antibodies to do battle. Cells are damaged; tissue swells. If skin tissue is affected, hives result. If the membranes in the nose and around the eyes become the battleground, there is sneezing and tearing.

The most effective remedy for an allergy is to identify the allergen and avoid contact with it. That isn't always possible, of course. Victims can often be desensitized by repeated injections of small amounts of the antigen, which reduces the severity of their reactions. Physicians may prescribe various kinds of drugs to relieve symptoms.

Hay Fever

Hay fever, or *allergic rhinitis,* afflicts about a tenth of all the people in the United States. The majority of the sufferers are adolescents and young adults. It is a direct reaction of the mucous membranes in the nose to specific allergens, usually pollens. Attacks occur during the seasons when plants are releasing their pollen into the wind. Substances, such as house dust, are sometimes responsible. In those cases, there is year-round suffering. Hay fever does not actually cause a fever. It is uncomfortable but hardly ever dangerous.

Asthma

Asthma, which occurs in about 1 percent of the population, is likely to be more serious. It affects the bronchial passages to the lungs, causes them to swell, and forces the victim to cough and gasp for breath. Prolonged attacks can be disabling or even fatal, although fatalities are rare. *Extrinsic* asthma is an allergic reaction to any of a number of substances. There is another kind, *idiopathic,* or *intrinsic,* asthma, which results from unknown causes.

Summary

The lungs feed oxygen into the blood and remove waste carbon dioxide. Air enters and leaves the lungs through the bronchial tubes. Chronic bronchitis, characterized by persistent coughing, narrows the tubes, encourages infections, and is associated with emphysema, a disabling and often fatal lung disorder. Cigarette smoking is believed to be a major cause of emphysema and chronic bronchitis.

The brain controls body functions by sending and receiving electrochemical impulses through the nerves. Its control can be disrupted by nervous system disorders including epilepsy, Parkinson's disease, and multiple sclerosis.

Exocrine glands secrete fluid including milk, sweat, tears, mucus, saliva, and digestive juices. Endocrine glands secrete hormones, often in response to emotions, and influence the personality as well as physical well-being. Results of glandular dysfunctions range from improper growth to diabetes.

Genetic diseases are transmitted in the genes from parents to offspring. Among them are Huntington's chorea and sickle cell anemia. Scientists hope eventually to be able to modify chromosomes to eliminate genetic disorders.

A group of painful and sometimes crippling diseases, affecting millions of Americans, fall under the general heading of arthritis. Osteoarthritis, really a degenerative joint disease, is the most common. Rheumatoid arthritis, also common, causes severe pain and can result in bone and joint deformities.

People develop allergies when their bodies create antibodies in response to contact with pollen or other substances. Hay fever and asthma are among the most common types of allergies.

References

p. 261   Genesis 2:7.

p. 272   Sheldon Paul Blau and Dodi Schultz, *Arthritis* (New York, 1974), p. xii.

PART VII
Well-Being

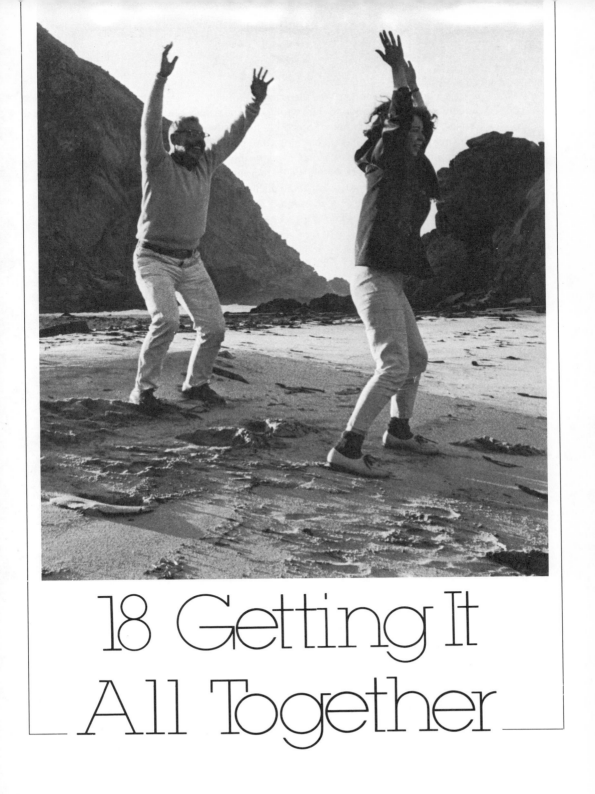

18 Getting It All Together

Jerry is a humanities student. His plans for the future are unsettled. He would like to do something to help the poor, to right wrongs, to make the world a better place. He would also like to get rich and famous. Sometimes he sees himself as a precocious politician, at once modish and dignified, charming and profound, bowing humbly to gratefully cheering masses from a dais he shares with the mighty. Once he envisioned himself graciously accepting the Nobel Peace Prize as his ideal mate (looking remarkably like a certain girl in Sociology 101) watched worshipfully. And then there are times when Jerry thinks he might chuck it all and go into forestry.

What he really likes to do is go rock-climbing with a pleasant companion (should he call the girl in Sociology 101?) or get together with friends to talk and listen to music or go to movies or take a girl someplace to eat hot-fudge sundaes and explore life's possibilities. He likes to do a lot of things, and he doesn't have enough time for all of them because study and work take so much of his time. He realizes, of course, that education is important and that he is going to have to make a living some way. And there are all those dreams of fame and fortune. But the future is vague and uncertain, and there is always *now*.

At the moment, Jerry is plodding through a reading assignment for a required health course, something that hasn't figured in any of his dreams. The book will probably suggest that he give up hot-fudge sundaes, live on raw carrots, and jog five miles a day so that even if he doesn't live forever it will seem that way.

Health, he reads, is a delicate balance. . . .

The Balancing Act

At the beginning of this book it was observed that health is a state of balance among numerous and diverse elements of our internal and external environments. That includes the social environment, which is both physical and mental. Everything is interrelated. Both physiological and psychological causes have both physiological and psychological effects. Which is a wordy way of saying that life is very complicated.

In practical terms, we have to balance things as best we can. Much of the time that means balancing immediate pleasure against potential consequences, palpable *now* against shadowy future, today's hot-fudge sundae against—well, where's the harm in a hot-fudge sundae? No harm, really, if one has only an occasional hot-fudge sundae. If Jerry has a hot-fudge sundae today, though, will that satisfy his sweet tooth? What about tomorrow? How many hot-fudge sundaes will he consume during the next ten years? How much sugar and cholesterol (possible contributors to heart attacks and other illnesses) will he consume? How fat will he get? How would obesity, in a culture that places a high value on slimness, affect his social life, his self-image? How would a damaged self-image affect his confidence, his performance? Could hot-fudge sundaes cost him his good grade average, the girl in Sociology 101, the Nobel Prize? What, on the other hand, is life without hot-fudge sundaes?

Fortunately, Jerry doesn't have to give up hot-fudge sundaes. What he has to do is strike a balance between now and the future. He has to have enough hot-fudge sundaes to keep him from becoming terribly unhappy without having so many that he sabotages his potential. If Jerry can't be reasonably happy without an unhealthy number of hot-fudge sundaes, then his life is out of balance somewhere. He may need professional counseling. Or he may just need some realistic self-examination. Does his life lack something for which he compensates by consumption of hot-fudge sundaes? What are his needs? What, really, are his goals?

Basic Needs

Abraham Maslow, the humanistic psychologist, postulated a hierarchy of human needs, beginning at the bottom with the most basic requirements for survival and ascending. According to Maslow, each of the needs emerges as an urgent motivating factor only after the needs lower in the hierarchy have been at least partially satisfied; to one who is starving and freezing, food and shelter are more important than companionship; and one who feels unloved puts, often unconsciously, acceptance ahead of achievement.

Not all psychologists accept Maslow's hierarchy in its entirety. The concept of self-actualization, which some consider so vague as to be indefinable, is particularly troublesome. There is no doubt, however, that some needs take precedence over others. Some needs, such as those for food and water, are clearly physiological; if they are not satisfied, the deprived one dies. Other needs are psychological in origin, based on values acquired from parents, peers, or society; their fulfillment may or may not be matters of survival, but, in any case, the happiness of the individual is at stake. Because of the inseparability of mind and body, organism and environment, and individual and

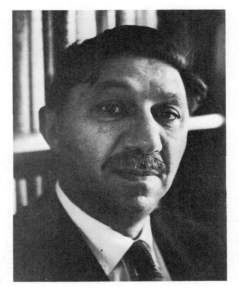

Abraham Maslow.

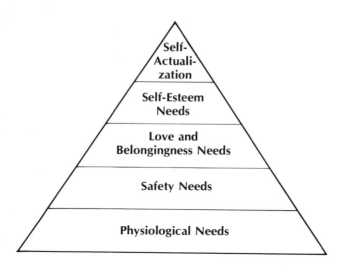

FIGURE 18-a *Maslow's hierarchy of human needs. The level of each class of needs must be reached and satisfied before the next higher level can begin to assume a dominant role in motivating the personality.*
Source: A. H. Maslow, *Motivation and Personality* (Harper & Row, 1954).

society, unsatisfied physiological needs affect emotions, and unsatisfied psychological needs often make people physically ill.

Higher Needs

As the more basic needs are fulfilled, higher needs assert themselves. Given food, warmth, and security, a person becomes aware of his or her loneliness. Provided with companionship and affection, people begin, inevitably, to yearn for something more. This new itch demands scratching, but sometimes the itchers cannot figure out just *where* they itch. Or they locate the itch but can't reach it, can't find a way to satisfy their needs. So they distract themselves by scratching in familiar, reachable places. They have another hot-fudge sundae. Hot-fudge sundaes are not primarily responses to the basic, physiological need for food. The chemical ingredients of a hot-fudge sundae, taken separately in powdered form from a laboratory shelf, would satisfy whatever physiological need there might be for those particular ingredients. But they wouldn't be as satisfying as an actual hot-fudge sundae.

A hot-fudge sundae might, to some extent, satisfy certain aesthetic needs. It might, possibly through conscious or unconscious association with a childhood experience, serve temporarily as a substitute for the satisfaction of some other need. But *what* other need? And does it matter, if the substitute works, if what is happening *now* is satisfying?

Preparation for the Future

The flower children of the 1960s tried to live completely in the present, the eternal now. They took drugs and were satisfied with whatever was happening at the moment. For them, there was no tomorrow. But tomorrow eventually came.

Everyone gets older. For many, that undeniable fact is difficult to accept. It isn't easy for today's football hero to see himself as a middle-aged man. He admits intellectually that he will age, but emotionally he doesn't believe it. The realization that it *has* happened dawns astonishingly, sometimes devastatingly, on the middle-aged. Deep down, they still feel like the same people they were in college, but the evidence of their mirrors, and of their aches and pains, their stiff joints, and their shortness of breath, proves that something has happened for which they were never quite prepared. "Oh to be twenty again," they exclaim, "and know what I know now!" They try to warn their children. The children listen impatiently to these older people, knowing secretly that *they* are different, that it will never happen to them.

Middle Age

One of the astonishing things about middle age is the realization by those who have arrived on that plateau that, however worn and ridiculous and boring they may look to their children, they are still very interesting to themselves. Life, rendered at least somewhat more intelligible by experience, yields new fascinations, new promise—if the bemused survivor remains in any sort of condition to take advantage of it.

A healthy young human is like a factory-fresh, custom-built car, every part

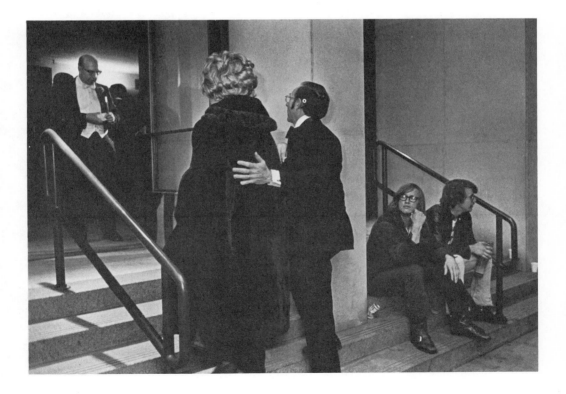

machined to perfection, a marvel of softly throbbing harmony. Lovingly maintained, thoughtfully driven, such a car can provide a lifetime of dependable, pleasurable service. Neglected, ill-used, it begins to squeak and rattle and balk, perhaps almost imperceptibly at first, then more and more alarmingly. Parts fail. Trips to the mechanic become increasingly frequent. With enough patching, the battered machine may keep running, but much of the pleasure is gone. A beat-up car can, of course, be traded in for a new model. A life cannot.

The trick with life, as with a fine car, is to enjoy it now *and* in the future. The secret of the trick lies at least partially in the pursuit of goals.

Establishing Goals

In her early twenties, Shirley MacLaine was already a famous movie star. At the age of forty she was an even more famous star. She was also involved in politics, was writing books, and was still being interviewed for her beauty secrets by writers for popular magazines. In one such interview, she described her preparation for a strenuous nightclub act:

> So there I was in a gym, day after day, working out with these god-awful exercises. The mental and physical discipline was horrendous. But I now realize that the reason it was horrendous was that I was impatient. You must give yourself time, make it yours, make it work for you. What you have to do is focus on, say, a six-month period ahead, when what you're working for, whatever it is, will be accomplished, and concentrate on *that*. If you keep visualizing what you want at that point six months ahead—like a skinny you on December 25—and have that constantly in your mind when those exercises hurt a little, or you have to turn down something delicious occasionally, you won't be so plagued with how difficult the present is. Temptation won't last more than four or five seconds. And, as a matter of fact, the struggle and denial while you're working toward your goal can be enjoyable. I'm certainly not a masochist, but I truly believe that if life is "pleasant" all the time, you get bored and restless. *I* do. I think that happiness is a struggle, if what you're struggling for is self-improvement. The little hard things you have to do to improve yourself are part of the happiness. And, if you're working to better yourself, your self-esteem will be higher. Purpose and self-esteem—now *that's* beauty, that's health, that's attractiveness. That's also women's liberation.

For most people, the "horrendous" kind of discipline described by Shirley MacLaine is neither necessary nor advisable. Shirley MacLaine's thoughts, however, serve to illustrate how goals can link present and future, how they can make getting through tonight without a hot-fudge sundae seem worthwhile. Instead of a negative approach—giving up tonight's hot-fudge sundae because otherwise something terrible might happen in the future—the goal inspires a positive attitude. This attitude justifies the sacrifice of the hot-fudge sundae in favor of the enjoyment of increased self-esteem and the probability that something good will happen in the future.

The fact is, of course, that most of the things we think of as goals are really only symbols. They are ways of visualizing the fulfillment of needs. The visualized goal may be a million dollars, a seat in the Senate, a one-person show at the Guggenheim; it may be spiritual enlightenment or a vine-covered cottage full of happy children. The true goal, however unconscious, is the satisfaction of needs such as security, love, esteem, knowledge, and beauty. And at least some of those needs can be satisfied, as Shirley MacLaine observed, in the *pursuit* of goals.

Having established as a goal a successful nightclub act, which symbolizes the fulfillment of various needs including increased self-esteem, the performer submits herself to discipline, which in itself increases her self-esteem. She thus obtains, as a benefit of *pursuing* a goal, at least part of what she is seeking. The goal, in a sense, brings the future into the present; instead of *now* versus uncertain *then,* life becomes a continuum, a reflection of one aspect of the wholeness that is the literal definition of health.

Developing a Perspective

If I were to put it into a very few words, my dear sir, I should say that our prevalent belief is in moderation. We inculcate the virtue of avoiding excess of all kinds— even including, if you will pardon the paradox, excess of virtue itself. . . .

Such was the philosophy of Shangri-La, that mysterious earthly paradise in which life was forever tranquil and, it seemed, almost immoderately satisfying. Shangri-La was, to be sure, a figment of a novelist's imagination, but the philosophy makes good scientific sense. The word moderation is rooted in the Latin *modus,* a measure. To moderate is to measure, to put things together in their proper proportions, to *balance.*

Balancing Your Life

This chapter has been concerned with the balancing of things that may not, considered separately, seem to have very much to do with each other; the relationships become evident only when the perspective shifts, when life is considered as a whole. In the following chapters, some important elements of life and health—food, physical exercise, and the management of stress—will be considered separately. It will be found, however, that each element creeps into discussions of the others, that they are interrelated in sometimes surprising ways.

Awareness of the interrelationships and of the importance of balancing all of the parts of the whole helps make more sense out of the business of dieting and exercising and, perhaps, even meditating. Such awareness is helpful, too, in avoiding the pitfall of "excess of virtue." And in this context, a health faddist who adheres grimly to tasteless diets and punishing exercise schedules, however boring and depressing they become, could be described as excessively virtuous.

As Shirley MacLaine put it, "Short range, I would say my goal is to try and get through tonight without having a hot-fudge sundae, because I really feel like one, and

I've been thinking about it for six days. Eventually, of course, I'll have one. I'm not going to ask *too* much of me.''

Summary

The balancing act necessary for good health may involve the weighing of today's pleasures against tomorrow's consequences. All of us have needs: some of them are matters of survival, some of pleasure. Higher needs assert themselves as the more basic needs are satisfied.

Your aim in life should be to enjoy it now *and* in the future. At least part of the secret lies in pursuing goals—and enjoying the struggle.

References

p. 287   James Hilton, *Lost Horizon* (New York, 1922).

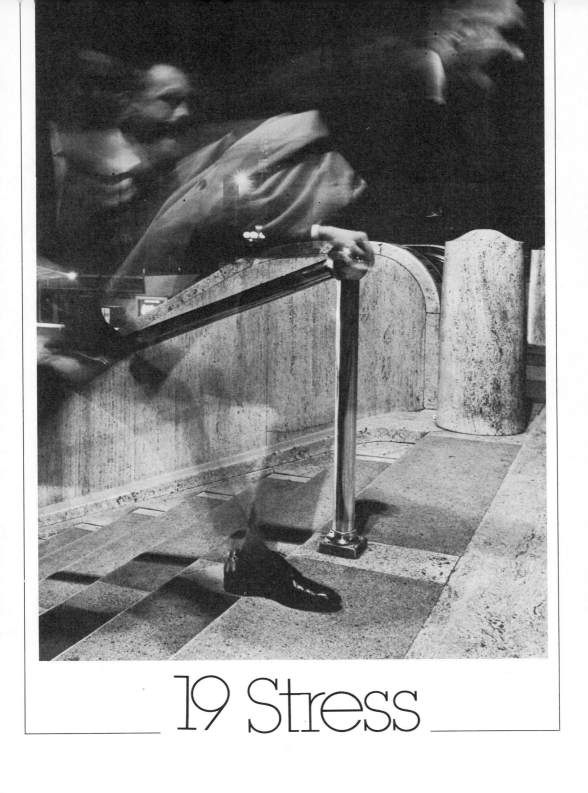

19 Stress

A guitar player tunes his instrument by applying just the right amount of stress to each string. If a string is too slack the notes turn sour. Stretch the string too tight and it snaps.

The human organism is also "tuned" by stress, but in much more complex ways. We have no handy knobs we can twist to adjust the amount of stress we experience. There are, however, methods that can be used to control human stress to some extent. Before we discuss these methods, we must define just what stress *is* in a human being.

Defining Stress

The literal definition of the word (from the Latin *stringere,* to draw tight) describes what people usually mean when they complain about stress; they are "under pressure," which makes them "uptight," "tied up in knots," "all wound up." As a scientific term, stress means something more. It is a continual, variable state of tension produced by the normal functioning of the body. Every demand on the body, whether for the extra energy needed to run up a flight of stairs or for the production of a particular enzyme by a single cell, results in some change in the balance of the internal chemistry. And every such change demands some additional response in order to restore the internal balance to normal. A great many such adjustments and readjustments are going on constantly inside each of us. Every change, however minute, produces some stress. Only if there were no activity of any kind—no breathing, no heartbeat, no brain functioning—would there be no stress. In the words of Hans Selye, a researcher in the field, "Complete freedom from stress is death."

Demands that produce stress are called *stressors.* Stressors may be either physical or psychological. A stressor may be pleasant, unpleasant, or neutral, so far as our subjective emotional reactions are concerned. A stressor may be a kiss, a promotion, a chill wind, a drug, a germ, a punch in the nose, the prospect of final examinations, or some unfelt, invisible exchange between molecules. Depending on the nature of the stressor, the response may be negligible or it may be literally hair-raising. What we usually mean when we talk nonscientifically about stress is *excessive* stress produced by psychological stressors, the kind that makes one feel tied up in knots. That kind of stress is always uncomfortable and sometimes disastrous.

The Modern Primitive

. . . Nor is it any wonder that we offend the stomach in our language, as it is the stomach which accounts for the offenses to our person. *I shall no longer stomach your insults* makes clear our outrage, and heralds, too, the production to excess of hydrochloric acid. Prodded by tension, rage, angst, the floodgates open and a veritable torrent of corrosion flows from the stomach lining to slosh in scalding puddles across membranes, inflaming, burning, eroding—finally ulcerating. . . . It is through such a punched-out hole that we plunge to escape the injustices of our lives, our lovelessness, business reverses, resentment of the mortal condition. . . .

It is a long-established fact that emotional strain often leads to stomach ulcers. We don't know just why anger or anxiety should cause the brain to send messages along the vagus nerves telling the stomach to release excessive amounts of hydrochloric acid, which, normally, is a necessary and harmless digestive juice. Perhaps it has something to do with the fact that when primitive people met up with a potent stressor it was likely to be something that they could eat, if it didn't eat them first. Perhaps, along with spurts of adrenalin to prepare them for action, the cave people's bodies, when confronted by a sabre-tooth tiger, gave them extra shots of digestive juices to prepare them for their potential meals. In any case, whether they were going to club the tiger or run from it, the cave people weren't required to do a lot of thinking. They were tuned for *physical* action. And once they had acted, assuming that they survived, they could go back to their caves and relax while their bodies returned themselves to their normal, balanced states.

As a continuous, automatic process, all of this tuning and retuning made primitive people highly adaptable organisms. They were able to put on bursts of speed when it was called for and relax when the demand was gone, without wasting a lot of energy and incurring unnecessary wear and tear during relatively idle intervals. Without some such mechanism, people wouldn't have survived the rigors of evolution. The problem is that modern people, having inherited this admirable tuning mechanism, encounter different kinds of stressors, and their primitive responses are sometimes inappropriate.

Stress Response

Confronted, for example, by an overbearing and angry boss, the body responds as it would respond to a sabre-tooth tiger. The electrical and chemical messages that speed through the body do not say *Boss!* or *Tiger!* but *Prepare for action!* And the body, as of old, prepares for *physical* action.

The civilized brain, however, tells the modern person that the boss is a boss, not a tiger, and that the rules say people cannot club other people, let alone eat them. The person can't even run away from the boss without risking serious consequences. So the chagrined employee accepts an unjust dressing-down and goes back to his or her desk with grinding teeth, a churning stomach, a pounding heart, and muscles tied up in knots.

Still knotted up, the employee goes home and tries to relax. Internally, the body is attempting to restore its normal chemical balance. But the person is worried—about the boss, the bills, his or her excess fat, the bomb, black holes in space, barracudas. And the body responds to all of these dire fantasies as to so many sabre-tooth tigers. Inside the body, a furious struggle for balance is going on. The stress builds up.

Anxious and depressed, the person suffers the aches and palpitations and fatigue brought on by excessive, unrelieved stress. The physical discomfort makes him or her *more* anxious and depressed, which increases physical distress, and so on, creating a vicious circle. The person is constantly anxious, constantly tired. Eventually, unless the stress is brought under control, the person may literally wear him- or herself out.

Chronic excessive stress can lead to some of those psychological states called mental illness; it can result in ulcers, or it may contribute to other serious conditions, including heart disease.

Type A and Type B Stress Theory

A controversial theory advanced by two cardiologists (heart specialists), Meyer Friedman and Ray H. Rosenman, suggests that excessive stress may be the most important factor in the development of premature heart disease. By premature, we mean heart disease that claims its victims before they reach old age.

After studying their own and other doctors' patients, Friedman and Rosenman divided people into two categories, Type A and Type B. The Type A people are hard-driving, aggressive, acquisitive, always fighting the clock, never having enough time for all the things they try to accomplish. The Type Bs are more relaxed, though not necessarily less ambitious or less successful; they take their work or play as it comes, and they do not suffer from a sense of the urgency of time, nor are they overly competitive.

The Type As, Friedman and Rosenman reported, have a far greater number of premature heart attacks than do Type Bs. In fact, the doctors said, "In the absence of Type A Behavior Pattern, coronary heart disease almost never occurs before seventy years of age, regardless of the fatty foods eaten, the cigarettes smoked, or the lack of exercise. But when this behavior pattern is present, coronary artery disease can easily erupt in one's thirties or forties."

Other researchers have disagreed with the Friedman-Rosenman theory, observing that many studies have produced evidence that faulty diets, smoking, and lack of exercise *do* contribute to premature heart disease. There is little dispute, however, about evidence that excessive stress is at least one of the factors associated with heart disease. The evidence is at least strong enough to suggest that everyone should examine his or her own life-style and consider whether stress-reducing changes could or should be made.

Learning to Relax

There is one sure way to relieve excessive stress of the kind suffered by modern people: Relax.

That isn't, of course, always easy. *Try to relax* is a difficult piece of advice to follow; trying is not relaxing. Many people seek relief in alcohol or other drugs, but the body

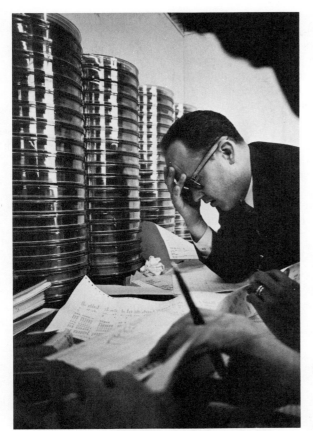

Two very different reactions to stress.

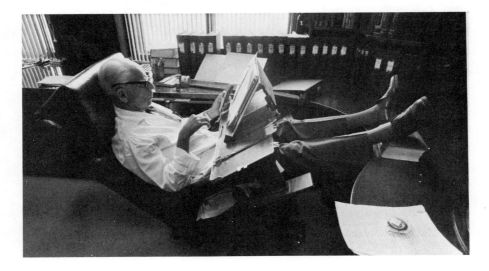

pays, often dearly, for such temporary surcease as these drugs can provide; the drugs themselves are potent stressors. The dangers of dependence on drugs, including alcohol and tranquilizers, are described elsewhere in this book.

What, then, is one to do? Fortunately, there are techniques by which numbers of people have learned how to relax without the aid of drugs. Since *trying* to relax, as a direct approach, doesn't work very well, these techniques employ various indirect approaches, some of which are described here.

Meditation

Meditation is a way of dealing with problems, in a sense, by ignoring them. There are numerous techniques for meditating. Usually, they involve sitting alone in a quiet, comfortable place for fifteen or twenty minutes once or twice a day and mentally chanting some particular word or phrase or syllable, or breathing slowly and rhythmi-

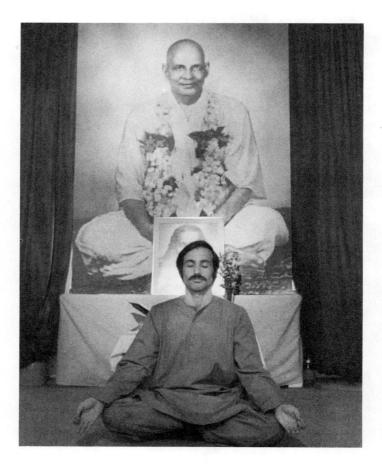

cally, or both. The mind seems to become concentrated on the chanting or breathing, and worries recede for the time being. Because of the intimate relationship between emotions and muscular tension, the body becomes relaxed as the mind relaxes. If the technique does its work, the meditator emerges from the session tranquil and refreshed, better able to cope calmly with the daily stressors.

One technique that has received a great deal of publicity is transcendental meditation, or TM, a name owned by a commercial organization called the International Meditation Society. TM involves the chanting of a word or syllable called a *mantra*. In Sanskrit, *mantra* means "instrument of thought." Many people have reported excellent results from using the TM technique. However, critics object to claims by TM practitioners that such results can be achieved only by the use of a *mantra* especially selected for each individual by a trained TM instructor during an expensive course of instruction. Some researchers say that the chanting of almost any word or phrase or syllable seems to serve the purpose. Herbert Benson, a Harvard Medical School cardiologist who has done extensive research into the effects of meditation, has reported that TM is only one of numerous techniques that can produce the desired results.

In one technique described by Benson, the meditator makes himself as comfortable as possible, closes his eyes, and breathes rhythmically through the nose, repeating the word "one" with each exhalation. For the metaphysically minded, according to Benson, words or phrases from the prayers of various religions can be substituted for the word "one" with equally good results.

Whatever technique is used, it is usually recommended that meditation be made a daily routine, to be practiced each morning and evening, or at whatever times seem to work best for the individual. For those who find that they are unable to discover an effective technique without personal instruction, some physicians and psychologists, among others, are prepared to teach meditation techniques.

Muscle Relaxation

Meditation attempts to relieve stress through the mind, but stress can also be tackled from another direction, through the muscles. Since *trying* to relax tense muscles does little good, the trick is to take the opposite approach, to *increase* the tension and then let the muscles relax themselves.

The subject sits in a quiet, comfortable setting, as one would for meditation. Then he begins at one or another of his extremities, the right hand, for example. The subject clenches his fist as tightly as possible, clenches it until it hurts, holds it clenched for a few seconds, then lets it go limp, as limp as possible, at the same time making himself mentally aware of just how his hand feels, observing the difference between tension and relaxation. The subject then repeats the process with the muscles of the forearm, then the upper arm. Then he or she goes through the same routine with the left hand and arm, the shoulders, neck, facial muscles and scalp, chest, stomach, buttocks, genitals, and so on down each leg in turn, until as many muscles as possible have been tensed and relaxed.

Throughout the exercise, the subject makes himself aware of the feelings of each muscle in turn, noticing how the tension seems to flow out of muscles when they are relaxed. Particular attention is paid to the facial muscles, which are very much involved in emotional states.

As quieting the mind through meditation also relaxes the body, so relaxation of muscles can help quiet the mind. The vicious circle of stress feeding on stress is interrupted. The organism is given a chance to restore its internal balance.

Biofeedback

In recent years some researchers have been exploring the stress-reducing potential of electronic equipment that provides "feedback," enabling the subject to monitor some of his own brain waves by listening to audible signals or watching dials. The signals are produced by special devices attached to an electroencephalograph (EEG). By means of electrodes affixed painlessly to the scalp, the EEG "listens" to electrical activity in the brain. The instrument can be adjusted so that only electrical waves of certain frequencies—those associated with relaxation—create the desired signals. After several training sessions with such equipment, many subjects are said to be able to produce the "alpha" waves associated with relaxation more or less at will. The subjects usually report that they feel mentally and physically relaxed after such sessions.

Biofeedback is still basically an experimental field, requiring expensive equipment and qualified operators. Researchers have reported that low-cost "feedback" machines

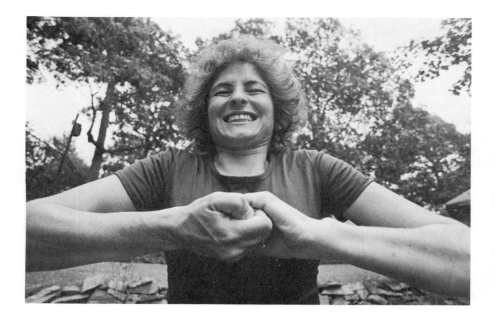

marketed commercially for use at home usually turn out to be ineffective money-wasters.

Exercise and Stress

Cave dwellers had no tranquilizers, EEG machines, or *mantras,* but they did get a lot of old-fashioned physical exercise. Many doctors believe that physical exercise is the best stress-reducer of all. Confronted by psychological stressors, as we have seen, the organism prepares for *physical* action. Running, swimming, and playing vigorous games enable the body to expend in healthy ways the energy that might otherwise go into the production of those uncomfortable symptoms associated with excessive stress. As the cave person "worked it off" by clubbing or running from the sabre-tooth tiger, we can work it off in play or in physical labor. People usually find that the pleasant tiredness that follows a strenuous swim is accompanied by a lifting of the spirits, once again accounted for by the inseparability of mind and body.

Summary

The ability to deal with stress is an essential component of good health. Stress is always with us—in the pressures of everyday life. Stress may be physical or psychological; the emotional reaction may be pleasant, unpleasant, or neutral.

Internal stress can produce physical discomforts that intensify the emotional distress. Stress must be controlled. Recommended stress reducers include meditation, biofeedback, and exercise.

References

p. 290   Hans Selye, *Stress Without Distress* (Philadelphia, 1974), p. 32.

p. 291   Richard Selzer, "The Belly," *Esquire,* Vol. 83, No. 3 (March 1975), p. 97.

p. 292   Meyer Friedman and Ray H. Rosenman, *Type A Behavior and Your Heart* (New York, 1975), p. 9.

p. 295   *The New York Times Book Review* (July 27, 1975), p. 21.

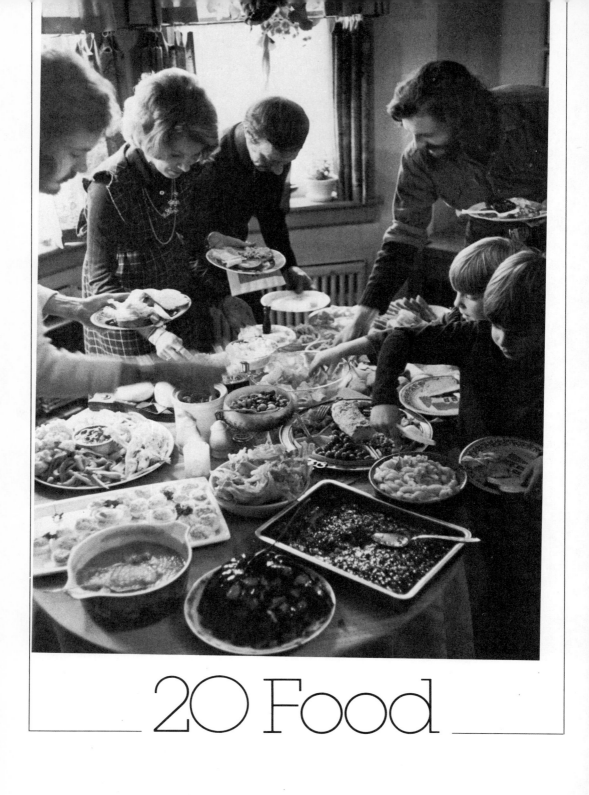

20 Food

Consider what happens when the organism we call a human being encounters the portion of its environment that is called a cheeseburger. The organism is made up of trillions of microscopic cells. Each carries on a complex life of its own: it reproduces itself according to its own genetic blueprint; it communicates with other cells; it performs a great many functions and contributes to the well-being of the community—the organism—as a whole.

An average cell manufactures hundreds of different compounds, each of which plays a part in some function of the body, and each requires specific building materials. The cell must obtain these materials from the external environment, but it is unable to reach out and get them itself. The acquisition of supplies is an enormously complicated community endeavor.

Humans and Food

When you eat a cheeseburger, it is not your stomach you are feeding but those individual cells. By the time the ingredients of the cheeseburger have been absorbed from the digestive tract, they are not anything that we would ordinarily think of as food. They are a lot of chemicals—elements and compounds—some of which will provide structural materials for enzymes, hormones, chromosomes, bones, skin, or hair, and some of which will be "burned" as fuel to provide the energy that drives the infinitesimal factories in all those cells. Through the organism's consumption of a cheeseburger, a community supply of materials has been acquired. Each cell can now select from the stockpile the particular materials it needs. But some essential materials may still be missing.

The Cell Factory

A cell may be thought of, very loosely, as a tiny manufacturing complex. Component parts are hauled in, products assembled, and orders shipped off to customers. Think of an automobile factory with cars in various stages of completion moving along an assembly line. Suddenly it is discovered that, through some management error, the assemblers have run out of fan belts. For want of a single part, the entire assembly operation is halted. The factory doesn't immediately go out of business. It sends out a rush order for more fan belts. If the order is filled promptly, work resumes with no great harm done. But if no fan belts arrive, the factory closes. Now suppose that all of the auto manufacturers ran out of fan belts at the same time, and all of their urgent orders for fan belts went unfilled. The entire auto industry would be shut down and the effects would spread rapidly to producers of component parts and raw materials. The economy would sink into depression; the community would suffer.

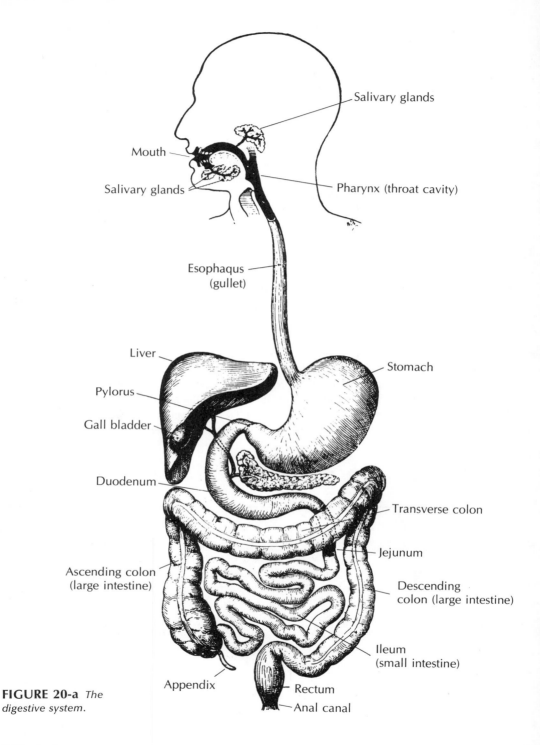

Salivary glands

Mouth

Salivary glands

Pharynx (throat cavity)

Esophaqus
(gullet)

Liver

Stomach

Pylorus

Gall bladder

Duodenum

Transverse colon

Jejunum

Ascending colon
(large intestine)

Descending
colon (large intestine)

Ileum
(small intestine)

Appendix

Rectum

Anal canal

FIGURE 20-a *The
digestive system.*

So it is with the organism, the community of cells, when a vital component is missing from the diet. The cells are unable to complete the assembly of some product needed to maintain the body's internal balance, and the whole system begins to falter. Lack of certain materials can lead to specific diseases, and resistance to diseases in general may be lowered. Stress increases as the body struggles to restore the balance. Both physical and emotional suffering may result.

The key to a healthy diet, then, is to select foods that provide both sufficient energy and *all* of the building materials the cells need to construct their innumerable products. The different kinds of building materials and fuels that we need to get from food are described in this chapter.

Proteins

About 80 percent of the human body is salty water, very much like the sea water in which, it is believed, life on this planet originated. Of the remaining 20 percent—the solids—about three-quarters consists of various *proteins* (from the Greek *proteios*, primary), the primary stuff of all living matter. The human body, in its various kinds of cellular "factories," manufactures more than 100,000 different proteins, which include the structural materials of the cells themselves, plus a great many enzymes and hormones that perform specific essential functions.

Amino Acids Proteins are complex molecules made up of smaller molecules called *amino acids.* When we talk of the need for proteins in our diets, we do not mean the plant or animal proteins, but their component amino acids. Proteins in foods are broken down in the digestive process, and the amino acids reach the cells separately, where they are reassembled into whatever kinds of human proteins are required. The human body uses only twenty different amino acids. But because of the many different ways in which they can be arranged in molecules, an almost infinite variety of proteins can be created—just as countless words can be formed out of the twenty-six letters in the English alphabet.

Ten of the amino acids that we need can be manufactured by the cells out of elements obtained from other food sources. They are called *nonessential* amino acids because it isn't necessary that they be included, as such, in our diets. The other ten amino acids cannot be assembled in the cells and must be included in the diet. They are the *essential* amino acids. Proteins that contain all of the essential amino acids are described as *complete,* and those that do not are *incomplete.* The importance of this distinction will be explained later in the chapter.

Carbohydrates and Fats

Our cells use the amino acids from protein foods primarily as building materials. All of that construction work requires a lot of energy. We usually get most of that energy from *carbohydrates* and *fats.*

Sugars and *starches* are carbohydrates. Fats are composed of *fatty acids* and other compounds. All carbohydrates and all fats are made up of different molecular arrangements of just three elements: carbon, hydrogen, and oxygen. In the cells, these elements react with additional oxygen that we inhale. Bonds between atoms are broken, releasing the energy that drives the cells. The atoms recombine to form water (hydrogen and oxygen) and carbon dioxide (carbon and oxygen). By a highly efficient arrangement we excrete the water and exhale the carbon dioxide.

Carbohydrates and fats, however, are not merely energy sources. Their constituent elements, along with some nitrogen from other sources, can be used by the cells in the assembly of some of those nonessential amino acids (all amino acids are composed of carbon, hydrogen, oxygen, and nitrogen). Furthermore, certain fatty acids, like some of the amino acids, are *essential* nutrients. And carbohydrates help break down some fats that otherwise would be incompletely metabolized.

Saturated and Unsaturated Fats   Later in the chapter you will read about *saturated* and *unsaturated* fats and why it is important to distinguish between them for dietary purposes. For the moment we will simply define these terms—for the benefit of those who wonder what they signify when they appear on food labels. The terms refer to the structures of the molecules. The molecules of unsaturated fats have empty spaces that could accommodate additional hydrogen atoms, while those of saturated fats do not. The molecule of a *monounsaturated* fat has room for one more hydrogen atom. The molecule of a *polyunsaturated* fat has room for more than one additional hydrogen atom. *Hydrogenated* fats are formerly unsaturated fats that have had hydrogen atoms added to make them saturated.

Micronutrients

Proteins, carbohydrates, and fats supply practically all of the structural materials and fuel needed by our cells, but small quantities of other materials are also essential. They are the *micronutrients,* so called because such tiny amounts of them are required by the body. The micronutrients are *vitamins* and *minerals.*

Vitamins were originally called vita-amines (*vita* is Latin for life) because scientists thought they were all amines, or ammonia compounds. When it was discovered that they were not, the word was shortened to its present form. Neither building materials nor fuel, vitamins appear to serve as tools in various cellular functions, such as assisting the enzymes in assembling and disassembling the amino acid links that make up proteins.

The essential minerals are common elements, such as iron, calcium, and phosphorus, which are used as structural materials (bones and teeth are largely calcium) and as components of many of the body's chemicals.

Sources of Essential Nutrients

The cheeseburger with which we opened this chapter, depending on its size and the quality of its ingredients, probably would satisfy at least a fourth of the daily protein

TABLE 20-1 U.S. Food and Drug Administration Recommended Daily Allowances for Certain Vitamins and Minerals

Vitamin or Mineral	Unit	Infants (0–12 Months)	Children Under 4 Years	Adults and Children 4 or More Years	Pregnant or Lactating Women
Vitamin A	IU	1500	2500	5000	8000
Vitamin D	IU	400	400	400	400
Vitamin E	IU	5	10	30	30
Vitamin C	mg	35	40	60	60
Folic acid	mg	0.1	0.2	0.4	0.8
Thiamine (B_1)	mg	0.5	0.7	1.5	1.7
Riboflavin (B_2)	mg	0.6	0.8	1.7	2.0
Niacin	mg	8	9	20	20
Vitamin B_6	mg	0.4	0.7	2	2.5
Vitamin B_{12}	mcg	2	3	6	8
Biotin	mg	0.05	0.15	0.3	0.3
Pantothenic acid	mg	3	5	10	10
Calcium	g	0.6	0.8	1.0	1.3
Phosphorus	g	0.5	0.8	1.0	1.3
Iodine	mcg	45	70	150	150
Iron	mg	15	10	18	18
Magnesium	mg	70	200	400	450
Copper	mg	0.6	1.0	2.0	2.0
Zinc	mg	5	8	15	15

Sources: FDA Drug Bulletin, 1975; National Academy of Sciences (National Research Council), Recommended Dietary Allowances, 8th Edition, 1975.

needs of an average-sized man. Assuming that it was served with the usual trimmings of tomatoes, lettuce, and pickles, the sandwich would also provide a good many other essential nutrients. The cheeseburger eater, however, would need to add a variety of other foods to his daily fare to meet all of the requirements of all of his cells for building materials and fuel. Nutritionists recommend that each day's meals include selections from each of the major food groups. Most foods are sources of some important nutrients, but it takes a number of different kinds of foods to furnish all of the nutrients we need.

Particular attention needs to be paid to protein sources. Meats, fish and fowl, milk and other dairy products, and eggs are the richest sources of complete proteins, although certain vegetables, as we shall see, are also good protein sources. Most nutritionists recommend that some source of complete proteins be included in every meal.

It is also generally recommended that several different kinds of fruits and vegetables—not just one or two—be eaten every day, since different plant foods provide different vitamins and minerals, as well as carbohydrates. Besides supplying many kinds of nutrients, vegetables and fruits serve another important purpose in the diet. Their cellulose fibers are made up of complex chains of starches that cannot be broken down by the human digestive system. Consequently they furnish bulk, or roughage, which helps keep the rest of the food moving through the digestive tract and aids in the disposal of wastes.

Food Supplements

Americans spend many millions of dollars every year on vitamin and mineral pills, protein concentrates, and other diet supplements, which are supposed to provide nutrients presumed to be missing from ordinary diets, or which are expected to give the users additional vigor or sexual potency or other special benefits. Nutritionists and physicians generally feel that most of that money is wasted. And, in fact, that the health of many people may actually suffer because they depend on such supplements instead of nourishing food.

Vitamins

The prevailing scientific opinion is that the kind of varied, well-balanced diet described in the preceding pages fills all of the nutritional needs of a normal, healthy adult. Additional vitamins or other supplements are required only in professionally diagnosed cases of deficiencies. As for pepping people up or improving their sex lives, vitamins

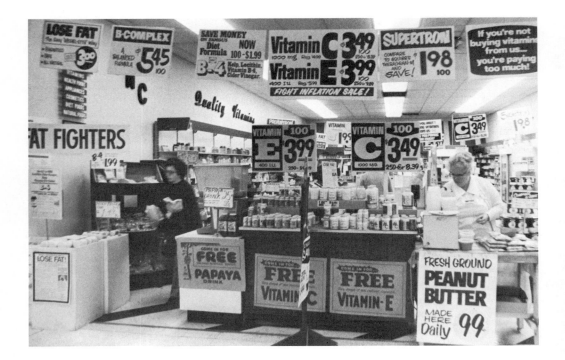

simply don't work that way, unless the person *has* been suffering from a deficiency. The cells will use only as much of each nutrient as they need for structural or other purposes, and additional quantities do no good at all. They may, in fact, do some harm; excessive amounts of certain vitamins, minerals, and even protein supplements can be toxic.

Vitamin C   Frequently a researcher reports that large doses of a particular vitamin appear to yield some special benefits. The news media make a fuss about the new "miracle" vitamin, and people rush to their drugstores to stock up. Usually, carefully controlled studies fail to substantiate the original findings. In recent years, for example, it has been claimed that massive doses of Vitamin C would prevent colds or minimize their symptoms. Some studies have indicated that Vitamin C may be somewhat effective in reducing cold symptoms, possibly because various kinds of infections increase the body's need for that vitamin. However, other researchers have concluded that Vitamin C's effectiveness against colds is nonexistent or negligible. In any case, many scientists are concerned about the possibility that ingesting unusually large amounts of *any* chemical may, over a period of time, have undesirable effects that cannot be foreseen. The question is not just, "What does this vitamin do?" The question is, "What *else* does it do?" Instead of taking a chance on the unknown, the cold sufferer is probably better off drinking some orange juice, which furnishes not only Vitamin C, but other nutrients, and at the same time replenishes body fluids that are depleted in fighting infections.

Vitamin E   Vitamin E is another example of a popular fad with no sound scientific basis. Its proponents claim, among other things, that it helps prevent heart disease and that it increases sexual appetites. Controlled studies have disproved such claims, but many people continue taking massive doses of the vitamin. Such dosing is fruitless, most authorities say, since Vitamin E is abundant in many different foods, and deficiencies are all but unknown.

Breakfast Cereals   Nutritionists are unenthusiastic, too, about breakfast cereals that are said to provide, in a single serving, all of the vitamins and minerals needed in the daily diet. The vitamins and minerals may be there, but the cereals, even with milk added, usually furnish only a small percentage of needed proteins. Instead of or in addition to cereal, a healthy breakfast includes some substantial source of complete proteins, as well as some fruits or vegetables, or their juices.

In general, nutritionists advise us to eat foods that are the natural sources of all of the essential nutrients, and to forget about additional vitamins or other supplements unless they are prescribed by a doctor.

Health Foods

During the past decade or so the health food business has grown into a large industry in the United States. So-called health food stores usually stock a variety of vitamin, mineral, and protein supplements, such foods as wheat germ, brewer's yeast, and blackstrap molasses, and some "organic," or "natural," fruits and vegetables. Just how much such merchandise does for anyone's health is questionable.

We have already observed that unprescribed vitamin, mineral, and protein supplements are likely to be a waste of money and could, in some cases, be harmful if taken to excess. Wheat germ, brewer's yeast, and the like are good sources of some nutrients, but they are no better than many other foods, and are often more expensive than other nutritious edibles. If they are used, the diet should still include a variety of other foods to make sure that no essential nutrients are missing. There are no miracle foods that can take the place of a varied, balanced diet.

Organic Foods

Claims about the supposed superiority of "organic" foods are often misleading. Usually, the term is taken to refer to vegetables and fruits that are grown without the use of commercial fertilizers or pesticides. The popularity of such foods seems to be based on a belief that fruits and vegetables grown with commercial fertilizers and protected by pesticides are somehow contaminated and that people who eat them may be poisoned. This idea reveals a lack of understanding of the way in which plants use the ingredients in fertilizers. In fact, the commercial preparations, as such, never get inside the plants. What they do is restore to the soil certain nitrates and other essential plant nutrients that have been depleted by farming of the land. Cow manure and other "organic" fertilizers do the same thing. The nutrients are taken from the soil by the plants as separate molecules, and there is no difference between a molecule of nitrogen from a commercial preparation and a molecule of nitrogen from cow manure.

The safety of certain pesticides has been questioned by authorities from time to time, and the use of some pesticides has been banned by the government. In general, however, there is no scientific evidence that the use of approved pesticides poses a serious threat to the health of consumers.

Food Additives   In the commercial preparation of foods, chemicals are often added as preservatives, coloring agents, or stabilizers. Such chemicals are tested for safety before use, and they are generally considered harmless in small quantities. With the growing use of such additives, however, some nutritionists have become concerned that the cumulative effects of taking a variety of nonessential chemicals into the body over a long period of time might eventually prove harmful in ways that are not now suspected. To be safe, nutritionists suggest that foods whose labels do not list unnecessary additives should be selected if such choices are available.

Vegetarianism

A person can obtain all of the nutrients needed from a vegetarian, or nonmeat diet, but the ingredients need to be chosen carefully. Most vegetables are low in protein content, and the proteins they do contain are often incomplete; they lack some of the essential amino acids.

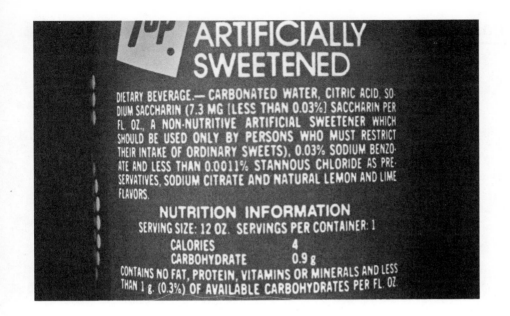

ARTIFICIALLY SWEETENED

DIETARY BEVERAGE.— CARBONATED WATER, CITRIC ACID, SODIUM SACCHARIN (7.3 MG [LESS THAN 0.03%] SACCHARIN PER FL. OZ., A NON-NUTRITIVE ARTIFICIAL SWEETENER WHICH SHOULD BE USED ONLY BY PERSONS WHO MUST RESTRICT THEIR INTAKE OF ORDINARY SWEETS), 0.03% SODIUM BENZOATE AND LESS THAN 0.0011% STANNOUS CHLORIDE AS PRESERVATIVES, SODIUM CITRATE AND NATURAL LEMON AND LIME FLAVORS.

NUTRITION INFORMATION
SERVING SIZE: 12 OZ. SERVINGS PER CONTAINER: 1

CALORIES 4
CARBOHYDRATE 0.9 g

CONTAINS NO FAT, PROTEIN, VITAMINS OR MINERALS AND LESS THAN 1 g. (0.3%) OF AVAILABLE CARBOHYDRATES PER FL. OZ.

Eggs, milk, and other dairy products are used by many vegetarians as sources of complete proteins. For those who eschew animal products altogether, soybeans, lentils, and other dried beans, dried peas, grains, and nuts are good protein sources. However, nutritionists usually recommend that a variety of such foods be eaten—some rice along with the beans, for example—so that amino acids missing from one may be supplied by the other. It should be remembered, too, that vegetable proteins are often less *available* than animal proteins for use by the body. Available proteins (a term often found on food labels) are proteins that can be broken down in the digestive process so that their amino acids can be absorbed by the body. Some of the proteins in vegetables are often locked into indigestible cellulose, and are therefore *unavailable;* so far as the cells are concerned, they are wasted. For this reason, people who depend entirely on vegetables for their proteins need to pay particular attention to their protein sources.

Zen Macrobiotic Diet

The late George Ohsawa, a Japanese writer, invented something he called the Zen macrobiotic diet, which, its name notwithstanding, has nothing to do with Zen Buddhism. Ohsawa did, however, draw on Oriental mysticism in designating foods as *yin* or *yang,* symbols that represent all of the opposites of the universe.

A proper balance of yin and yang foods, according to Ohsawa, would guarantee perfect health and cure everything from mental illness to cancer. There is no scientific basis for such claims. In its most extreme form, the macrobiotic diet consists almost entirely of brown rice. Nutritional deficiencies resulting from this diet have led adherents to the diet to a variety of diseases and to some deaths.

Food and Heart Disease

One of the puzzles that scientists have been trying for decades to solve is the relationship between the *cholesterol* in our foods and heart disease, the leading cause of death in the United States.

Cholesterol is a waxy substance, resembling the fats, but chemically a member of the alcohol family. The body, specifically the liver, manufactures cholesterol. We get still more cholesterol when we eat certain foods, particularly animal fats. It helps hold the walls of our cells together, acts as a sort of insulator between cells, and serves other important purposes in our bodies. We could not live without it. Yet it is also involved in the development of atherosclerosis (hardening of the arteries), the condition that leads to most heart attacks and strokes. Scientists are trying to answer several questions concerning this: Is it the cholesterol we eat that causes atherosclerosis? Would reducing the amount of cholesterol in our diets help prevent heart disease? Much of the evidence collected so far suggests that a high-cholesterol diet *does* promote atherosclerosis, but there are some baffling contradictions, and a definitive answer may be years in coming.

While waiting for that answer, cardiologists generally feel that the prudent course is to limit cholesterol intake, especially if blood tests reveal an above-normal amount of cholesterol in the blood. Blood samples are commonly taken during routine physical examinations, and if the cholesterol level is high, the doctor may recommend a low-cholesterol diet. Even if blood tests do not reveal elevated cholesterol levels, it seems advisable to avoid cholesterol-rich diets.

High Cholesterol Foods

Foods that contain particularly large quantities of cholesterol include egg yolks (not the whites), whole milk and products made from whole milk, beef, pork, mutton, lamb, and organ meats—such as liver and kidneys. All saturated fats seem to contribute to elevated levels of cholesterol in the blood. Saturated fats usually come from animals, but certain vegetable fats are also saturated. The latter include coconut and palm oils and, perhaps surprisingly, chocolate. Unsaturated fats do not raise blood cholesterol levels. Unsaturated fats, which are also the best sources of essential fatty acids, usually come from vegetables such as corn, safflower, cottonseed, soybeans, sesame, and sunflowers. Some researchers have reported that polyunsaturated fats actually seem to *reduce* blood cholesterol levels.

One of the problems in reducing cholesterol intake is that the richest sources of cholesterol and saturated fats include some of the best sources of complete proteins. Cholesterol intake can be reduced, however, without eliminating those protein sources from the diet. Use skim milk or low-fat milk instead of whole milk and cheeses made from skim or low-fat milk instead of those made from whole milk. Substitute fish or chicken, which are relatively low in cholesterol content, for other meats. When other meats are eaten, make sure they are as lean as possible, and trim off visible fat.

Good ways to cut down on saturated fats include the substitution of margarine

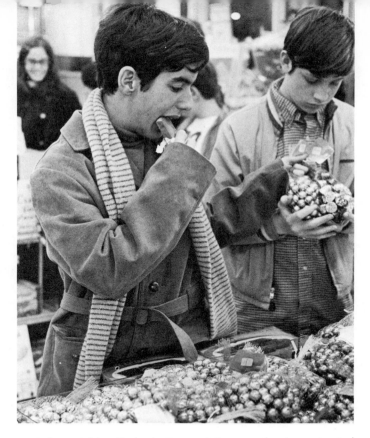

made from polyunsaturated vegetable oils for butter, and the use of polyunsaturated cooking oils instead of lard or other animal fats. It should be remembered, too, that the saturated fat content of processed meats such as frankfurters, bologna, and salami is quite high.

Suspicions About Sugar

America is a nation of sweet-teeth. Our sugar consumption averages about one hundred pounds a year for every man, woman, and child. This statistic takes on an ominous tinge when we consider the fact that sugar, like cholesterol, is suspected by many of contributing to the high incidence of heart disease.

When a person consumes more carbohydrates than his or her cells need for their immediate purposes, most of the excess carbohydrates are converted into fats, called *triglycerides,* and stored in the body. While it has not been proven that triglycerides are involved in the development of atherosclerosis, various studies have shown a statistical relationship between heart disease and high blood levels of triglycerides. Some researchers have suggested that triglycerides may affect artery walls and thus enable cholesterol deposits to build up. However, the body needs carbohydrates, both to provide energy and to help break down fats. What is to be avoided are *excessive* amounts of carbohydrates that will become possibly harmful triglycerides. Some carbohydrates could be eliminated from the diet by giving up fruits, vegetables, and grains, but these foods are also sources of many essential nutrients and of the roughage needed in digestion. Refined sugar, on the other hand, supplies (like alcohol) only empty calories—nothing but energy. Even raw and brown sugars and honey provide no significant quantities of important nutrients. Since we can get all of the energy we need from carbohydrate sources other than sugar, it is obvious that cutting down on sugar consumption is the best way to avoid triglyceride build-ups in the body.

Glucose   The sugar one eats, incidentally, is not the essential blood sugar from which the cells finally get their energy. Blood sugar is *glucose,* which is manufactured by the body from all kinds of carbohydrates and fats and even, if necessary, from proteins. Refined sugar, raw sugar, brown sugar, and honey are all forms of *sucrose,* which the body must convert into glucose before it can be used by the cells. Since the conversion takes a little time, the idea that eating sweets provides instant energy is fallacious. Eating any kind of food seems to yield a certain amount of instant energy because the liver releases additional glucose into the blood to furnish the energy needed for digestion. But that energy comes from the body's stores, not from the food we have just eaten.

If nutritionists and cardiologists frown on sugar as such, they frown even more on rich desserts containing whole milk, eggs, and cream, since such concoctions add cholesterol and saturated fats to large amounts of sugar. They are even more disapproving if the desserts also contain chocolate, adding still more saturated fat. To some nutritionists and cardiologists, ice cream is anathema, and such a thing as a hot-fudge sundae is unspeakable.

There are, however, psychological factors to be considered. On some occasions the sweet tooth must be satisfied. Too much self-denial can lead to excessive stress. If one can't make do with nutritious fruits, or with sugarless soft drinks as a less desirable alternative, the example offered by Shirley MacLaine in an earlier chapter may serve: Build up self-esteem by resisting temptation until an excess of virtue becomes unbearable, and then thoroughly enjoy the *occasional* hot-fudge sundae.

Hypoglycemia

Among the health fads that sweep the country from time to time, the recent popularity of *hypoglycemia* as a self-diagnosed disease has caused concern among nutritionists and physicians. Hypoglycemia, or low blood sugar, results when the pancreas secretes too much insulin (as opposed to diabetes, a condition in which the pancreas secretes too little insulin). Insulin is a hormone required by the cells for the metabolism of sugar. Too much insulin lowers blood sugar levels. The many possible symptoms of low blood sugar range from fatigue to irritability to anxiety to, in extreme cases, apparent mental illness.

Most physicians agree that hypoglycemia is not one of the more common ailments. Some cases are caused by tumors in the pancreas. But "functional" hypoglycemia, caused by some unexplained malfunction of the pancreas, has seldom, if ever, been diagnosed by most doctors.

Nevertheless, some doctors have claimed that millions of Americans suffer from hypoglycemia, and these claims have received widespread publicity. A great many tired, irritable, and anxious people (whose symptoms could be caused by any number of things) have decided that they probably have hypoglycemia, and have put themselves on "hypoglycemic" diets recommended in popular books, newspapers, or magazines.

One reason for concern is the fact that such diets, for complicated and scientifically controversial reasons, usually call for the elimination from one's diet of most foods high in carbohydrates. There are, as we have seen, good reasons for cutting down on some nonessential carbohydrates, but one shouldn't go too far; we need some carbohydrates.

Another cause for concern is that by self-diagnosing their vague complaints as hypoglycemia, and "treating" themselves with low-carbohydrate diets, people may be dangerously postponing professional diagnosis and treatment of some other illness. Self-diagnosis of any severe or persistent ailment is always hazardous; if a person thinks he or she is sick, the prudent course is to see a physician.

Why People Get Fat

It's unlikely that there were very many fat cave dwellers. Cave people did not regularly eat three meals a day, or even two. They ate what they could find, when they could find it. Their diets probably consisted largely of nuts, fruits, berries, and other vegetable matter, supplemented by bird's eggs and such animals as they could catch and kill with their crude weapons.

Sometimes, in draught or in winter, when there was no fruit and the hunting was poor, the cave people probably went hungry for days or even weeks. They no doubt suffered, at such times, from vitamin deficiencies and other penalties of poor nutrition. But they could go for a long time without starving to death because evolution had provided them with a means of storing in their bodies surplus fuel, which would, at least, supply their cells with enough energy to keep them functioning through a temporary famine.

Storing Fats

Along with other survival apparatus, which, though still necessary, often seems to do civilized people more harm than good, we inherited from the cave people their fuel storage system. It consists of a large number of specialized cells, unevenly distributed throughout the body. These cells contain compartments in which surplus fuel, in the form of triglycerides and other fats, can be stored for lean days. These *adipose* (from the Latin *adipis,* soft fat) storage cells are always with us. When their fuel compartments are empty, they are like collapsed ballons, taking up little space. When full, however, they bulge. When too many of them become too full, we are fat.

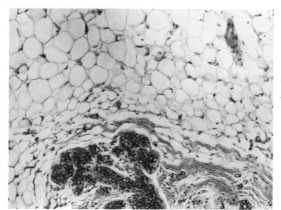

A cluster of fat cells (adipose tissue).

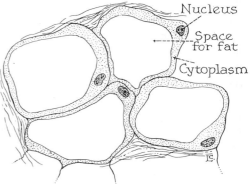

High magnification of adipose tissue showing spaces for fat.

Appestat

The cave people were unlikely to get fat, not only because their food supplies were uncertain and seldom overabundant, but because another internal mechanism, provided by evolution, regulated their food intake. In the hypothalamus, a primitive part of the brain, modern researchers have discovered two areas that together make up what is sometimes called the *appestat.* As a thermostat controls temperature, the appestat controls appetite. One part of it responds to the organism's need for food by setting in motion what behavioral scientists call food-seeking behavior. When the need for food has been satisfied, the other part of the appestat "turns off" the appetite, and the organism stops eating. That is, unless the appestat isn't working properly, in which case the organism may go right on stuffing itself with surplus supplies to be stored in bulging adipose cells.

We don't know why, but proper functioning of the appestat seems to be related to physical exercise. Most animals, in their natural habitats, never become overly fat, however much food is available. This has been attributed, at least in part, to the fact that the animals get plenty of exercise, which keeps their appestats in good working order. They "know" when to stop eating. It can be assumed that the cave people, what with hunting for food, fleeing from predators, and fighting with other cave people, got plenty of exercise and therefore had well-tuned appestats. Even when food was plentiful, they probably didn't eat much more than their bodies needed.

Then, over the millennia, the cave people became farmers, built cities, established universities, opened delicatessens, and created many sedentary occupations. More and more of them got less and less exercise. At the same time, for more and more people, food supplies became constant, varied, and abundant. Eating became as much a matter of aesthetic pleasure and social ceremony as of satisfying hunger. Unexercised appestats broke down, or were overridden by psychological urges ("I'm already stuffed, but I just can't pass up a hot-fudge sundae"). People ate for fun, or because they were depressed, or just because the food was there. They ate a lot more than their bodies needed. And all those adipose cells, provided by nature for emergency use only, bulged and bulged.

Obesity and Mortality

Until a few generations ago, fat was beautiful. It was a sign of prosperity and, people thought, good health. Successful businessmen draped gold watch chains across vast expanses of protruding abdomen, and the reigning female beauties were amply proportioned. They may, however, have been literally eating themselves to death. Although the cause-and-effect relationships are still unclear, it has now been established statistically that fat people are far more likely than others to suffer from a variety of serious conditions including heart disease, high blood pressure, kidney ailments, and diabetes.

Nowadays, avoiding accumulation of excess fat is considered both cosmetically desirable and medically prudent. It is not, however, easy—and the fault lies at least partly in habits and customs passed on by our fat-loving predecessors.

Good Eating Habits

All through high school and college, Red was as skinny as the well-known rail. He grew, as they say, like a weed, and was always ready to eat. He took second helpings of everything, snacked between meals on cream puffs and chocolate bars and hot-fudge sundaes, drowned his occasional sorrows in extra-thick milkshakes, and remained as skinny as ever. It wasn't until his late twenties that Red, now settling into a desk job, began to notice that all of his clothes seemed to be shrinking. By the time he had reached his mid-thirties, Red's waistline, among other things, had expanded alarmingly. He went on a crash diet, one of those high-protein, low-carbohydrate fads popularized by a succession of best-selling books. He shunned his favorite desserts, pushed aside the bread, butter, and potatoes, barely nibbled at most of his vegetables, lived for weeks on steaks and low-fat cottage cheese and not much else.

Red quickly shed a dozen pounds, and for a while he was buoyed by self-congratulations on his unshakable "will power." It wasn't long, however, before virtue grew stale. Red noticed that he tired easily, often felt weak, sometimes had dizzy spells. He was suffering from the effects of an unbalanced diet, but he didn't know that because his "scientific" diet book assured him that his steak-and-cottage-cheese diet was quite safe. All Red knew was that life had turned grim and the sight of a steak was becoming stomach-turning. He dreamed about coconut cream pies, banana splits, hot-fudge sundaes. He became irritable and depressed. Finally, he caved in—he went on an eating binge and soon was fatter than ever. He also had a new feeling of guilt about his lack of "will power," a feeling that deepened over the years as he tried one crash diet after another, always falling off the wagon and winding up fatter than before.

Poor Red, stuck on a feast-or-famine merry-go-round familiar to multitudes of once-slender people, might have been spared some misery if he had learned and heeded certain facts about eating habits and about the ways in which the body changes as it becomes older.

Food and Culture

Red is a member of a culture that feeds babies to keep them quiet, teaches children to associate candy and ice cream with good times—and deprivation of such delights with punishment—makes eating to the point of satiety a ritualized part of holidays and casual social gatherings, and uses food as a substitute for the fulfillment of all kinds of psychological needs, which have nothing to do with physiological hunger. In early childhood, Red had become *habituated* to the use of food as pacifier, tranquilizer, antidepressant, mood elevator. Food, in a sense, had become to him an all-purpose drug—and a drug whose use was approved by society.

When he was growing up, Red's eating habits didn't seem to pose a problem. No matter what he ate, or how much, he didn't get fat. His body *needed* a lot of food then because it was constantly increasing in size, and because Red, like most children and adolescents, burned up a lot of energy playing, running, jumping, fidgeting. Most males go on growing into their early twenties (females usually complete their growth a little earlier). Their bodies continue to fill out even after they have stopped growing taller.

Post-Adolescent Weight Gain

Red finished growing just about the time he graduated from college and began his career. Now he was tied to a desk most of the day, and he seemed to have less and less time for physical exercise. His body no longer needed as much food as before, but, unaware of that, Red continued to follow the same eating habits, gobbling sweets and taking extra helpings even when his stomach felt full. His appestat didn't stop him because he no longer got enough exercise to keep it working. And by now his eating habits were so much a part of him that psychological promptings, which he interpreted as physiological hunger, could have overridden the delicate appestat mechanism anyway. His adipose storage cells were filling up, but he didn't notice for a long time that he was accumulating excess fat because it happened so gradually. The scales didn't tip him off at first because all his life he had been used to gaining weight.

By the time Red realized that he was becoming unhealthily fat, he had a number of problems. Simply maintaining his current weight was no longer enough; he needed to *lose* weight and not regain it. And while his deeply rooted eating habits hadn't changed, he had lost the habit of exercise. Exercise, in fact, had become an unpleasant strain; he just didn't seem to have enough energy. Some of his energy was being expended in *stress* as his body worked to adjust imbalances resulting from overconsumption of food. Excessive stress from overeating may have had emotional effects to which he responded, according to habit, by eating still more. And when Red plunged into a crash

TABLE 20-2 Daily Intake of Proteins and Calories Needed to Maintain Normal Growth

	Age (years)	Weight		Height		Total calories	Protein (g)
		kg	**(lb)**	**cm**	**(in.)**		
No difference by sex	0–⅙	4	(9)	55	(22)	kg × 120	kg × 2.2
	⅙–½	7	(15)	63	(25)	kg × 110	kg × 2.0
	½–1	9	(20)	72	(28)	kg × 100	kg × 1.8
	1–2	12	(26)	81	(32)	1100	25
	2–3	14	(31)	91	(36)	1250	25
	3–4	16	(35)	100	(39)	1400	30
	4–6	19	(42)	110	(43)	1600	30
	6–8	23	(51)	121	(48)	2000	35
	8–10	28	(62)	131	(52)	2200	40
Males	10–12	35	(77)	140	(55)	2500	45
	12–14	43	(95)	151	(59)	2700	50
	14–18	59	(130)	170	(67)	3000	60
	18–22	67	(147)	175	(69)	2800	60
	22–35	70	(154)	175	(69)	2800	65
	35–55	70	(154)	173	(68)	2600	65
	55–75	70	(154)	171	(67)	2400	65
Females	10–12	35	(77)	142	(56)	2250	50
	12–14	44	(97)	154	(61)	2300	50
	14–16	52	(114)	157	(62)	2400	55
	16–18	54	(119)	160	(63)	2300	55
	18–22	58	(128)	163	(64)	2000	55
	22–35	58	(128)	163	(64)	2000	55
	35–55	58	(128)	160	(63)	1850	55
	55–75	58	(128)	157	(62)	1700	55
	Pregnant					+200	65
	Lactating					+1000	75

Source: James Crouch and J. Robert McClintic, *Human Anatomy and Physiology*, 2nd Edition (Wiley & Sons, 1976), p. 654.

diet, drastically altering lifelong habits overnight, the stress became unbearable. His "will power" crumpled, making him feel guilty and inadequate, adding still more stress.

The guilt was unwarranted, because Red's problems weren't his fault. He had simply done what was normal in his culture.

Keeping Slim

Red is a fictitious but not untypical character. Generation after generation, millions of people go through the same unhappy metamorphosis, from slender youth to rotund middle age. Many resign themselves to getting fat (with the attendant risk of life-threatening diseases) as an inevitable part of the aging process. But middle-age weight-gain is not inevitable.

The still-slender young person who cultivates healthy eating habits and who makes a regular routine of vigorous exercise has a good chance of remaining slender throughout his or her life. Exercise is discussed in the next chapter. We are concerned here with eating habits. We will now, with authorial omnipotence, give Red a second chance, put him back in college, still young, still slim. What can he do to keep his youthful figure and lessen the risk of disease?

Being Aware of What You Eat

He can begin by making himself aware of what he eats and how much he eats and, to some extent, *why* he eats. It might be helpful if, every day for a full week, he made a written note of everything he ate and drank, including snacks, the odd pat of butter, and the sugar and cream in his coffee. Any alcoholic beverages, with their "empty" calories, and sugary soft drinks should be listed. Red should not, for purposes of this exercise,

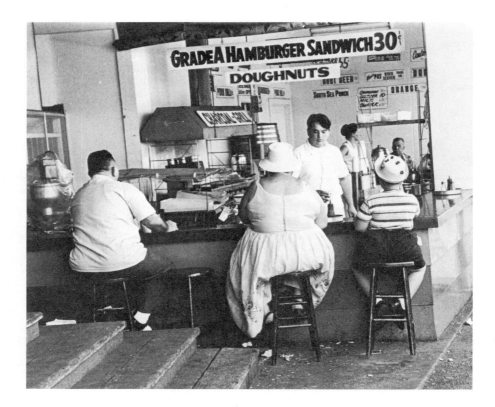

change his previous eating habits; his object, at this point, is *awareness,* not change. Alongside each item on his list, he should make a note of what, in his opinion, was his reason for consuming that particular item. Did he take the second serving of meat because he was still hungry, or just to clean the dish, or simply because it was there, or because he wanted that comfortably stuffed feeling? Did he have the hot-fudge sundae because he was hungry or because he wanted to experience the taste and textures?

Red shouldn't expect, in listing his reasons, to uncover all of the hidden motives he might have for eating this or that. His purpose, at present, is only to start himself thinking about his eating habits. This should cause him to reflect for a moment before taking second helpings or buying sugary concoctions.

Sensible Dieting

Now that he has begun to take more notice of what he eats, Red's next step is to put himself on a controlled diet. This will not be a weight-reducing diet, since Red doesn't need to lose weight. It will be a multipurpose diet, the first purpose being to make sure that Red is supplying his cells with all of the essential nutrients. This is of primary importance; lack of important nutrients can, among other things, cause increased stress, fatigue, and depression. Many people respond to such symptoms by giving up exercise or eating more for the psychological lift it gives them—doing exactly the wrong things.

Using the information provided earlier in this chapter, Red should make a point of eating each day some foods from each of the important food groups. He should try to include some complete proteins in every meal and a variety of fruits and vegetables; he should use unsaturated instead of saturated fats whenever possible and eliminate from his basic diet all ice cream, candy, and pastries. (He doesn't have to be too alarmed; some sweets are going to be permitted later.)

Since Red doesn't usually do his own cooking, he may encounter some problems in getting all of the right kinds of foods into his daily fare. However, the more ingenuity he has to use, the more aware he will become of his eating habits, and increased awareness is another purpose of the diet. Eventually, the new way of eating should become as habitual as the old, but in the meantime Red may need frequent reminders to keep his guard up.

Having put himself on a nutritionally sound diet, Red can now turn his attention to the *amount* of food he eats. At his age, Red still needs quite a lot of food. It won't do for him to starve himself, to go around hungry all the time. What he needs is to learn to eat enough, and no more; but there are no firm rules by which he can determine just how much is enough. He is going to have to learn to pay attention to his appestat (it is assumed that Red is getting enough exercise to keep his appestat working), as well as what his stomach and his taste buds and his eyes tell him. He needs to learn to tell the difference between satisfying hunger and stuffing himself, to think twice about extra servings and snacks, to turn down food he doesn't feel he really needs.

Red should remember that as he grows older his body will probably need less food, and he will gradually have to reduce his normal food intake to avoid getting fat.

Learning to cut down now may save him a lot of trouble later in life. It might help if he cultivated a habit of reciting to himself before each meal a little reminder that he should stop when he is no longer hungry, and before he is stuffed.

After he has been on his new diet for a few weeks, Red may be glowing with virtue, but he may also be experiencing some distressing symptoms—nervousness, irritability, difficulty in concentrating—not unlike symptoms experienced by people who try to quit smoking. These "withdrawal" symptoms may be partly physiological—the body adjusting its internal chemistry to the new regimen—and partly psychological; deeply rooted habits *will* assert themselves.

Red can make some interesting observations at this point. Since his diet now includes all of the essential nutrients, and since he is not starving himself, the cravings that beset him must result from something besides physiological hunger. By trying to discover just what it is he craves, and how strongly he craves it, Red may learn something about the extent to which he has been controlled by habit, rather than by physiological need. Now Red may have to ease up on himself a little. However much he may pride himself on his "will power," he is not made of steel. He is dealing with powerful urges. If he tries too hard to resist all temptation; he may do himself more harm than good; to be healthy is to be reasonably happy as well as physically sound.

Red should allow himself some of his favorite foods, but try to be satisfied with, for example, a spoonful or two of ice cream now and then instead of a dishful every day. Such nonessentials should become treats to be anticipated and savored, rather than routine rations. He should allow himself just enough of the nonessentials to make life reasonably comfortable, without slipping back into his indiscriminate eating habits. He should try, in other words, to learn to *balance* today's cravings against his future well-being. This is, after all, not an endurance test but an attempt to develop healthy habits that can serve for a lifetime.

Fad Diets

Several times a year, another book about some new "miracle" diet hits the best-seller lists, often to the accompaniment of much publicity in newspapers and magazines. Usually the author has impressive credentials and offers a very scientific-sounding explanation of why his or her pet theory works better than others. The titles of the books often include words such as "fast," "quick," and "easy."

Many people do lose weight, at least temporarily, on these fad diets, but in some cases they suffer from nutritional deficiencies as a result. Whatever the popular publications may say, most physicians and nutritionists agree that no one has yet discovered a quick, easy way to remove excess fat and *keep* it off without sacrificing good nutrition.

Any diet that calls for a drastic departure from the normal balance, such as eliminating most carbohydrates and living almost entirely on proteins and fats, should be avoided. And no one, we emphasize again, should embark on any crash diet that calls for the loss of more than a pound or two a week without the approval of his or her personal physician.

Calories

Weight-conscious Americans have long been accustomed to thinking of food in terms of calories, although many have only the vaguest notion about what a calorie is. The general idea seems to be that a calorie is something that makes people fat.

In physics, a calorie is a unit of heat, the amount needed to raise the temperature of a gram of water from 15 to 16 degrees centigrade. The unit used by nutritionists is actually a *kilocalorie,* a unit of energy one thousand times as great as the physicist's calorie. Nutritionists call kilocalories calories for short, and so shall we.

Foods do not *contain* calories. They have the *potential* to provide the body with so many calories of energy. As a rule, fats provide more calories than carbohydrates, and carbohydrates more than proteins. A person expends a varying number of calories of energy each day, the number depending on various factors, including the individual's age, size, sex, and the kinds of activities engaged in. (See Table 21–1.) The body uses a considerable amount of energy to keep the cells and organs functioning even when there is no other activity; the number of calories used for these basic functions is called the *basal metabolism* rate. The basal metabolism rate varies among similar individuals, and generally tends to decline with age.

Potential energy is stored by the body in the form of adipose tissue, or fat. If a person eats nothing at all, fat is burned to release energy, and the person loses weight at the rate of about one pound for every 3,500 calories of energy expended, including the energy used in maintaining the basal metabolism. If the person eats foods that provide approximately the same number of calories expended, his or her weight should remain stable. If a person's diet provides more calories than he or she expends, weight is gained (fat is stored up) at the rate of about one pound for every 3,500 unexpended calories.

Counting Calories

In theory, it should be simple to determine just how much a person should eat in order to lose weight at the rate of one pound a week. He or she merely looks at one table to find out how many calories the average person answering his or her general description expends in an average day, then uses another table to select foods that will provide about 500 calories a day (3,500 a week) less than the dieter can expect to use up.

It sounds easy, but in practice that kind of calorie-counting isn't very reliable. For one thing, few individuals are "average." Basal metabolism rates for people of the same age, weight, and sex may differ by hundreds of calories a day. And unless a person does all of his or her own food shopping and cooking, carefully weighs and measures everything he or she eats, and is a good judge of the quality of meats and such, the "average" figures for the numbers of calories provided by "average" servings of different kinds of foods don't mean much. For someone who eats regularly in restaurants or coffee shops or cafeterias, accurate calorie-counting is all but impossible; it is difficult to determine how much fat there is in the meat, how many calories in the sauce, and what that stuff *is* in the soup, anyway.

People who are put on reducing diets by their doctors for medical reasons may be required to count calories as closely as possible. For others, calorie charts may be useful as rough guides in comparing the relative calorie potentials of different kinds of foods. It should be remembered, however, that no particular group of foods should be eliminated from the diet simply because the charts indicate that they are high in calories; good nutrition demands a variety of foods, and the best rule for would-be weight losers is to eat less of everything.

Exercise and Calories

The importance of physical exercise in keeping the body's appetite-control mechanism working properly has been emphasized in this chapter. Exercise also contributes to weight control by using up energy that might otherwise be stored as fat. As Table 21–1 indicates, however, it takes a lot of vigorous exercise to lose a pound at the rate of 3,500 calories for each pound.

It should be remembered, too, that if the exerciser doesn't control his or her food intake, he or she can easily consume more potential calories than is expended. For most people, exercise alone is not sufficient to remove excess fat; a combination of diet and exercise is the key.

The Ideal Weight

Table 20–3 shows average weights, by age, sex, and height, of people who are considered neither too fat nor too thin. Each category provides for considerable variation in weights to allow for individual differences in bone structure and musculature.

Usually, anyone whose weight exceeds the maximum shown in the table for his or her category is considered to be overweight, but there are exceptions. Someone who has large bones, a broad frame, and big muscles may weigh more than the maximum shown for his or her category without being fat. And a person with small bones and a narrow frame could be carrying quite a bit of excess fat without being overweight according to the figures in the table.

Individuals can usually tell if they are too fat by looking at themselves in a full-length mirror and by feeling their bodies. One rough test is to bend an arm at the elbow and pinch together the layers of skin and fat (not muscle) on the back of the arm, midway between elbow and shoulder; if the fold is more than an inch thick, the person probably needs to shed some fat.

While height-and-weight tables are useful as general guides, it is the amount of fat on the body rather than a certain number of pounds that should be the final guide.

The Underweight

Since most Americans tend to be too fat rather than too thin, people who are underweight get relatively little attention. A number of disorders can result in inability to gain

TABLE 20-3 Desirable Weights for Persons 25 and Over*

	Height (with shoes on, 1-inch heels) Feet	Inches	Small Frame	Medium Frame	Large Frame
Men	5	2	112–120	118–129	126–141
	5	3	115–123	121–133	129–144
	5	4	118–126	124–136	132–148
	5	5	121–129	127–139	135–152
	5	6	124–133	130–143	138–156
	5	7	128–137	134–147	142–161
	5	8	132–141	138–152	147–166
	5	9	136–145	142–156	151–170
	5	10	140–150	146–160	155–174
	5	11	144–154	150–165	159–179
	6	0	148–158	154–170	164–184
	6	1	152–162	158–175	168–189
	6	2	156–167	162–180	173–194
	6	3	160–171	167–185	178–199
	6	4	164–175	172–190	182–204

	Height (with shoes on, 2-inch heels) Feet	Inches	Small Frame	Medium Frame	Large Frame
Women[†]	4	10	92– 98	96–107	104–119
	4	11	94–101	98–110	106–122
	5	0	96–104	101–113	109–125
	5	1	99–107	104–116	112–128
	5	2	102–110	107–119	115–131
	5	3	105–113	110–122	118–134
	5	4	108–116	113–126	121–138
	5	5	111–119	116–130	125–142
	5	6	114–123	120–135	129–146
	5	7	118–127	124–139	133–150
	5	8	122–131	128–143	137–154
	5	9	126–135	132–147	141–158
	5	10	130–140	136–151	145–163
	5	11	134–144	140–155	149–168
	6	0	138–148	144–159	153–173

*Weight in pounds according to frame (in indoor clothing)
†For girls between 18 and 25, subtract 1 pound for each year under 25.

Source: Metropolitan Life Insurance Co., *4 Steps to Weight Control.*

weight, and anyone who feels excessively thin and who is unable to gain weight no matter how much he or she eats should consult a physician. Usually, thinness is an inherited characteristic, and the skinny person can take comfort from the thought that he or she is less likely than others to suffer from the diseases associated with excess fat.

Summary

When you eat a snack or a hearty meal, you're doing more than just feeding your stomach: you are nourishing billions of specialized and diversified cells—with sharply varying needs. That delicate matter of balance intrudes again here: your diet must provide all the energy you need, and all of the building materials those cells need. Virtually all of those needs are met by the proteins, fats, and carbohydrates in your food.

Different foods provide different quantities and combinations of these essentials. Many people supplement their diets with vitamins, minerals, and other pills, but doctors insist that no pills will ever supplant a good, balanced diet.

A diet heavy in fats may produce excess cholesterol, which is often blamed for atherosclerosis and heart disease. Excess sugars are carbohydrates that are stored in the body as fats and may contribute to the same diseases. People who tend to be overweight should readjust their eating habits and get regular exercise. The healthy objective of the overweight person is to be slim—and stay slim.

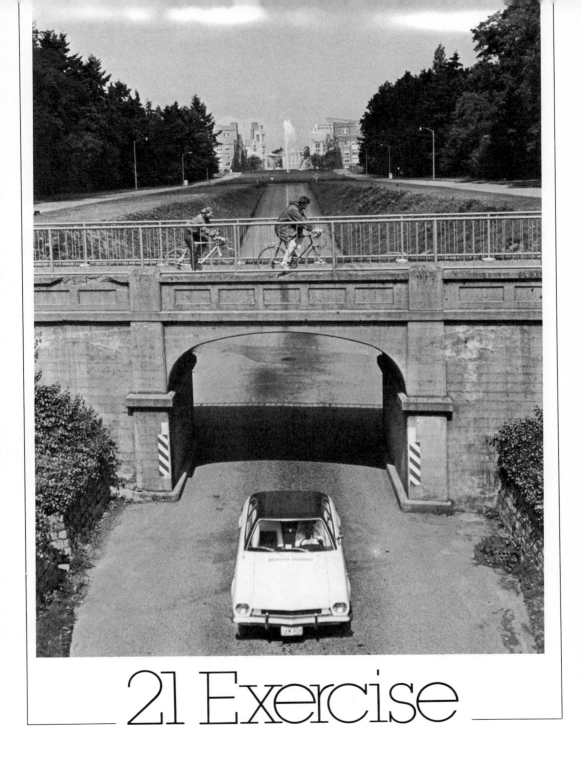

21 Exercise

At this point in the history of civilization, it is evident that technical progress may backfire unless it is matched by a balancing regard for human health and well-being. In its broadest sense, the question is whether man can prosper in the technological environment he has created. He must learn to protect the natural resources that sustain his life. He must learn to clean up the air and the water, and to preserve the land. But first of all, he must protect his own body against the ravages imposed by modern life.

Sally, sprawled on the sofa, is dividing her attention between the Sunday funnies and the televised tennis match (she vaguely regrets having given up tennis, but then who has the time, not to mention the energy?). For the past half hour she has been trying to ignore DeGaulle, the poodle, who keeps racing from the sofa to the front door and back again, pawing, whining, begging. Finally, Sally sighs and drags herself to her feet, fetches the leash from the closet, and snaps it onto DeGaulle's collar. Tucking the Sunday magazine section under her arm, she allows the poodle to half-drag her to the door.

The elevator is slow to come. Sally glances at the stairs, thinks about walking the two flights down to the ground floor, and decides to wait. Eventually she and the near-frantic poodle reach her car, which is parked precisely opposite the entrance to her apartment building. She had to circle the block six times last night to secure that spot. Otherwise she might have had to leave the car a block away and walk. Sally drives the eight blocks to the park. She has to cruise around for twenty minutes before someone vacates a parking space near her favorite tree. At last, she releases DeGaulle from the leash, and, as the dog goes bounding off ecstatically, Sally collapses at the foot of the tree and buries herself in her magazine.

For the next hour DeGaulle runs, leaps, chases his shadow, rolls in the grass, wiggles, dances, and cavorts. Now and then he picks up a piece of bark and brings it to Sally, who, without getting up, halfheartedly flings the bark just far enough to show the poodle that she means well. Sally is trying to concentrate on an article about a new diet, which, she imagines, just might, without too much effort on her part, help remove that extra inch that has somehow added itself to her hips. She is feeling a bit noble about interrupting her day of rest to bring DeGaulle out for a romp in the park. She'd much rather have remained sprawled on the sofa, but she knows that DeGaulle has to have his exercise.

The truth is that Sally, like a lot of other people, wouldn't dream of neglecting her dog the way she neglects herself.

Mixed Blessings of the Modern Age

In previous chapters we have emphasized more than once that the human body is an organism that evolved long before the beginning of civilization, an organism adapted to the cave dweller's life of strenuous physical activity, an organism that *requires* physical exercise to keep some of its processes functioning properly.

Most healthy animals get ample exercise if they are given the opportunity. They exercise either out of the necessities of finding food and protecting themselves from enemies, or, like DeGaulle the poodle, they frolic for the sheer joy of it. Exercise comes naturally. But humans, endowed with the blessings of civilization, tend to lose track of the knowledge that they are still a part of nature. We have seen how modern life frustrates and abuses natural survival mechanisms in ways that cause excessive stress and excessive fat, both associated with numerous destructive diseases. And physical exercise, one of the best ways of countering those destructive forces, is itself discouraged by modern technology.

DeGaulle's owner Sally, who never walks if she can ride, is more typical than exceptional. The automobile takes people off their feet. Television keeps them indoors. All kinds of labor-saving machinery has taken most of the exercise out of even formerly strenuous occupations. For most people, no more than a minimal amount of physical activity is necessary to make a living or to get from place to place. Leisure hours are often whiled away with no more effort than it takes to shuffle to the refrigerator during television commercials.

Under these conditions, getting a healthy amount of exercise, like staying on a diet, demands considerable self-discipline. Old habits may need to be broken and new ones developed. The cave people couldn't avoid exercise; modern humans need to make a point of it.

Kinds of Exercise

The roles played by exercise in relieving stress, regulating the appetite, and controlling weight have been described in earlier chapters. Physical exercise of various kinds can also improve the body's performance by strengthening muscles, by increasing their flexibility, and by building endurance.

Isometric Exercise

Generations of men and boys have been fascinated by those advertisements in which the ninety-seven-pound weakling, humiliated by a muscular bully, signs up for the Charles Atlas body-building course, develops a Mr. America physique, takes his revenge on the bully, and wins the girl. The Charles Atlas technique involves a system of *isometric* (from the Greek *isos,* equal, and *metron,* measure) exercises. Isometric exercises involve the contraction of muscles without stretching them. For example, the palms of the hands are pressed together as hard as possible (the muscles of both arms exerting pressure in equal measure) without bending the joints. Such exercises, if practiced regularly over a period of time, can enlarge and strengthen certain muscles. They do not, however, provide all of the benefits of certain other forms of exercise.

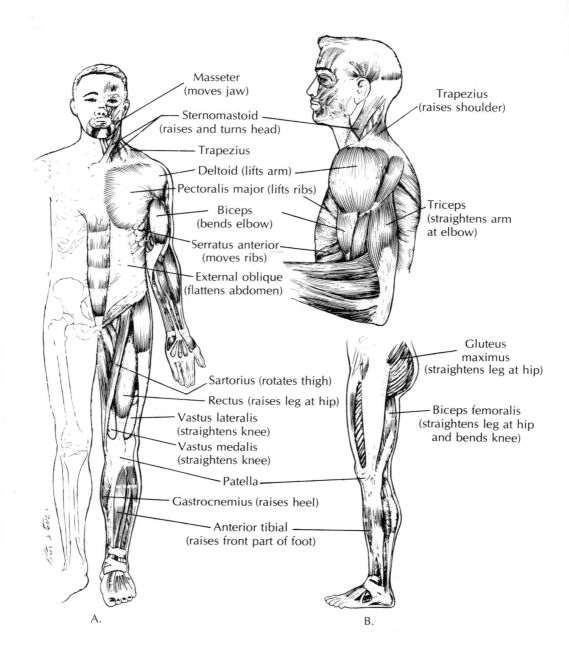

Masseter
(moves jaw)

Sternomastoid
(raises and turns head)

Trapezius

Deltoid (lifts arm)

Pectoralis major (lifts ribs)

Biceps
(bends elbow)

Serratus anterior
(moves ribs)

External oblique
(flattens abdomen)

Trapezius
(raises shoulder)

Triceps
(straightens arm
at elbow)

Gluteus
maximus
(straightens leg at hip)

Biceps femoralis
(straightens leg at hip
and bends knee)

Sartorius (rotates thigh)

Rectus (raises leg at hip)

Vastus lateralis
(straightens knee)

Vastus medalis
(straightens knee)

Patella

Gastrocnemius (raises heel)

Anterior tibial
(raises front part of foot)

A.

B.

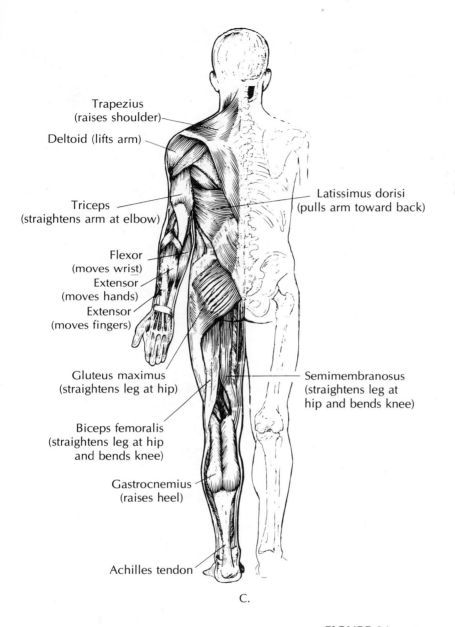

Trapezius
(raises shoulder)

Deltoid (lifts arm)

Triceps
(straightens arm at elbow)

Flexor
(moves wrist)

Extensor
(moves hands)

Extensor
(moves fingers)

Gluteus maximus
(straightens leg at hip)

Biceps femoralis
(straightens leg at hip
and bends knee)

Gastrocnemius
(raises heel)

Achilles tendon

Latissimus dorisi
(pulls arm toward back)

Semimembranosus
(straightens leg at
hip and bends knee)

C.

FIGURE 21-a *The structure and location of the superficial muscles. A. Anterior view; B. Lateral view; C. Posterior view.*

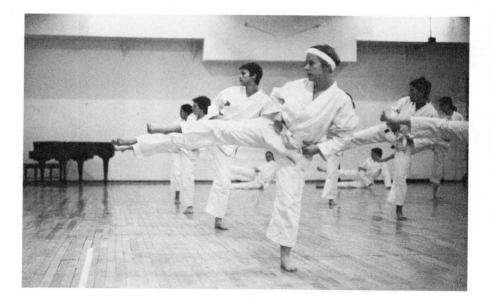

Isotonic Exercise

Isotonic (from the Greek *tonikos,* soundness) exercises involve movement, the bending of joints, and the stretching of muscles. They contribute to flexibility as well as to strength. Walking, running, swimming, and bicycling are isotonic exercises, as are some forms of yoga. Isotonic exercises are generally more beneficial than isometric, although some people may prefer a combination of the two.

For maximum benefits, exercise should be strenuous enough to noticeably speed up the heartbeat and breathing, increasing the capacity of oxygen that the heart, blood vessels, and lungs deliver to all the cells. This builds endurance, enabling the body to perform strenuous work over longer periods of time without becoming exhausted. A champion weight lifter may have enormous muscles but be unable to run any considerable distance unless he has built up his endurance through some form of exercise other than weight-lifting.

Strenuous Exercise

Although the theory is somewhat controversial, many authorities believe that regular, strenuous exercise, because it strengthens the cardiovascular system, helps prevent premature heart attacks and strokes. There is much statistical evidence that people who exercise regularly are less likely than others to be afflicted early by diseases of the cardiovascular system. But whether or not exercise contributes to longevity, there is no

TABLE 21-1 Energy Expenditures for Various Activities

Activity	Calories per Hour
Archery	312
Bowling	264
Chopping Wood	294
Cleaning Windows	180
Climbing	732
Cycling	396
Dancing	325
Driving a Car	168
Football Playing	534
Horseback Riding	400
Jogging	636
Polishing Furniture	140
Resting, Lying Down	90
Skiing	594
Sleeping	68
Squash Playing	612
Swimming	660
Sweeping Floor	100
Table Tennis Playing	360
Tennis Playing	426
Walking	336
Writing, Sitting at Desk	132

Source: Physiological Reviews 35:801, 1965.

doubt that it can—by relieving stress, by increasing endurance and reducing fatigue, and by generally improving the body's performance and the individual's sense of well-being—elevate the *quality* of life.

Choosing a Form of Exercise

The choice of a particular form of exercise is a matter of individual likes and dislikes. Some people enjoy jogging; others find it boring. Some like swimming. Some prefer games, such as handball. The important thing is for each individual to find a form of vigorous exercise that he or she enjoys, or at least doesn't find too burdensome, and to exercise frequently and regularly—daily if possible, three or four times a week as a minimum. And during the intervals the individual can do him- or herself much good by walking or bicycling instead of driving a car or riding in a bus, by using the stairs instead of the elevator, by learning to depend more on his or her body and less on machines.

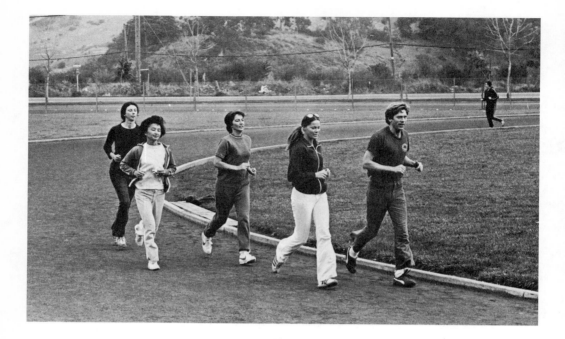

Precautions

From time to time the news reports include an item about someone who suffered a heart attack while jogging. Investigations have shown that in most cases such victims have been people, usually older men, who had suddenly taken up strenuous exercise after years of idleness; most had preexisting coronary artery disease. Research, however, has shown that many people can benefit from exercise programs, under proper medical supervision, even after they have had heart attacks. Whether or not strenuous exercise is safe depends largely on the individual's age, medical history, and general physical condition.

For people under thirty years old, any form of exercise is generally considered safe, provided that the individual has had a physical examination within the past year, is not grossly overweight, and has no obvious medical problems. Excess weight puts additional strain on the body, and anyone who is very much overweight should trim off some fat through dieting and moderate exercise before undertaking really strenuous activity.

No one, regardless of his or her youth and how healthy he or she might think him- or herself, should push too hard. Anyone who suffers extreme discomfort in the form of fatigue, pain, shortness of breath, dizziness, or nausea while exercising should stop and should not resume such strenuous activity until he or she has built up endurance gradually. People over thirty years old who have not been exercising regularly are advised to have a complete physical examination and the doctor's approval before beginning an exercise program. Unless the doctor disapproves, most people, regardless of age, can benefit from some form of physical exercise.

Summary

A regular and sensible program of physical exercise is necessary for the body if it is to function smoothly and at peak efficiency. But many people today tend to forget or ignore that simple fact. They loll around the house, reading or watching television, and almost never walk anyplace if they can drive or ride instead.

Exercise, like proper dieting, requires the breaking of old, bad habits; it requires self-discipline. Isometric exercises pit muscle against muscle and can build strength. Isotonic exercises involve movement, joint bending and muscle stretching. They include walking, running, swimming, and bike-riding, and are regarded as more beneficial than the isometric. But although regular, vigorous exercise is beneficial, it shouldn't be overdone—and people who are out of shape should build up their endurance gradually.

References

p. 322   Kenneth H. Cooper, *The New Aerobics* (New York, 1970), p. 171.

PART VIII
Caring for Your Health

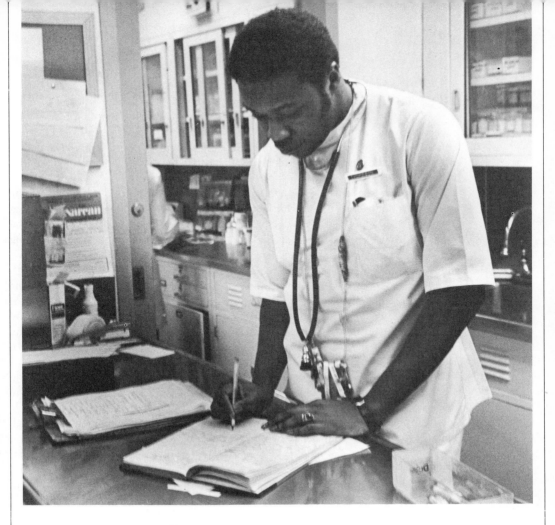

22 People in Health Care

Dr. Samuelson wrapped the heavy strap snugly around Harry's upper arm and snapped it in place. He put his stethoscope on Harry's arm just below the cuff, and started squeezing a rubber bulb connected to the cuff by a narrow tube. Harry could feel the cuff fill with air and tighten around his arm. He watched the doctor's face. The doctor was watching the mercury pressure-gauge attached to the cuff and mounted on the wall behind Harry.

Dr. Samuelson let some air out, then stopped. Harry could feel his pulse thumping strongly inside the cuff. The doctor let more air out and stopped again. He frowned at the gauge. Harry frowned at the doctor. The doctor shook his head. "Still too high," he said. "Lie down on your back and relax." Then they went through the whole thing again—pumping the air in, letting it out, frowning. "Still too high." This time the follow-up comment was: "I want to try another medication."

The whole scenario had begun a week earlier when Harry had come in for the routine checkup he'd been promising himself—but postponing—for several years. He'd finally made an appointment and had the checkup because he'd been bothered by recurring headaches and occasional dizziness. Dr. Samuelson had clamped on the *sphygmomanometer,* read the gauge, listened to his stethoscope, and announced that Harry's blood pressure was "dangerously high." The doctor had prescribed some pills to help bring it down, had ordered X-rays and an electrocardiogram, and had had the laboratory take samples of blood and urine for analysis. Today he told his patient the results.

Harry was suffering from "essential hypertension," the most common kind of high blood pressure, one with no known organic cause. The lab tests had ruled out the possibility that it was caused by a kidney disorder, for instance, or some other physical malfunction.

Dr. Samuelson prescribed some antihypertension pills and told Harry to take them regularly, without fail. He also ordered his patient to reduce his salt intake (he suggested a dietary salt substitute for flavor), to cut down on liquor, lose some weight, eat sensibly, get more exercise. He would have ordered Harry to quit smoking, too, if Harry had not already stopped several years earlier. The doctor minced no words about Harry's affliction: hypertension can kill. It can cause crippling, or fatal, strokes or heart attacks. But essential hypertension can be controlled with proper diet and medication. It took several return visits before the doctor was satisfied that he had Harry on the right dosage of the right medicine. The blood pressure was under control and normal, for a man Harry's age, forty-three. Harry was delighted. He also felt a lot better. And he admitted that he'd learned something about the value of routine checkups. In his case it had become a "routine recheck" every three months.

The Physician

The prime mover in medical care—in diagnosing, prescribing, testing, treating, healing—is, of course, the physician. By accepted definition and by law, a physician is a person who has received a Doctor of Medicine degree from an accredited medical school, and has served the required apprenticeship as an intern and as a resident physician at accredited hospitals. The physician must also be licensed to practice medicine in his or her state, following examination by a board of professional standards.

There are many kinds of physicians, but here we will consider them in two groups: those who serve as family doctors, and those who practice one of the many specialized medical disciplines recognized by the American Board of Medical Specialties. A specialist who is "board certified" must be found qualified by the professional standards board for his or her particular specialty—be it pediatrics, obstetrics, psychiatry, or something else.

The Family Doctor

The gruff but kindly old family physician often portrayed on television and in the movies hasn't really disappeared, but his numbers have diminished in this age of medical specialization. In recent years, the medical generalist has become a specialist in his or her own right: Medicine has developed a new, image-changing family practice specialty in the hope that many medical school students will choose that instead of some other specialty. The prevailing reasoning is that there is a strong need for a family doctor and that, in fact, *all* medical care should start with a family doctor.

The family physician is, by definition, a doctor who treats the whole family. He diagnoses and treats illness, performs routine surgery, delivers babies, and calls in

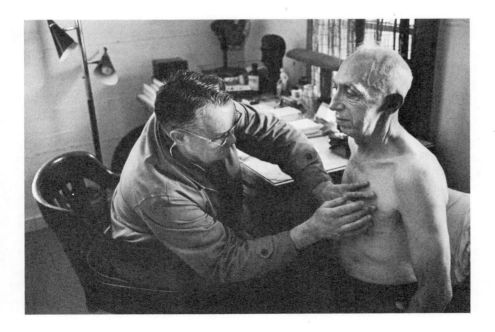

specialists for more complicated problems. His new image is that of a "board certified" family physician, which means he's met the requirements of, and been duly certified by, the relatively new American Board of Family Practice (founded in 1970). Probably, he's also a member of the American Academy of Family Physicians.

The physician who functions as the family doctor might also be an *internist*—a specialist in internal medicine who diagnoses and treats illness and injury but usually does *not* perform surgery, deliver babies, or treat injuries or diseases of the eye. He calls in specialists for those areas of treatment. (The pediatrician does most of the things the internist does, but his practice is limited to children.)

These rather generalized specialists function as what the medical profession calls *primary care physicians.* They see the patient first, initiate and carry out programs to cure his ailments or simply keep him well, and summon the right specialist when health conditions require one. Perhaps the most important function of the primary care physician is that he sees the patient regularly—and as frequently as age, general condition, and medical history dictate.

Ideally, the entire family should be treated by either a family practice specialist or an internist. Over a period of years, such a doctor gets to know everyone in the family group, and is well informed about their collective eating habits, emotional states, exercise habits, and general physical condition. This kind of approach, and its continuity, should develop an easy rapport between doctor and patients. But the age of specialization still dominates medicine. The American Academy of Family Physicians (AAFP) and the American Board of Family Practice (ABFP) were created to help counter that trend. General practitioners, as family doctors were long known, constituted two-thirds of the U.S. physician population in the early 1940s. Today about 15 percent of U.S. doctors are in family practice.

The Specialist

Medicine hasn't just been divided into specialties—it has subdivided those specialties into subspecialties. For instance, the internist might want to limit his practice to a specific internal ailment such as heart disease, gastro-intestinal problems, or pulmonary disorders. Each of these specialties and subspecialties requires certain kinds and periods of postgraduate education to satisfy the requirements of the appropriate certifying board.

Specialists usually charge higher fees than generalists for a number of reasons—including the time and expense they've invested in specialized training and, in some cases, the investment they've made in expensive and sophisticated equipment. Some specialists will accept only those patients referred to them by other physicians. The value of the family doctor is doubly demonstrable here: He will decide, on the basis of his medical training and his knowledge of your health and medical history, whether you need a specialist at all. And if he decides that you do, he can choose a competent person in the right specialty (or give you a list of several from which to pick) and give you a referral.

There are nearly as many medical specialties and subspecialties as there are parts of the body. Some of those you're more likely to encounter include the following.

The Obstetrician / Gynecologist   These two specialties are commonly combined. The gynecologist is concerned with the health of the female reproductive system, and the obstetrician cares for a woman during pregnancy and delivers her child.

The Pediatrician   This physician is concerned with the health of the growing child. The specialist advises the parents on nutrition and general health and oversees "well baby" programs including regular checkups and immunizations.

The Dermatologist   Treats diseases of the skin.

The Neurologist   Deals with physical diseases of the brain and central nervous system.

The Psychiatrist   Deals with emotional illness.

The Ophthalmologist   Treats ailments of the eyes.

The Anesthesiologist   Administers local and general anesthetics to patients undergoing surgery.

The Otolaryngologist   Treats the ear and throat.

The Radiologist   Uses X-rays, radium, and radioactive isotopes to diagnose and treat disease.

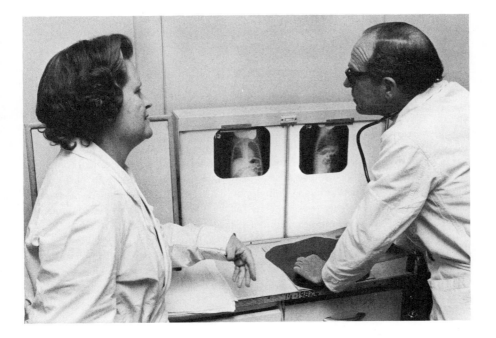

The General Surgeon   Performs all kinds of surgical procedures, but may call in a specialist when necessary. Specialists include the *thoracic surgeon* (chest), the *neurosurgeon* (brain), and the *orthopedic surgeon* (bones and joints).

Other Medical Practitioners

The Osteopath   Osteopathy is a branch of medical practice which has, since its founding in the 1870s, placed particular emphasis on the role of the musculoskeletal system in health and disease. Osteopathic physicians must complete a postgraduate education similar in most respects to a standard medical school course, and they use all of the medical, surgical, psychological, pharmacological, immunological, and hygienic procedures of modern medicine.

Osteopaths, like medical doctors, generalize (many are family doctors) and specialize (many are surgeons). Recognition of osteopathy as a legitimate kind of medical practice was slow in coming—and in some states osteopaths still can't practice in medical hospitals. But in 1961, California became the first state to license osteopathic physicians and surgeons as medical doctors, and the former osteopathic colleges in the state now confer the M.D. degree on their graduates. Several other states have since followed suit.

The Chiropractor   The *chiropractor* is a widely known practitioner whose basic premises are regarded as medically unsound by organized medicine in general. The underlying theory of chiropractic is that disease is caused by impaired nerve functions—and that these impairments are caused by pressure, strain, or tension on the spinal cord and its nerve network. Chiropractors work for cures by manipulation of bones, particularly the vertebrae. Chiropractors must pass professional examinations and obtain state licenses in order to practice.

Group Practice

Often, generalists and specialists in medicine will work together in private *group practice*. An internist or family practitioner might share office and equipment space and expenses with a number of specialists—perhaps a general surgeon, an obstetrician/gynecologist, and a pediatrician. Sometimes their office space includes a medical laboratory, which conducts tests ordered by the various physicians; sometimes the medical group has a working arrangement with a nearby lab.

There are larger and more comprehensive groups that include a wider range of medical specialties and laboratory equipment and facilities. They are sometimes operated in conjunction with a hospital. These groups include Health Maintenance Organizations (HMOs), and often are operated as part of a prepaid medical and surgical plan financed by employers, employees, or both.

The need for good dental care is something most of us hear about, with great regularity, throughout childhood: Brush after every meal, see the dentist twice a year, and so on. Repetitive, yes, but true—and of great importance to our general health and mental outlook. Aching or rotting teeth can have an adverse effect that's more than just physical.

In dentistry as in medicine, there are generalists and specialists. A practitioner of *general dentistry* examines, diagnoses, and treats. If you visit your dentist twice a year, you'll get a thorough cleaning and, probably, X-rays (both of those functions are often perfomed by an assistant to the dentist). If X-rays show cavities, the general dentist will drill and fill them. He extracts teeth and replaces them with bridges or dentures. He also treats various ailments of the mouth and gums.

Specialists in dentistry include the *oral surgeon,* who limits his practice to surgical procedures involved with diseases, injuries, or deformities of the mouth and teeth. He performs complicated extractions, which might be too complicated for the general dentist. The *orthodondist* uses braces and other devices in programs to correct deformities that develop during the growth of the teeth and jaw. The *prosthodondist* specializes

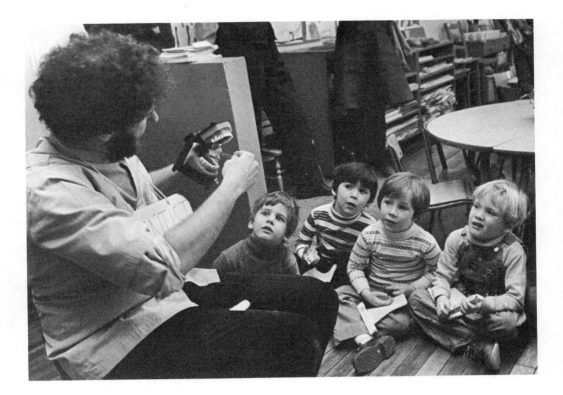

in the replacement or repair of lost or damaged teeth, using artificial bridges, crowns, and dentures. The *periodondist* treats ailments of the gums and the parts of the jaw that support the teeth.

Most dentists recommend that children use *fluoridated* toothpastes, and in many communities, artificial fluorides have been added to the water supplies. (Fluorides occur naturally in some water.) The use of fluorides is invariably a matter of controversy.

Choosing a Doctor or Dentist

If you are new in a community and want to find a physician or dentist, you can get the names of qualified generalists or specialists from the local medical society or dental society. In most cities, both organizations maintain twenty-four-hour telephone services for emergencies and referrals—but both stress that you should find a family doctor or dentist while you are well, and not wait until an emergency confronts you.

If you are moving to another city, your present family doctor might be able to recommend some qualified physicians in your new area. Or, after you move, you might call the nearest accredited hospital in the new city for a list of doctors on its staff of attending physicians. If there is a medical school in the area, it might be another source of names. Sometimes a friend or relative can provide valuable leads. In a small town or a rural area, the choices obviously won't be as wide as in a city. You'll probably find more generalists in a small town—in both medicine and dentistry—and hospital facilities may be limited.

Paramedical Health Professionals

Many family doctors work at the head of teams of professionals who do many phases of the doctor's work but aren't trained or licensed as physicians. These trained specialists are called *paramedics* because they work alongside doctors. They include nurses and a variety of other health personnel.

The Nurse

The *registered nurse* is a skilled, highly trained professional who assists the physician or dentist in office, clinic, or hospital care of patients, and in surgery. Most nurses work in hospitals where, among other things, they administer medicines to patients as directed by the responsible physicians. Most other nurses work in medical or dental offices or clinics. But there are also visiting nurses, who go to the homes of the ill, and nurses employed in factories, schools, stores, and on transportation facilities.

Practical Nurses Not as extensively trained as registered nurses, the practical nurse performs many routine duties that free the registered nurse for duties requiring more specialized training. *Nurses' aides,* who are sometimes students, also perform some of the routine nursing chores in hospitals, clinics, offices, and rest homes.

Nurses are but one of many paramedical specialties organized to work in support and under the direction of doctors and dentists. Among the other paramedical health professionals are laboratory technicians, physiotherapists and occupational therapists, and social workers. Ambulance drivers and attendants use telemetric equipment to transmit an injured person's vital life-sign readings to the hospital. Doctors then instruct the ambulance personnel, by radio, in the emergency treatment to administer, when to transport the patient to the hospital, and so forth. Paramedical personnel assisting the dentist include the dental hygienist who cleans teeth, the dental assistant who helps when the dentist works on a patient, and the dental technician.

Preventive Medicine

The regular checkup is considered the surest way to continued good health. A family physician might want to see a particular patient just occasionally—perhaps three or four times a year—for a general checkup. The frequency would depend on the patient's general health and medical background. Depending on these and other factors, the family doctor will want a thorough physical examination about once every year or so.

Multiphasics

Some medical groups offer comprehensive examinations called *multiphasics*. They are usually conducted in special facilities offering clusters of specialized examinations and laboratory procedures. A patient taking a typical multiphasic will give blood and urine specimens to be tested for a variety of possible problems. Hearing, vision, and lung-capacity are also tested, and the patient is given an electrocardiogram and a blood-pressure check. Some multiphasics also include a simple psychological test.

The computerized results of the multiphasic are given to the family physician, who analyzes them to see if they show any special problems—present or potential—that might require additional treatment or medication. The multiphasic is followed by a thorough office physical exam by the family doctor.

Medical Quackery

Dictionaries variously define the quack as "a fraudulent or ignorant pretender to medical skill," or "an untrained person who pretends to have medical knowledge." The words "charlatan" and "mountebank" are sometimes used. But the most pertinent synonym listed probably is "phony." *Quackery* is the word for what the quack does, and it "thrives most in those areas of human illness for which there is no cure," in the opinion of Consumers Union, a nationally influential consumer organization. "When legitimate expertise fails, patients often turn to other sources," the organization says in its book *The Medicine Show*. "Whether in continuous pain, suffering from varying degrees of disability, or just experiencing vague discomfort, these patients may become prey to outright quacks, as well as to licensed doctors on the fringe of organized medicine. Both of these types promise relief from symptoms—for a price. They also sell hope . . ."

Quackery is believed to stem from the medicine shows (they began with entertainment and ended with the hawking of a surefire nostrum) that were so much a part of the scene a generation or so ago. The nostrum, of course, would cure anything from fallen arches to terminal dandruff. The quacks are still peddling their cure-alls today, and desperate people are still trying every nostrum they can get their hands on. New laws against selling or advertising fraudulent "cures" have been enacted and are being vigorously enforced. But the quack has a big thing going for him: People who are desperate are liable to grab at any straw.

Summary

Continuing good medical care is probably best provided by a physician who serves as your family doctor. He might be a family practice physician or an internist who will learn your medical history and that of your family. He will practice preventive medicine by regular checkups, and will cope with various illnesses. A family doctor will also refer you to a specialist when and as needed. Sometimes family doctors and specialists combine their talents and facilities in a group practice.

Dentists, too, are both generalists and specialists. In medicine and dentistry alike, regular checkups are essential. To find a doctor or dentist in a new city, you might consult the local medical or dental society, an accredited hospital, or a nearby medical school. Or you might make a selection on the advice of trusted friends or relatives.

Family doctors and dentists often head teams of highly trained paramedical professionals—including nurses, lab technicians, therapists, ambulance attendants.

Quackery is a term applied to the fraudulent practitioners who claim skills they don't have, and often offer relief and recovery from incurable illnesses.

References

p. 340   Ernest W. Saward, "The Organization of Medical Care," *Scientific American* (September 1973), pp. 169–75.

p. 342   *Consumer Reports* Editors, "How to Look for a Family Doctor," *The Medicine Show: Some Plain Truths about Popular Products for Common Ailments* (Mount Vernon, N.Y., 1974), pp. 323–35.

p. 344   *Consumer Reports* Editors, "The Quacks," *The Medicine Show,* pp. 170–77.

p. 344   Warren G. Magnuson, *The Dark Side of the Market Place* (Englewood Cliffs, N.J., 1968).

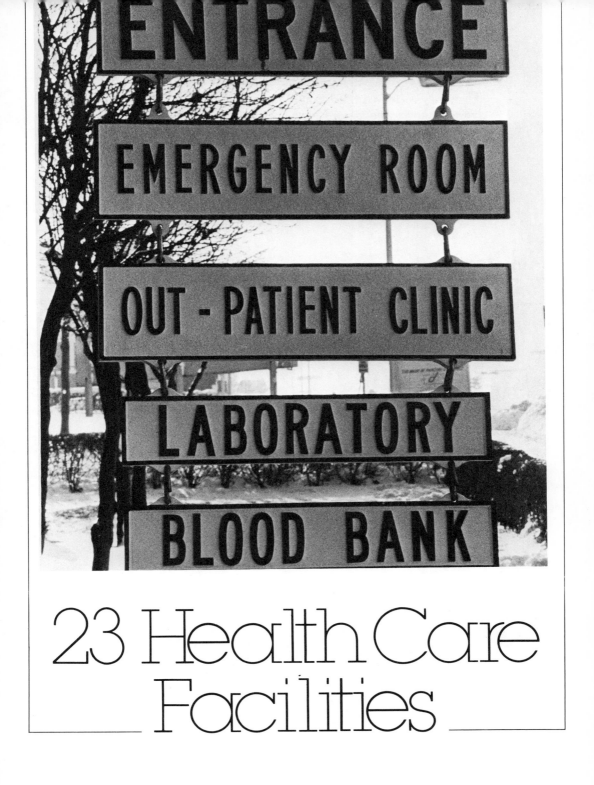

23 Health Care Facilities

The family doctor has been described as a *primary care* physician. The facilities for providing *primary health care* are the physician's office and the *clinic*. The two other levels of care are *secondary*, involving more specialized treatments and techniques and conducted in a *community hospital*, and *tertiary*, which involves highly specialized, technologically sophisticated, intensive care and is conducted in a *regional hospital* or medical center. In some countries, medicine is precisely organized on a regional basis, and these three levels of health care are performed within a rather clearly defined structure. In this country, the regional structure exists in some places, but not in others.

Primary Health Care

For most people, primary health care is associated with the family doctor's office or the clinic, which sometimes evolves into a *neighborhood health center*. In many U.S. counties, the health care personnel involved in clinics go to selected rural areas on regular schedules. This sort of service usually is provided by the county government, and financed by tax revenues.

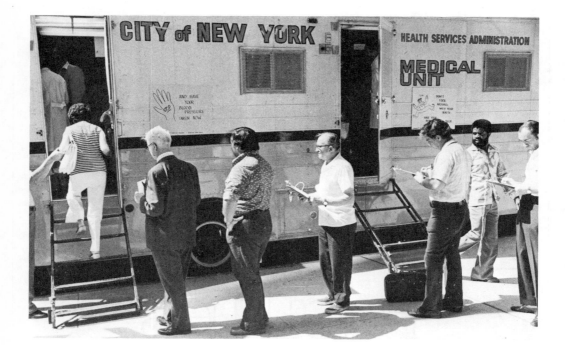

Clinics abound in most big cities and many smaller ones—although they vary considerably in nature: some are publicly financed, some are run by private nonprofit agencies. Many of the participating physicians and paramedics are unpaid volunteers, or are paid minimal salaries. Often, health-care professionals provide their services on an unpaid basis—putting in perhaps a day every week, two days a month.

Some clinics are general in nature, that is, they are staffed by generalists who will cope with routine problems and refer the patient elsewhere for specialized attention to more complex problems. Many other clinics are single purpose, working in a particular field such as birth control, fertility, abortion, or drug-related problems. Many other clinics—and this seems to be a growing trend, often financed by government—are rather large, and multipurpose. They are staffed by general medicine physicians, and sometimes a number of specialists. Clinics and medical centers are not hospitals. These are the neighborhood health centers. They are centers for *outpatient care,* and they treat people who are ambulatory, not confined. Some of them charge nothing; some ask contributions. Others charge fees, and the fees are usually payable by the various kinds of health insurance the patients might have.

Secondary Health Care

The Community Hospital

Secondary health care is the kind that requires procedures and facilities that are only available at a hospital. A hospital is, by definition, "an institution providing medical or surgical care and treatment for the sick and injured." The things a hospital offers include beds for the ill, equipment for surgery and the delivery of babies, kitchen and dietary facilities, X-ray and other diagnostic equipment, medical laboratories, and around-the-clock nursing and medical staffing.

A community hospital may be quite small or rather large, depending on the city, towns, and surrounding region it serves. The typical community hospital is a nonprofit "voluntary" institution set up by a religious or charitable institution or the community itself. Other kinds of hospital ownership are governmental and proprietary (profit-making, commercial).

The Regional Hospital

The regional hospital or medical center can offer a wide choice of sophisticated diagnostic and treatment facilities, and may provide a broad selection of medical specialists. This depth and versatility simply aren't available in the typical small community hospital. Regional hospitals and medical centers are of great value for the ailments requiring specialized medical knowledge and sophisticated (and expensive) equipment.

Large public hospitals—usually operated by a city or county—offer the most extensive emergency medical and surgical facilities, and provide services to indigent patients, in addition to functioning as general hospitals. Some of the best equipped and staffed hospitals are those operated in conjunction with university medical schools.

Accreditation Most but not all hospitals are "accredited"—which means they've met the exacting standards of the Joint Commission on Accreditation of Hospitals (JCAH). The JCAH derives most of its financial support from its member organizations—the American College of Physicians, the American College of Surgeons, the American Hospital Association, and the American Medical Association.

JCAH teams conduct intensive examinations of a hospital's physical plant before deciding on accreditation. Among other things, they are concerned with the organization, competence, and performance of the medical staff, and the kind and quantity of medical records maintained. They review records of the medical staff's own "peer review" committees. A hospital is accredited for a specific period of time, and its qualifications are regularly reexamined.

Nursing Homes

Nursing homes are sometimes also called rest homes or convalescent hospitals. Essentially, they provide necessary health services to people who must be cared for as patients, but who don't need the kind of attention, care and, medical services they would get in a hospital. Although some of these institutions specialize in the care of persons recovering from major illness or surgery, most are devoted to the elderly.

Nursing homes must obtain state licenses and are supposed to maintain specified standards of care—in terms of regular care by physicians and nurses, and the quality of medications, food, and other services. There is often dramatic contrast between the extremes of nursing home care: Some offer excellent care in pleasant surroundings and some are dismal in all respects. Those who believe a nursing home is the proper place for an aged relative or friend should check all possibilities carefully, and consult with people who know about them—including the family physician.

Health Care Agencies

There are many other health care organizations and agencies, public and private, operating in most cities and in many smaller communities. Public or governmental agencies include city and county public health departments that enforce health and sanitation laws for bars, restaurants, hotels, and apartment houses. Public health agencies also inform the public about possible epidemics and, if necessary, organize and oversee immunization programs.

Sometimes private organizations are involved in health care. For instance, the Planned Parenthood agencies operate birth control clinics at which men and women can receive advice and obtain medical examinations, birth control products and

TABLE 23-1 Percentage of the Population of the United States with Private Health Insurance for Various Services, 1974

	Under 65 Years	Over 65 Years
Hospital Care	79.9	57.9
Surgical Services	78.3	54.0
X-Ray; Lab Exams	77.5	31.7
Office and Home Visits	62.3	35.5
Dental Care	17.4	1.9
Prescribed Drugs	73.2	16.9
Nursing-Home Care	35.2	15.8
Visiting Nurse Service	70.1	21.0
In-Hospital Visits	77.5	40.3
Private Duty Nurse	72.9	16.8

Source: U.S. House of Representatives, Ways and Means Committee, *Basic Facts of the Health Industry,* 1972; *Statistical Abstract of the United States,* 97th ed., 1976, p. 74.

prescriptions for the contraceptive methods requiring them. Some organizations, such as the Heart Association, the American Cancer Society, and the National Council on Alcoholism, specialize in certain ailments, solicit contributions for research, and conduct public information programs. Volunteer agencies operate in many areas. The Red Cross, for instance, is best known for its disaster relief mobilization efforts, but the organization also operates community blood banks, and trains and supplies the nurses' aides and "gray ladies" who assist in hospitals, clinics, and nursing homes.

Paying for Health Care

Everybody involved in health care agrees that its costs are quite high—and getting higher. The Department of Health, Education and Welfare (HEW) estimates that, of every $9 a typical American earns, $1 is spent for health care. In 1975, according to HEW figures, total expenditures for health care in this country were $118 billion, 8.3 percent of the gross national product, or $540 for each man, woman, and child in the country. Even if Congress finally approves the kind of compulsory national health insurance long advocated in some quarters, HEW says the total health care price-tag in the U.S. will rise to $224 billion a year by 1980.

Someone who has a good salary and maintains a careful budget presumably can pay for routine medical and dental care—checkups and the like—on a pay-as-you-go basis. But even for the fairly affluent, prudent planner a major illness—something requiring prolonged hospital care and specialized treatment—can be a financial disaster. Today most people—approximately 95 percent, according to HEW estimates—are covered by some kind of health and hospital insurance, much of it woefully inadequate.

Some plans simply fail to cover some of the most vital—and costly—kinds of medical treatment, and others consistently lag behind the spiralling costs of living in general and health care in particular.

Health Insurance

Insurance programs that pay all or part of your medical and hospital care come in a number of sizes and shapes. There are public plans financed (at least in part) by the government, and private plans for the group or the individual, prepaid or pay-as-you-go. Some of them are discussed here.

Prepaid Group Plans   A prepaid group plan is simply a contract between a group of people and a health care organization, providing that the group will receive comprehensive health care for a fixed annual payment. In most cases, the group is made up of employees of a particular firm; sometimes the employees pay for the coverage, sometimes the employer pays, and sometimes both contribute.

The other party to this kind of contract is a group practice organization consisting of physicians—the family doctor and some specialists—along with necessary backup personnel. The medical group provides hospital care as part of the contract. Medical practice organizations involved with prepaid care may be large or small. One of the biggest and most successful in the United States is the Kaiser Foundation Plan in California, Hawaii, and the Pacific Northwest. Kaiser employs its own doctors, in a wide range of specialties, along with all the needed backup medical personnel and administrative staff. It operates its own pharmacies, medical and optical laboratories, clinics, and general hospitals. Kaiser offers several classes of coverage—geared to the amount paid in by the employee and/or employer. The top coverage includes all examinations, consultations, X-rays and other lab services, prescription drugs, and up to 365 days a year in the hospital—*everything,* in other words—at no extra cost to the family.

The *Health Maintenance Organization (HMO)* program established by Congress is patterned after the Kaiser plan. HMOs provide comprehensive care for a set, prepaid fee. Also drawing federal funds is the *Neighborhood Health Center* program, which is designed to provide comprehensive medical care to the urban poor. The centers are managed in part by the people in the neighborhood.

TABLE 23-2 Medical Care Prices in the United States, 1950–1975

Components	1950	1960	1970	1975
Physicians' Fees	55.2	77.0	121.4	169.4
Dentists' Fees	63.9	82.1	119.4	161.9
Hospital Daily Service Charges	28.9	56.3	143.9	236.1
Drugs and Prescriptions	88.5	104.5	103.6	118.8

Figures represent millions of dollars.

Source: Statistical Abstract of the United States, 97th ed., 1976.

Health Insurance and Income

The lower a person's income, the less likely he or she is to have health insurance. In 1970, only 39 percent of persons in families with incomes under $3,000 had hospital insurance coverage. In contrast, an overwhelming proportion—90 percent—had hospital coverage in the $10,000-plus group. In general, the proportion of the population with hospital insurance coverage increases as income increases.

Similarly, income is probably the most important factor in determining whether a family has surgical insurance. Only about a third of the poor, compared with almost nine-tenths of those in the highest income bracket, had this type of coverage.

TABLE 23-3 Income Level and Type of Insurance

| Income Level | Percent of Population Under Age 65 With: | |
	Hospital Insurance	Surgical Insurance
Under $3,000	39.3	36.7
$3,000–$4,999	53.1	50.2
$5,000–$6,999	74.5	71.8
$7,000–$9,999	84.3	81.9
$10,000 or more	90.1	88.3

Source: Social Security Administration, *Medical Care Expenditures, Prices, and Costs: Background Book* (Washington, D.C., 1975).

Other Private Plans   Private health-care plans that offer *coverage* but don't perform the *services* are available to groups or individuals on a kind of elective-coverage basis. Basically, you pick the coverage you want (or feel you need) and pay accordingly. The more extensive the coverage, the higher the premium you (or your employer) must pay. The biggest and best-known plans of this kind are those of *Blue Cross* and *Blue Shield*. Some people pick a plan that emphasizes *major medical* coverage—the really serious, expensive illnesses—but does little, if anything, to pay for routine medical care. A more expensive plan is *comprehensive* coverage, which pays for all or part of routine care as well as the major medical problems.

Many general insurance companies offer different kinds of health care plans for individuals and groups.

Public Health Care Plans

Government-financed plans which pay for part of a patient's basic medical, dental, hospital, and pharmaceutical needs have been established by the federal government and some states. Best known are the two main federal programs, Medicare and Medicaid.

Medicare A health care plan for the elderly, operated under the Social Security system, which pays for benefits under the compulsory hospital-care part of the program. The recipient and the government share the costs of the companion medical-coverage plan, which is voluntary and covers part (but not all) of a patient's doctor bills and other medical expenses. The recipient must be age 65 or older.

Medicaid Supplements the welfare system, paying for some of the health care needs of people who are poor—regardless of age. Medicaid consists of federal grants to the states enabling them to provide health care assistance to people already on welfare, and to those others who might not otherwise be able to meet their medical expenses.

Proposed Compulsory Plans

Experts in health care and its financing problems believe that some kind of nationwide compulsory, comprehensive, medical and hospital insurance program is inevitable. Different approaches to this problem have been proposed, only to be modified, compromised, and finally defeated. But the general feeling among those close to the problem is that a compulsory program is on the way, and that it must make it possible for all citizens to obtain the health care they need, at prices they can afford. Compulsory comprehensive national health care is opposed by the important segments of organized medicine.

Summary

The family doctor provides primary medical care in his office or clinic. Secondary care usually is provided in a community hospital, and tertiary care—the kind involving intensive specialization and sophisticated facilities and equipment—is best done in a large regional hospital or medical center. These are often operated in conjunction with medical schools.

Accreditation is important to hospitals—and to the patients selecting them—whether the hospital is a public facility (run by a government agency), a nonprofit "voluntary" facility, or a profit-making "proprietary," commercial venture. Health care for the aged is provided in nursing homes.

Everything in health care—from the routine office visit to the most complicated surgery—costs more these days, and the costs continue to rise. Most people simply can't afford good medical and hospital care on a pay-as-you-go basis—particularly where major illness and prolonged hospital stays are involved. Consequently most Americans today are covered by some kind of health-care insurance—although much of it is inadequate.

Some organized health-care institutions provide comprehensive coverage, including hospitalization, on a prepaid basis for a fixed annual sum to patient groups. Private health care for groups and individuals is available through specialized organizations such as Blue Cross, or through commercial insurance companies. Government plans include Medicare, for the elderly, and Medicaid, for the poor. Various plans for prepaid, comprehensive coverage on a compulsory national basis are repeatedly debated in Congress, and enactment of some such plan is believed to be inevitable.

References

p. 346 *Consumer Reports* Editors, "What Makes a Good Hospital," in *The Medicine Show: Some Plain Truths about Popular Products for Common Ailments* (Mt. Vernon, N.Y., 1974), pp. 336–47.

p. 348 John H. Knowles, "The Hospital," *Scientific American* (September 1973), pp. 128–37.

p. 353 Ernest W. Saward, "The Organization of Medical Care," *Scientific American* (September 1973), pp. 169–75.

Illustration Credits

Drawings

Figures 5a, p. 54; 5b, p. 55; 15b, p. 236; 15c, p. 240; 15d, p. 245; 17a, p. 262; 17b, p. 264: Illustrations by Edith Tagrin from *Human Design: Molecular, Cellular and Systematic Physiology* by William S. Beck. © 1971 by Harcourt Brace Jovanovich, Inc. Reproduced by permission of the publishers.

Figures 5e, p. 64; 15a, p. 234; 17c, p. 267: From *Life: An Introduction to Biology*, Shorter Edition, by George Gaylord Simpson and William S. Beck. © 1969 by Harcourt Brace Jovanovich, Inc. Reproduced by permission of the publishers.

Figure 5e Adapted from W. F. Pauli, *The World of Life*, Houghton Mifflin, 1949.

Figure 5c, p. 56–57: Adapted from R. W. Kistner: *Gynecology, Principles and Practice*, Second Edition. Copyright © 1964 and 1971 by Year Book Medical Publishers, Inc. Chicago. Used by permission.

Figure 5d, p. 63: from *Health*, Second Edition, by Benjamin A. Kogan, M.D. © 1974 by Harcourt Brace Jovanovich, Inc. Reproduced by permission of the publishers.

Figure 14a, p. 223: Adapted from *Explain It To Me, Doctor* by L. K. Ferguson, M.D. © 1970 by J. B. Lippincott Company. Reprinted by permission of the publisher.

Figure 17d, p. 273: From *Gray's Anatomy of the Human Body*, 29th Edition, edited by C.M. Goss. Lea and Febiger, Philadelphia, 1973.

Figure 20a, p. 300: From *The Human Body*, Fourth Edition, Revised, by Logan Clendening. Copyright 1927, 1930, 1937, 1945 by Alfred A. Knopf, Inc. and renewed 1955, 1965 by Mrs. Alfred B. Clark. Reprinted by permission of the publisher.

Figure 21a, pp. 326–27: Reprinted with permission of Macmillan Publishing Co., Inc. from *The Human Body; Its Structure and Physiology* by Sigmund Grollman. Copyright © 1974 by Sigmund Grollman.

Photographs and Cartoons

Key to abbreviations
t: top
b: bottom
c: center
l: left
r: right

Part I: p. 3, Flip Schulke/Black Star; 6, Wayne Miller/Magnum; 11, photo by Ben Ross

Part II: p. 21, © Elihu Blotnick/BBM Associates; 26, Erika Stone/Peter Arnold; 29, Nacio Jan Brown/Black Star; 31, John Laundis/Black Star; 33, Wide World; 38, Benyas-Kaufman/Black Star; 41, Eve Arnold/Magnum; 44, United Press International

Index

Moniliasis, **90,** 200
Monogamy, 101, 102
Mononucleosis, **215**–16
Monounsaturated fats, **302**
Mons pubis, **55**
Mons veneris, 59
Morning sickness, 71
Morphine, *120–21,* 156, 157, 160, 164
Mouth, *300*
    cancer of, 138
Multiphasics, **343**
Multiple-drug abusers, 154
Multiple orgasms, 62
Multiple sclerosis, **267–68**
Mumps, **210,** 211, *213,* 213–14
Muscles, *326–27*
    relaxation of, 295–96
Mutations, genetic, 67–68, 250
Myelin, 146, **265,** *267*
Myocardial infarction, **237**

Narcolepsy, 136
Narcotics, **156**–65
Nasal cavity, *262*
National Commission on Marihuana and Drug
    Abuse, 118–19, 182, 183, 185
National Institutes of Health, 215
Natural abortion, 84
Natural childbirth, 72–73
Natural immunity, 211
Natural methods of birth control, *77–78,*
    80–81
Needs, hierarchy of, 283–84, *284*
Neighborhood health centers, 346, 350
Nephrons, **244**
Nephrosis, **246**
Nerve cells, 265–66, *267*
Nervous system
    alcohol and, 145, 146
    central. *See* Brain; Central nervous system
    disorders of, 266–70
Nerves, 265, **266**
Neuritis, **146**
Neurologist, 339
Neurons, **265**–66
Neuroses, 32, **36**–37, 39
Newborn baby, 72, 73
Nicotine, 119, 137–40
Nipple, *55,* **56,** 59, 71
Nitrous oxide, 165
Nodes, lymphatic, *240*

Nonessential amino acids, **301**
Nongonococcal urethritis, **200,** 202
Nuclear family, **102**
Nucleoli, **67**
Nucleus of cell, **67**
Nurses, 342
Nurses' aides, 342
Nursing, 73
Nursing homes, 348
Nutrition. *See* Food
Nyctophobia, **36**

Obesity, 311–13
Object permanence, 28
Obsession, **37**
Obstetrician / gynecologist, 339
Oedipal phase of personality development,
    22–23, 24
Ohsawa, George, 307
Old age, 43–46
On Death and Dying (Kübler-Ross), 47
Ophthalmologist, 339
Opiates, 155–65. *See also* Heroin
Opium, **155**–56, 157, 160
Opium derivatives, 156–59, 160. *See also*
    Heroin
Oral cancer, *251, 254, 256*
Oral cavity, *262*
Oral contraceptives (the Pill), *75–76,* 81–82,
    108, 195, 196
Oral sex, 59–60
Oral stage of personality development, 22
Oral surgeon, 341
Organelles, **67**
Organic foods, 306
Organic psychotic disorder, **37**
Organic solvents, inhaling, 165
Organisms, **7–8**
Orgasm, **61**–62, 108
Orthodontist, 341
Osteoarthritis, 272, **274**
Osteopath, 340
Otolaryngologist, 339
Outpatient care, 347
Ova, **57**–58, 63, *64,* 65, 67, 68, *70*
Ovaries, **57,** *57, 64, 67,* 197
Overpopulation, 9–12
Overreacting, 35
Oviduct, *64*
Ovulation, **57,** 63, 65

Trichinosis, **219**
Trichomoniasis, **90,** 200, 202
Trichomonas vaginalis, 90
Tricuspid valve, *234*
Triglycerides, **309**
Trust, 23–24, *25*
Tubal ligation, *78,* 83, **84**
Tumors, 250
Turn-arounders, 119, 170–83
 LSD, 116, 119, *122–23,* 171–76
 marijuana, 115, 119, *120–21,* 122, 176–83
 mescaline, 119, *122–23,* 170, 173

Ulcers, 39, 225, 291, 292
Umbilical cord, *64,* **69**
Underweight persons, 320, 322
U.S. Food and Drug Administration, 303
U.S. Public Health Service, 241
Unsaturated fats, **302**
"Uppers." *See* Stimulants
Uremia, **246**
Urethra, **54,** *54, 57, 245*
Urinary bladder, *54, 57*
Uterine cavity, 57
Uterus, 56–**57,** *57, 64,* 72, 83
 cancer of, *251, 254,* 256
 gonococcal infection of, 197

Vaccines, **211**–14
Vacuum aspiration, **85**
Vagina, 55, *57,* 62
Vaginal deodorants and douches, 58
Vaginal spermicides, 79, 83, 196, 201
Valium, 117, 154
Vas deferens, **54,** *54,* 84
Vasectomy, *78,* 83–**84**
Vegetables, 303–04, 306
Vegetarianism, 306–07
Veins, *234, 236, 245, 262*
Veneral diseases. *See* Sexually transmitted diseases
Ventricle, *234*
Vertebral column, *264*

Vestibule, **55**
Virulence, **206**
Viruses, **206,** *208*
 antibiotics and, 217–18
 cancer and, 252
 diseases caused by, 210–11, 215–17, 261–62
 genetic code and, 207–09
 immunization and, 211–14
 interferon and, 218
 natural immunity and, 211
 replication of, 208–09
 response of body to, 209–10
Vitamin C, 217, 227, *303,* 305
Vitamin E, *303,* 305
Vitamins, **302,** *303,* 304–05
Vollmer, August, 184
Voyeurism, **94**
Vulva, **55,** 59

Warts, genital, **91,** 200
Well-being, 282–88
 basic needs, 283–84
 establishment of goals, 286–88
 preparation for the future, 284–86
 See also Exercise; Food; Stress
White blood cells, 207, 209–11, 250
Whiteheads, 222
Whooping cough, *213,* 213–14
Withdrawal syndrome, **118**
Witte, John J., 213
Wolfe, Tom, 12
Womb. *See* Uterus
World Health Organization, 5, 118, 211

X-ray arteriogram, 243
X-ray radiation, overexposure to, 71
Xanthines, **126**–29
Xenophobia, **36**

Zen macrobiotic diet, 307
Zona pellucida, **65**
Zygote, **65,** 66, 67, 69

A 8
B 9
C 0
D 1
E 2
F 3
G 4
H 5
I 6
J 7